MW00569511

# EVERYWOMAN'S GUIDE TO NUTRITION

# EVERYWOMAN'S GUIDE TO NUTRITION

JUDITH E. BROWN, R.D., M.P.H., Ph.D.

UNIVERSITY OF MINNESOTA PRESS
MINNEAPOLIS
OXFORD

Published by the University of Minnesota Press
2037 University Avenue Southeast, Minneapolis, MN 55414
Printed in the United States of America on acid-free paper

**Library of Congress Cataloging-in-Publication Data**

Brown, Judith E.
Everywoman's guide to nutrition / Judith E. Brown.
p. cm.
Includes bibliographical references and index.
ISBN 0-8166-1500-4
1. Women—Health and hygiene—Popular works. 2. Women—Nutrition—Popular works. 3. Women—Diseases—Prevention—Popular works.
I. Title.
RA778.B879 1991
613.2—dc20 89-20473
CIP

A CIP catalog record for this book is available from the British Library

The University of Minnesota is an
equal-opportunity educator and employer.

▶ *William Brown, this book is for you.*
*You're the best, Dad.*

# Contents

# Acknowledgments

▼ To get to you, this book has undergone multiple layers of review by scientists and health professionals at Minnesota and other universities. It has been examined by women who are part of its intended audience. The process is a source of great strength for the book, and a heartfelt thanks goes out to the reviewers who helped put its contents on target. My thanks are extended to Margaret Reinhardt and Barbara Turgeon of Nutrition Plus, Inc., for their development and testing of the recipes that are included in this book.

To Beverly Kaemmer, copy editing and production manager, Jack Ervin, the distinguished former director of the University of Minnesota Press, and all the other talented people who worked on this project, thanks for your guidance and for taking such a strong interest in the book. Working with you and Mary McKee Lopez, the copy editor, has been a joy. It is my pleasure to include a thank you to Esther Schak, the woman who edited and typed the manuscript.

There are three other people who are very important to me that I would like to acknowledge: my husband Joe, my daughter Amanda, and my son Max. Thanks for the good times of days gone by and those to come.

# Preface

## *The "Healthier" Sex*

*"Hmm," Joan wondered aloud to her friend. "We're called the weaker sex, fragile females, and the more emotional sex. On top of that, I just read in today's paper that we're also sick more often than men. So tell me, how is it we're also known as the healthier sex?"*

*"Well," Joan replied after a moment's thought, "we simply must be stronger. You know, like the flowers that make it through the small cracks in the pavement."*

▼ Women are the tougher sex. On average, women live to be seventy-eight years old, seven years longer than men. By the year 2000, it's expected that most women will live to be eighty-six.[1,2] Women are tougher not only because they live longer, but because they survive more bouts of illness and serious health problems than men.[3] Although you'll often hear that it's a woman's hormones or genes that protect her, that notion is a great exaggeration of the facts. There was little difference in the life expectancy of men and women in the early part of this century.[1] Women don't naturally live longer than men; they earn it.

Women generally are more careful about their health. They smoke and drink alcoholic beverages less than men and pay more attention to their diet. When they aren't feeling right, women are more likely to seek medical attention than men.[3] Women do plenty that's right for themselves and their families, and credit is due. Because women are oriented toward action when it comes to health, there is no better place to put nutrition information than in their hands. They are in a strong position to make good nutrition happen for themselves and their families.

This book is intended to meet the needs of women who want more information about nutrition but can't find it, who want to eat healthfully but aren't sure what that means or how to do it. It's hard to solve a puzzle when you don't have all the pieces. I have tried to include all the pieces of the nutrition puzzle in *Everywoman's Guide to Nutrition*.

After the introductory section, which highlights the importance of nutrition for health, you'll be asked to take a nutrition test. This test will help you identify strengths and weaknesses of your existing diet—no grades are assigned. The results can serve as a starting point for improving your diet and for leaving well enough alone. Chapter 3 provides basic, but hard-to-find, information about nutrition. It was written to help you find answers to a wide variety of questions about nutrition that come up over time. Practical advice about planning nutritious meals is given in chapter 4. If you've been looking for a list of the best food sources for fiber, potassium, calcium, omega-3-fatty acids, or the leading sources of sugar, saturated fats, cholesterol, sodium, or beta-carotene, you'll find them and many others in this chapter. Chapters 5 and 6 provide in-depth, no-nonsense information about nutrients: a look, in turn, at carbohydrates, proteins, fats, vitamins, and minerals.

Although women live longer than men, there are serious concerns about the quality of women's lives. The higher rates of health problems among women compared to men mean that women may lead less comfortable and satisfying lives. They are more restricted in what they can do because of illnesses and disabilities. The "healthier" sex doesn't feel healthier. Fewer women think they are in "excellent" health than do men, and they simply don't feel well as often.[4] Women lose more workdays and spend more days sick in bed or hospitalized than do men. These statistics hold up even after pregnancy-related issues are excluded. Surviving is no substitute for thriving. The advantages of a longer life may be soured by the realities of living it. The nutrition of women is directly linked to appearance and level of stamina. It affects the likelihood of developing osteoporosis, diabetes, cancer, gall stones, and arthritis—problems that occur more commonly in women than in men.[2] It is becoming clear that dietary characteristics that contribute to a woman's health and those that predispose her to disease are not always the same as they are for men. Yet, what research has identified as being good for men is frequently recommended for women as well. Women have sufficiently different biological systems and live under different enough social circumstances to make it important that nutritional recommendations for women are based on research studies with women.

Information about diet and disease risks based on studies of women is presented in chapter 7. This chapter addresses nutrition and heart disease, cancer, hypertension, osteoporosis, diabetes, and obesity. The information given represents the condensation and translation of thousands of scientific studies on diets that help prevent or manage disease. Practical guidance is provided on achieving diets that reduce the risk of developing disease and that foster recovery from it.

Women are naturally smaller and fatter, need fewer calories, and have higher nutrient needs per pound of body weight than men, but they eat less. Because of their relatively low calorie intake, women are more likely to have inadequate diets. In addition, body weight and body image become a preoccupation for many females starting at an early age. Books abound advocating one weight-loss diet or another, but nutritionally sane guidance is definitely lacking. The method for controlling weight described in chapter 8 is a sensible alternative to the punishing and short-lasting approaches commonly offered. An extensive listing of the calorie-burning value of physical activities is also provided.

Nutrition, physical fitness, and performance are highlighted in chapter 9. If you are involved in a physical-fitness program or competitive sports, or if you are gearing up for an exercise program, you may find the information on aerobic and anaerobic exercise, glycogen loading, and sports aids useful.

Although women spend more time on weight-control diets, they are less satisfied with their body weight than men.[4] They are far more likely to develop the eating disorders of anorexia nervosa and bulimia, the subject of chapter 10.

Chapter 11 addresses three areas of particular importance to women: fertility, pregnancy, and breast-feeding. The reproductive system of women and the hormones that support it have a major influence on women's nutritional health. This statement holds true for women who don't reproduce, as well as for those who do. Hormones that primarily exist to support reproduction influence mood, appetite, body temperature, bone formation and breakdown, body composition of fat, muscle, and water, blood-cholesterol levels, and the need for iron and other nutrients. Because of their body's setup for reproduction, women live with fluctuating levels of hormones and the periodic changes they produce for about forty years. (That equals approximately 520 menstrual cycles and their side effects!) About 30 percent of women monthly experience some of the effects of PMS.[5] Many women are given hormones to control fertility or to treat the symptoms of menopause. These extra doses of hormones also affect physical health and emotional well-being.

There is much more nutrition misinformation than sound information available to consumers. How to recognize and separate the two is the subject of chapter 12. Since individuals ultimately make decisions about what to eat, which supplements to take, and what information about nutrition is accurate, it's important to get the facts straight. Reading this chapter may save you time and money, and spare your health in the future.

The last chapter is a very practical one. It provides menus and recipes for good eating. The tested recipes are accompanied by a summary of their caloric and nutrient content. In general, they take less than thirty minutes to prepare.

In the appendixes you'll find a glossary that defines scientific terms used in the book—I have attempted to keep it free of jargon and to define terms as they appear—a list of reliable sources of nutrition information on topics ranging from child nutrition to food allergies, a grocery-shopping guide for balanced diets, and a weight-volume equivalents table.

On the last page of the book you'll find a form for ordering DAS™ (Diet Analysis and Assessment Software). DAS allows you to take an in-depth look at the quality of your diet and to monitor the results of dietary changes aimed at lowering fat, cholesterol, or sodium intake, or to increase fiber, vitamin C, or calcium intake—to name just a few of the possibilities.

Although the volume of research on nutrition and health is more extensive for men than for women, increases in the number of women scientists and an appreciation of the practical importance of distinguishing female from male health risks have led to an explosion of research projects involving women. It is clear that the greatest improvements in the health of women will likely come not from medical advances, pills, or transplant surgery. Rather, they will come from changes we make in the way we care for and feed our bodies.

Enjoy your journey into nutrition. Have fun reading this book; I enjoyed writing it.

JEB

# EVERYWOMAN'S
GUIDE TO
# NUTRITION

# Chapter 1

## *Health and the U.S. Diet*

***There are no secrets to a long and healthy life. How healthy you are and how long you live depends on four factors: your lifestyle, the environment to which you are exposed, your genetic makeup, and your access to quality health care (see figure 1). Of the lifestyle factors that affect health, food may be the most important. This situation is indeed fortunate. Our diet is within our control.***

▼ Well-maintained bodies, like well-maintained cars, last longer and need fewer repairs than bodies or cars that are neglected. Healthy eating is a requirement for body maintenance and extends the warranty on your health that was awarded to you at birth. The number-one advantage of a good diet is that it helps keep you healthy. Good diets benefit your health in many ways.

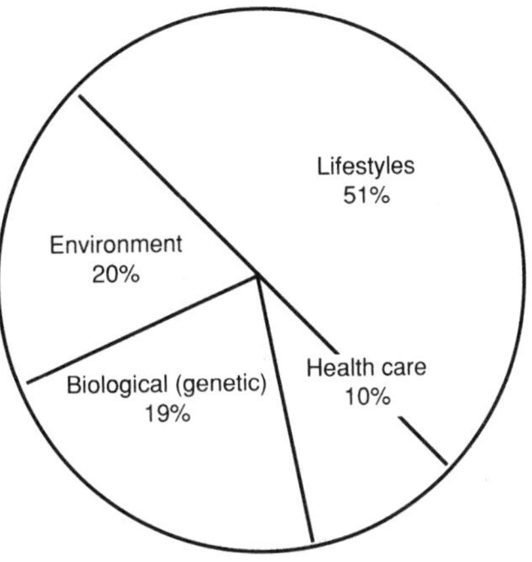


**FIGURE 1. FACTORS THAT CONTRIBUTE TO PREMATURE DEATH AMONG ADULTS UNDER THE AGE OF 75 YEARS IN THE UNITED STATES**

*Source: Centers for Disease Control, Center for Health Promotion and Disease Prevention, Atlanta, 1989*

It has been known for a hundred years that what we eat is related to the development of vitamin and mineral deficiency diseases, to compromised growth and mental development in children, and to our ability to fight off infectious diseases. We are sixty years beyond the days when pellagra, rickets, and other deficiency diseases filled children's hospital wards and contributed to serious illnesses and death in the United States. We are in the midst of an era, however, when dietary excesses are filling hospital beds and contributing substantially to a lower quality of life and premature death among millions of Americans.

Today, the major causes of illness and death of Americans are long-term or chronic diseases such as heart disease, cancer, and diabetes (table 1). Heart disease and cancer alone are responsible for 60 percent of all deaths in the United States, and dietary factors associated with their development have received a great deal of attention. Characteristics of diets have also been identified for a variety of other diseases and disorders; a number of these relationships are shown in table 1. The information presented gives a good indication of the broad influence of nutrition on the development of health problems.

Although generally noninfectious, the increasing incidence of chronic diseases in the United States is related to "contagious" changes in lifestyles. The manner in which we live our lives day to day has the greatest influence on chronic disease development. Lifestyle factors such as what we eat, how much we eat, if we smoke

TABLE 1. ESTIMATED TOTAL DEATHS AND PERCENTAGE OF TOTAL DEATHS FOR THE 10 LEADING CAUSES OF DEATH: UNITED STATES, 1987

| RANK | CAUSE OF DEATH | NUMBER | PERCENTAGE OF TOTAL DEATHS |
|---|---|---|---|
| 1[a] | Heart diseases | 759,400 | 35.7 |
| | (coronary heart disease) | (511,700) | (24.1) |
| | (other heart disease) | (247,700) | (11.6) |
| 2[a] | Cancers | 476,700 | 22.4 |
| 3[a] | Strokes | 148,700 | 7.0 |
| 4[b] | Unintentional injuries | 92,500 | 4.4 |
| | (motor vehicle) | (46,800) | (2.2) |
| | (all others) | (45,700) | (2.2) |
| 5 | Chronic obstructive lung diseases | 78,000 | 3.7 |
| 6 | Pneumonia and influenza | 68,600 | 3.2 |
| 7[a] | Diabetes mellitus | 37,800 | 1.8 |
| 8[b] | Suicide | 29,600 | 1.4 |
| 9[b] | Chronic liver disease and cirrhosis | 26,000 | 1.2 |
| 10[a] | Atherosclerosis | 23,100 | 1.1 |
| . . . | All causes | 2,125,100 | 100.0 |

*Source: National Center for Health Statistics 1988.*
[a]*Causes of death in which diet plays a part.*
[b]*Causes of death in which excessive alcohol consumption plays a part.*

NUTRITION RISK FACTORS ASSOCIATED WITH THE DEVELOPMENT OF DISEASES AND DISORDERS

| CHRONIC DISEASE OR DISORDER | NUTRITION RISK FACTORS |
|---|---|
| Coronary heart diseases | High total fat, saturated fat, and high-cholesterol diets |
| | Obesity |
| Cancer[a] | High-fat diet |
| | Obesity |
| | Low intake of vitamin A and beta-carotene |
| | Low intake of vegetables (?) |
| | Low intake of vitamins E and C (?) |
| Stroke | Excess sodium intake |
| | High-fat, high-cholesterol diets |
| Atherosclerosis ("hardening of the arteries") | Obesity, high-fat and high-cholesterol diets |
| Diabetes (in adults) | Obesity |
| Cirrhosis of the liver | Excess alcohol intake, malnutrition |
| Infertility | Underweight |
| | Obesity |
| Abnormalities in pregnancy | Underweight |
| | Obesity |
| | Malnutrition |
| Low-birth-weight infants | Low-pregnancy-weight gain |
| | Prepregnancy underweight |
| | Excess alcohol consumption |
| Growth retardation in children | Malnutrition |
| Tooth decay | Frequent consumption of sweets |
| Iron deficiency anemia | Low fluoride intake |
| Constipation | Low fiber, low fluid intake |
| Obesity | Caloric intakes that exceed the need for calories |
| Hypertension | High sodium intake |
| | High alcohol intake |
| | Obesity |
| Osteoporosis | Low calcium, low vitamin D intake |

[a]*Most types of cancer, notably excluding leukemia, have been associated with habitual diet.*

or drink excessive alcohol, if we are physically active or psychologically stressed, or whether we get enough sleep largely determine if we are promoting our health or chronic disease.[1]

The impetus for chronic-disease prevention through dietary and other measures is stronger today than ever before. The costs of poor health in terms of illness care, reduced human productivity, and quality of life are becoming higher than can be afforded in this and many other countries. Since 1960, national expenditures for health care have increased twelvefold and are continuing to increase at a high rate.[2] Life expectancy, however, has increased by only five years, or by 7 percent since 1969.[3] Reductions achieved in infant and early-childhood death rates accounted for most of the gain in life expectancy.[4] Life expectancy in the United States now averages seventy-eight years for women and seventy-one years for men. We are outlived by people in a number of other countries such as Switzerland, Japan, Norway, and Australia.[5] Rather than through increased availability of modern health care, the greatest gains in health and longevity have been primarily achieved through improved nutrition, economic status, education, housing, and sanitation. Historically, nutrition has been perhaps the most important contributor to successes against disease and disability.[6]

There is a good deal of evidence to indicate that the chronic diseases now prevalent in the United States and other western countries have their roots in dietary and other changes that accompanied civilization. Our bodies are biologically the same as those of our early ancestors. But our common biological system may not be coping very well with the drastic changes that have occurred in what we feed it.

## OUR DIETS HAVE CHANGED BUT OUR BODIES HAVEN'T

Biologically modern humans have walked the earth for about forty thousand years. For thirty thousand of these years, humans survived by hunting wild animals and gathering plants. Early humans were constantly on the move either pursuing wild game or following the seasonal maturation of fruits and vegetables. Animals and plants obtained from successful hunting-and-gathering journeys spoiled quickly, so they had to be consumed in a short period of time. Feasts would be followed by famines that lasted until the next successful hunt or harvest. Sugar, salt, alcohol, food additives, and fats such as oils, margarine, and butter—common components of diets today—were not a part of the diets of early humans. These ingredients came with civilization.

The bodies of biologically modern humans, adapted to exist on a diet of wild game, fruits, and vegetables, to survive periods of feasts and famines, and to sustain a physically demanding lifestyle, are now exposed to a different set of circumstances. The foods modern humans eat bear little resemblance to the foods available to our early ancestors. Periods of feasts are generally not followed by famines or periods of strenuous physical activity.

The human body developed other survival mechanisms that are not the assets they used to be. Mechanisms in place that stimulate hunger in the presence of excessive body stores of fat, that conserve the body's supply of sodium, that confer an innate preference for sweet-tasting foods, and a digestive system that functions best on a high-fiber diet were advantages for early humans but are not for many humans today. Yet those mechanisms persist because they are part of the human genetic makeup. Although the human body has a remarkable ability to adapt to changes in diet, health problems of modern civilization such as heart disease, cancer, hypertension, and diabetes are thought to result partly from diets that are vastly different from those of our biological ancestors, the hunter-gatherers.[7,8]

There appears to be no end to the changes in diets that our forty-thousand-year-old biological systems encounter. Our food supply and our diets are changing all the time.

Changing food habits toward healthy diets appears to be within the range of normal behavioral changes of adults, regardless of their age. In a study of 100 women and men over the age of sixty, 100 percent had made some change in food choices in the recent past. They changed for health, tastes, convenience, or social reasons.[9] Food choices and intake clearly change throughout life and can change acceptably for the better.

## DIETARY RISK FACTORS

Characteristics of diet and nutritional health that are known to be associated with the development of a disease or disorder are called "risk factors." The presence of risk factors increases the likelihood that a person will develop a particular disease or condition. For example, diets habitually high in fat increase the risk of developing heart disease and certain types of cancer. People who consume a high-fat diet may not develop heart disease or cancer, but their chances of developing one or the other will be higher than for people who consume less fat. An analogy can be made with the use of seat belts. If you don't put on your seat belt, you may not get injured if you end up in a car crash; you're simply more likely to get injured if you don't wear one.

Most risk factors can be reduced or eliminated. When the risks for developing a particular disease or disorder are reduced, the associated health problems develop less frequently. The declining incidence of heart disease in the United States represents a primary example of the benefits of nutrition risk-factor reduction. The actual rates of death from heart disease in the United States since 1960 are considerably lower than expected. Reduced intakes of animal fat and cholesterol over the past thirty years are strongly associated with a lowering of risk for heart disease development and with the drop in heart disease death rates.[10] Whereas the treatment of heart disease has improved, more importantly, the percentage of people at risk of developing heart disease has declined. The death rate from heart disease is still declining in this country, but it remains the leading overall cause of death in women and men.

The dietary habits that contribute to the high rate of heart disease in the United States are unfortunately being adopted by other industrialized countries. Since 1964, the rates of heart disease in the Soviet Union and a number of eastern European countries have increased. The increased incidence of heart disease in these countries is associated with higher animal fat and cholesterol intakes, and an increasing use of tobacco.[11]

Achieving dietary changes that reduce nutrition risk is a major goal of health programs in this country and elsewhere. In view of current dietary practices, it is an ambitious but important goal. Dietary habits linked to diseases such as overeating, excessive consumption of fat, high intake of cholesterol, excessive salt intake, and inadequate consumption of fiber represent the all-American diet. We are not talking about isolated cases of nutritionally high-risk individuals, but of risk factors shared by the majority of Americans.[12]

## ESTABLISHING THE LINKS BETWEEN NUTRITION AND HEALTH

The links between diet and heart disease, cancer, hypertension, and other conditions under investigation do not generally represent cause-and-effect relationships as did the earlier vitamin and mineral deficiency disease studies. Rather than directly causing today's chronic disorders, dietary characteristics are one of a number of factors associated with their development. Vitamin C deficiency, for example, *causes* scurvy, the vitamin C deficiency disease. On the other hand, high-fat diets, as well as high blood pressure and smoking, contribute to the development of heart disease. None of these factors by themselves causes heart disease, but each is *associated* with its development.

Most foods we eat contain hundreds to thousands of different chemical components and there are thousands of different foods. There are about forty thousand edible plants, for example, and most contain chemical components yet to be identified. Each chemical component of food may have different effects on body processes. Inside the body, there are between 2 and 10 billion chemical reactions that take place, and each reaction could play a role in how the food we eat ultimately affects health. Along with these considerations, the potential influence of existing disease, physical activity, psychological factors, genetic characteristics, age, occupation, and other factors on nutritional health needs to be assessed. Further complicating the search for definitive knowledge about nutrition-and-health relationships are the facts that nutrition-related health problems take many years to develop, and human nutrition research is generally very expensive to conduct and must be limited in scope so as to not endanger the health of the human research participants.

Given these constraints, it is highly unlikely that we will be able to explain with absolute certainty how dietary factors cause health problems. Action, in the form of nutrition guidance and programs, has to be taken before all the details are known. If not, if we did wait for absolute certainty, there could be no recommended action for change.

The method used for deciding nutrition "truths" is that of scientific consensus. The process entails deciding if changing diets, to be consistent with the results shown in multiple, scientifically controlled studies, would have a greater chance of improving rather than harming health. Most dietary changes recommended as public health policy have the support of 90 percent or more of the nutrition science community.[13] By and large, the system for basing nutrition action on scientific consensus has worked. Far more people have benefited from, for example, the enrichment of grain products, reductions in fat and salt intake, and increased fiber intakes than have been harmed.

## THE LOW-RISK DIET FOR AMERICANS

**Fred and Sue Smith Reduced Their Saturated Fat Intake and Won the Battle against High Cholesterol**

Ever read such a headline? The bitter news about the U.S. diet receives a good deal more attention than the sweet. The headlines and news reports about nutrition and health often ignore the fact that eating is *supposed* to be good for you. The type of diet that takes the risks out of eating is rarely featured, yet it represents perhaps the most important information people who are interested in nutrition could get.

We end this first chapter with an initial set of guides about low-risk, high-health eating. The prescription is generic—it is intended to promote overall health and to help protect individuals from a variety of chronic diseases. Later on we'll present ideas for dietary changes that may help eliminate or reduce existing risk factors such as high cholesterol or blood pressure levels, and we'll discuss foods and diets that contribute to the treatment of diseases.

### *Characteristics of Low-Risk, High-Health Eating*

1. Diets that are good for health include a variety of basic foods. *Variety* means a wide assortment of foods from the categories of vegetables and fruits, whole grain breads and grain products such as pastas and cereals, low-fat milk and milk products (cheese and yogurt), and meat and meat alternates (for example, beans, tofu, and seeds). The more simply prepared the food, the better. For example, oatmeal beats out granola bars as a source of whole grains, fresh fruits provide a better profile of vitamins and minerals than fruit drinks or fruit bars, and broiled fish is a better choice than deep-fried fillets. In the United States, women are most likely to consume too little of milk and milk products, and both men and women are likely to consume too little of vegetables and fruits.

2. Good diets are lean. Fat enters our diets in many ways. We add butter or margarine to vegetables and breads, we fry foods, consume high-fat meats such as bacon, sausage, hamburger, and hot dogs, and go for the rich sauces and desserts. Many Americans dine regularly on fast foods, which often contain high levels of fat. Healthy diets have the fat trimmed out of them. Cholesterol intake generally declines substantially when dietary fat intake is reduced.

3. Healthy eating is low on *empty-calorie* foods. Empty-calorie foods are those that provide calories and little else. Stellar examples of empty-calorie foods include sugar and sweets, fats, and alcohol. It's hard to get all the nutrients you need if too many calories are wasted on foods that supply little but calories.

4. Healthy diets contain a moderate amount of sodium. Nearly all of the salt we consume is added to foods during processing,

preparation, or at the table. Unprocessed, fresh foods are all naturally low in sodium.

5. Eating right tastes good. A key to a healthy diet is eating foods you enjoy that are also good for you. The balance can and must be struck if good diets are to persist. This is not the last word you'll read on this topic. The how to's are ahead in chapter 4.

Each woman reading this book will likely have a unique starting point of strengths and weaknesses in nutrition practices and knowledge. The purpose of the next chapter is to identify them. The process should make clear what areas need to be focused upon and where to affirm strengths and leave well enough alone.

How does your nutrition rate?

# Chapter 2

## *The Nutrition Test*

*It was the sort of event that sticks forever in the back of a nutritionist's mind. The year was 1976 and the Honorable Hubert H. Humphrey was delivering the opening address to a large conference on nutrition education. To show that he was personally concerned about what he ate, Senator Humphrey proudly announced that he starts each day with a nutritious breakfast: fried eggs, bacon, and toast.*

*Most of the dietitians and nutritionists in the audience were taken back by this statement. One had the gumption to go up after the address and talk with him about his choice of breakfast. The senator listened carefully and promised to give muffins, juice, and skim milk a try.*

*Two weeks later the nutritionist received a very kind thank-you note from the senator. It ended with: "I've got to run now. The muffins are just coming out of the oven."*

▼ The snapshot of Senator Humphrey's diet was enough to know he wasn't eating the breakfast of champions. But then, it's hard to know if your diet is on the right track if you haven't checked it out. This chapter gives you a chance to evaluate your diet and other factors linked to health such as body size, vitamin and mineral supplement use, and levels of physical activity and stress. PLEASE, AVOID ANY TEMPTATION TO GLOSS OVER THIS CHAPTER! Thank you. You may find you're in for some pleasant surprises. Even if you aren't, you'll identify your starting point. It will place you in a position to focus on the areas that need change and those that don't.

The self-appraisal starts with a look at your usual diet. You can examine it in two ways. The first option is to answer the questions about your diet given here. The other is to use the dietary analysis software for which a coupon is provided at the back of this book. Directions for using the program and interpreting the results are provided with the software. You could, of course, examine your diet using both approaches.

DOES YOUR DIET INCLUDE ENOUGH VARIETY?*

| How often do you usually eat: | *Daily* | *4 to 6 times/week* | *1 to 3 times/week* | *Less than weekly* |
|---|---|---|---|---|
| 1. At least four servings of breads, crackers, cereals, rice, pasta, or other foods made from grains? | ☐ | ☐ | ☐ | ☐ |
| 2. Foods made from whole grains such as whole wheat bread or whole grain cereals? | ☐ | ☐ | ☐ | ☐ |
| 3. At least two servings of vegetables? | ☐ | ☐ | ☐ | ☐ |
| 4. A serving of a vitamin-A-rich vegetable such as carrots, broccoli, spinach, green peppers, collards, or sweet potatoes? | ☐ | ☐ | ☐ | ☐ |
| 5. At least two servings of fruit or fruit juice? | ☐ | ☐ | ☐ | ☐ |
| 6. A serving of a vitamin-C-rich fruit or vegetable such as oranges and orange juice, tangerines, kiwi fruit, grapefruit and grapefruit juice, cantaloupe, or green peppers? | ☐ | ☐ | ☐ | ☐ |
| 7. At least two servings of milk, cheese, or yogurt? (Make that four servings if you're a teenager, pregnant, breast-feeding, or postmenopausal.) | ☐ | ☐ | ☐ | ☐ |

8. At least two servings of lean pork, poultry, or beef; seafood, dried beans, tofu, peanut butter, nuts or seeds? ☐ ☐ ☐ ☐

**Questions concerning diet quality have been adapted from USDA Home and Garden Publication Nos. 232–1, 232–2, 232–3, and 232–4, Washington, D.C., 1986.*

If you answered "daily" to all of the questions, you've done a good job applying the variety principle to your diet. Varied diets like yours generally provide the amount of protein, fat, carbohydrate, fiber, vitamins, and minerals people need for health.

If any of your answers were "less than daily," take a close look at the foods you're short on and decide which of them you like most. Then, try to find a spot for them in your diet. For example, if you only consume two servings of milk, cheese, or yogurt one to three times a week, think about where you could fit additional servings into your diet. Maybe your favorite yogurt (if you have one, that is) would serve nicely as a bedtime snack. Perhaps it could replace foods like cookies or chips that you snack on at night.

Diets that provide the minimum number of servings of foods in each of the basic food groups addressed in the questions usually supply 1,000 to 1,400 calories. (Concentrated sources of calories, such as margarine and butter, salad dressing and mayonnaise, pastries and sweets, aren't included in these eight questions. We will get to them in a minute.) A diet that includes the right number and variety of basic foods isn't high in calories. In fact, most people would lose weight if they ate the amounts and types of foods indicated in the questions. And, they would be getting a nutrient-dense diet, or more nutrients per calorie than if high-calorie foods were consumed.

The design of nutritious, health-promoting diets is an important topic and the discussion of what it is and why it's like that continues later in the book.

A person's diet usually consists of more than basic foods and these, too, need to be considered in an evaluation of a person's diet. The next three sets of questions focus on the other ingredients that make up diets. The questions address the fat, sugar, and salt content of your diet.

RATING FAT INTAKE

| How often do you eat: | *Daily* | *4 to 6 times/week* | *1 to 3 times/week* | *Less than weekly* |
|---|---|---|---|---|
| 1. Foods fried in fat such as french fries or fried onion rings, fried chicken, fish or shrimp, or other foods that are deep fried? | ☐ | ☐ | ☐ | ☐ |
| 2. Regular hamburger, juicy steaks or pork, bacon, sausage, hot dogs, bologna, or other non-low-fat luncheon meats? | ☐ | ☐ | ☐ | ☐ |
| 3. Ice cream, whipped cream, cream cheese, or sour cream? | ☐ | ☐ | ☐ | ☐ |
| 4. Whole milk or non-low-fat cheeses and yogurt? | ☐ | ☐ | ☐ | ☐ |
| 5. Butter, margarine, salad dressing, mayonnaise, gravy, or rich sauces? | ☐ | ☐ | ☐ | ☐ |
| 6. Nuts, potato chips, corn chips, taco chips, or cheese twists? | ☐ | ☐ | ☐ | ☐ |
| 7. Cookies, cake, pie, sweet rolls, or other pastry? | ☐ | ☐ | ☐ | ☐ |

First look at your responses to questions 1 and 2. If you don't include those types of foods more often than once or twice a week, you've already taken a lot of fat out of your diet. If you include them daily, your diet is probably on the fat side. "Daily" responses to questions 3 through 7 means that you may be piling up fat in your diet and it's very likely your diet is too high in fat. Whether the foods add too much fat to your diet will depend on how much you eat as well as how often you eat them. Please use your own judgment on this one. Eating three cups of ice cream every other day will put more fat in your diet than a cup of ice cream eaten daily.

SIZING UP YOUR SUGAR INTAKE

| How often do you usually eat: | *Daily* | *4 to 6 times/week* | *1 to 3 times/week* | *Less than weekly* |
|---|---|---|---|---|
| 1. Presweetened breakfast cereal or cereal with two or more added teaspoons of sugar? | ☐ | ☐ | ☐ | ☐ |
| 2. Regular soft drinks, sweetened seltzers, fruit drinks, presweetened powdered drink mixes, or chocolate milk? | ☐ | ☐ | ☐ | ☐ |
| 3. Candy, cookies, cake, sweet rolls, pie, sherbert, or sweetened fruit ices? | ☐ | ☐ | ☐ | ☐ |
| 4. Two or more teaspoons of sugar or honey, or two tablespoons or more of syrup, jelly, jams, or sweet sauces? | ☐ | ☐ | ☐ | ☐ |

The main problem with sugar is that it is a dud source of nutrients and it promotes tooth decay. Sugar adds only calories to our diet, and foods that contain a lot of sugar tend also not to be very nutritious. Sweets may, however, add enjoyment and good taste to diets and it's not necessary to exclude them totally. Sugary foods become a problem if they replace more nutritious foods in our diets or if they are eaten regularly as snacks.

THE SALT OF YOUR DIET

| How often do you usually: | *Daily* | *4 to 6 times/week* | *1 to 3 times/week* | *Less than weekly* |
|---|---|---|---|---|
| 1. Salt foods at the table? | ☐ | ☐ | ☐ | ☐ |
| 2. Eat processed foods such as luncheon meats, bacon, hot dogs, sausage, canned soups, spaghetti, broths and gravy, pot pies or TV dinners, or smoked fish? | ☐ | ☐ | ☐ | ☐ |
| 3. Eat pickles, green olives, chips, pretzels, cheese twists, salted crackers? | ☐ | ☐ | ☐ | ☐ |

| | | | | |
|---|---|---|---|---|
| 4. Use soy sauce, garlic salt, steak sauce, or catsup in recipes or on foods? | ☐ | ☐ | ☐ | ☐ |
| 5. Add salt to cooking water or to foods you're preparing? | ☐ | ☐ | ☐ | ☐ |

The nutrient we're trying to get at here is really sodium. Salt is by far our leading source of sodium in foods. Nearly all of the sodium we consume is added to foods during processing, in the kitchen, and at the table. People in the United States generally eat two to three times more sodium than they need—and you may be too, if you answered "daily" or "4 to 6 times per week" to several of the questions. Moderating salt intake is particularly important for people with hypertension or a family history of it.

### VITAMIN AND MINERAL SUPPLEMENTS

Do you take vitamin or mineral supplements? If yes, this next set of questions applies directly to you. To answer some of the questions, you may need to refer to the label on your supplement bottles.

| | *Yes* | *No* |
|---|---|---|
| 1. Do you spend over two dollars a week on supplements? | ☐ | ☐ |
| 2. Do you prefer "organic" or "natural" supplements? | ☐ | ☐ |
| 3. Does your daily intake of any of the supplements exceed 200% of the U.S. RDA? (You'll find this information on the supplement labels.) | ☐ | ☐ |
| 4. Are you taking supplements because you think they'll make up for a poor diet? | ☐ | ☐ |
| 5. Do the supplements you take include enzymes, bioflavonoids, PABA (para-aminobenzoic acid), lecithin, or inositol? | ☐ | ☐ |

If you answered "no" to each of these questions, you scored 100. If you're spending over two dollars a week on supplements, you're probably making some overly expensive choices about what to buy and use. Vitamins are vitamins and minerals are minerals. No one form is superior to any other. It doesn't matter if they come with a dull generic label or if you buy the kind that's labeled "natural" or "organic." You may pay more for brand names or "natural," but you won't be getting a superior supplement. You are also paying too much, regardless of the cost, if you buy supplements that contain enzymes or pseudovitamins like inositol or PABA. These substances have never been shown to benefit health.

For supplemental vitamins and minerals, there clearly is "too much of a good thing." Supplements should provide no more than 200 percent of the U.S. RDA because of problems that can be associated with taking higher amounts. Nearly 100 percent of the vitamin and mineral overdoses that occur result from taking excessive amounts of supplements.

Above all, keep in mind that the best place to get the nutrients you need is from the foods you eat. You need forty nutrients, and supplements generally contain just a few. Because a majority of adults in the United States take supplements, and because they can be both helpful and harmful to health, we'll get back to this subject in chapter 5.

## A STRAIGHT-ON LOOK AT BODY WEIGHT

Most adults aren't entirely happy with their body weight. (When was the last time you complimented someone on their weight and you received this response: "Thank you. My body weight is exactly what I want it to be.") It is common for adults (especially women) to think they weigh more than they should, even though their weight may be perfectly compatible with a good figure and health. Fashion or perceptions of what we should weigh are usually not the best guides for judging our weight status. The rational standards for weight are based on health; these are the standards you will use to assess your weight status.

If it were possible to do so with this sort of self-assessment, it would be preferable to assess body weight on a determination of body fat. How much of your weight consists of fat is a better indicator of health and fitness than weight for height. For example, you can be ten pounds overweight by the chart, but you wouldn't qualify as overweight unless you were overly fat too. Athletes or exercise enthusiasts may weigh in overweight because muscle weighs more than fat. But they really aren't. Some "normal-weight" people are really too fat. You're only overweight if your body contains too much fat.

There is a "quick and dirty" method for grossly estimating body fat composition. It goes like this: Take a pinch of your skin and the fat layer that lies underneath it about one inch above your navel. If the thickness of the pinch is less than three-fourths of an inch, you may be too lean. If it's about an inch thick, you may have about 25 percent body fat. If the pinch is over an inch and one-fourth, you may have over 30 percent body fat. Nutritionists consider about 25 percent body fat as normal for women. Body fats under 20 percent are considered too lean and those over 30 percent too fat. For men, a body fat content of less than 12 percent is considered under fat and a content of over 20 percent is classified as too high.[1] Please don't place bets on the results of your "pinch-an-inch" test. Even skilled technicians using calipers have trouble measuring fat fold thicknesses accurately.

Now to the weight-status assessment using the standard approach. Use the information in table 2 to identify your weight-status. Your best place to be as far as health is concerned is in the normal weight range. There is special information coming up for those who may be on the light or heavy side of this range.

TABLE 2. "NORMAL" BODY WEIGHTS BASED ON LIFE INSURANCE DATA[a]

| HEIGHT (WITHOUT SHOES) | | RANGE OF "NORMAL" WEIGHTS (WITHOUT CLOTHES) | |
|---|---|---|---|
| FEET | INCHES | WOMEN POUNDS | MEN POUNDS |
| 4 | 9 | 94–106 | |
| 4 | 10 | 97–109 | |
| 4 | 11 | 100–112 | |
| 5 | 0 | 103–115 | |
| 5 | 1 | 106–118 | 111–122 |
| 5 | 2 | 109–122 | 114–126 |
| 5 | 3 | 112–126 | 117–129 |
| 5 | 4 | 116–131 | 120–132 |
| 5 | 5 | 120–135 | 123–136 |
| 5 | 6 | 124–139 | 127–140 |
| 5 | 7 | 128–143 | 131–145 |
| 5 | 8 | 132–147 | 135–149 |
| 5 | 9 | 136–151 | 139–153 |
| 5 | 10 | 140–155 | 143–158 |
| 5 | 11 | 144–159 | 147–163 |
| 6 | 0 | | 151–168 |
| 6 | 1 | | 155–173 |
| 6 | 2 | | 160–178 |
| 6 | 3 | | 165–183 |

*Source: Adapted from Metropolitan Life Insurance Company, Statistical Bulletin No. 40, New York, 1959.*
*[a]Weight of insured persons in the United States and Canada associated with the longest life expectancy. Listed are values for persons with a medium frame, aged 25 years and over.*

EXERCISE

How much physical activity do you get?

1. Check the category that best describes your usual and overall daily activity level. DO NOT consider activities that are part of an exercise program.*

☐ Inactive: Sitting most of the day, with less than two hours of moving about slowly or standing.

☐ Average Activity: Sitting most of the day, walking or standing two to four hours each day, but not involved in strenuous activity.

☐ Active: Physically active four or more hours each day. Little sitting or standing, involved in some physically strenuous activities.

2. I exercise vigorously at least three times a week for at least thirty minutes a time. ☐ Yes ☐ No

*Source: Adapted from Harris and Benedict: Washington, D.C., Carnegie Institute, 1919; and Food and Nutrition Board, Recommended Dietary Allowances, 1974. Washington, D.C.: National Academy of Sciences, 1974.

For those who answered "active" to question 1, and "yes" to question 2, congratulations! You qualify as a mover and shaker. Good work. Keep it up. If your results spell *inactive* or *underactive* (a "no" response to question 2), what's keeping you from the exercise program you've intended to start for a while? Besides helping you feel hearty, regular exercise can help beat stress, overweight, high blood pressure, and chronic fatigue.[2]

As is the case with most things in life, enough is as good as a feast. Exercising to excess to keep body weight below a healthy level is going too far.

PACK YEARS

Do you smoke? If you do, continue on with this set of questions.

1. How long have you smoked? ☐ years
2. Have you set a quitting date? ☐ Yes ☐ No

People are bombarded with advice about smoking and the problems with it won't be repeated here. There is an up side to the story, however. Nearly half of all adults who start smoking quit, and in general the more attempts a person makes to quit, the more likely it is that she or he will eventually quit for good.[3]

STRESS

| | *Yes* | *No* |
|---|---|---|
| 1. Do you fail to fall asleep shortly after going to bed because worry or anxiety keeps you tossing and turning? | ☐ | ☐ |
| 2. Do you have trouble relaxing, even when you get a chance to relax? | ☐ | ☐ |
| 3. Do you spend most of your day doing things you don't enjoy? | ☐ | ☐ |
| 4. Do you always feel like you're "running behind"? | ☐ | ☐ |
| 5. Do you enjoy a laugh or two every day? | ☐ | ☐* |

*If you checked this box, refer to the last page of this chapter immediately! A prescription meant for you is waiting there.

Although imprecise, the answers to these questions may help you decide if there's too much stress in your life. Everybody has to deal with stress. What makes the difference to health and well-being is the level and how we cope with it. It appears that stress can affect nutritional health in several ways. It can lead to weight gain or loss, indigestion, increased plaque formation in arteries, and abnormal blood-glucose levels. Finally, stress can elevate your blood pressure.[4,5]

There are no special foods, vitamins, or mineral supplements that will combat stress. Those who would sell you "stress tabs" are selling you less than it takes. A balanced and adequate diet and exercise may, however, help give you a sense of well-being and the stamina it takes to overcome day-to-day stress.[5]

SLEEP

Do you get your recommended daily allowance of sleep? Do you get between seven and nine hours of sleep daily? ☐ Yes ☐ No

How much sleep a person needs to wake up feeling refreshed and ready to go varies considerably among people. However, most of us do best on seven to nine hours of sleep. Losing sleep has a way of catching up with people. If you cut it short, you pay the price of exhaustion, increased susceptibility to illness, irritability, and bags under the eyes. Have you ever tried to cheat sleep? Who won?

If you find you often need more than nine hours of sleep to feel right, and you are healthy, you might become energized by increasing your physical activity level.

OTHER IMPORTANT AREAS TO CONSIDER

There is a group of miscellaneous assessments that directly relate to women's health. They are too important to ignore.

| | *Yes* | *No* |
|---|---|---|
| 1. Do you self-examine your breasts monthly? | ☐ | ☐ |
| 2. Do you have your yearly Pap smear taken? | ☐ | ☐ |
| 3. If over thirty-five, have you had a baseline mammogram taken? | ☐ | ☐ |

We're hoping for three "yes" answers here. Perhaps "no" responses can serve as gentle reminders.

| | *Yes* | *No* |
|---|---|---|
| 1. Is your blood-cholesterol level under 200 mg/dl? | ☐ | ☐ |
| 2. Is your HDL-cholesterol level over 50 mg/dl? | ☐ | ☐ |
| 3. Is your ratio of total cholesterol/HDL-cholesterol less than 4.5? | ☐ | ☐ |
| 4. Is your LDL-cholesterol level less than 150 mg/dl? | ☐ | ☐ |
| 5. Is your hemoglobin level over 12 mg/dl? (If male, it should be over 11 mg/dl.) | ☐ | ☐ |
| 6. Is your blood pressure less than 140/90 mm mercury? | ☐ | ☐ |

Not everyone will have these results loaded into their memory and some people have never had one or more of these measurements taken. For those people, the values reported in the questions can be used as needed. (They apply to both women and men.) The values reported represent those considered normal and healthy. The surgeon general would like to see a "yes" answer to each question.

Five of the six questions asked in this part of the Nutrition Test have to do with your risk of developing heart disease. There is much more to be said about nutrition, blood-fat levels, and heart disease—and it's said in chapter 7.

Thanks for your attention and active involvement in this self-appraisal. You now have your starting point. You likely know enough about your nutritional status to focus on areas addressed in the rest of the book that apply particularly to you.

PRESCRIPTION: A DOSE OF LAUGHTER

This section is for people who don't get their Recommended Daily Allowance of Laughter. *Directions*: Read one of the following jokes every hour till you've read them all. The best response is laughter, but a chuckle may do.

*Dose 1*: Johnny comes home after school to find that his aunt is visiting. Interested in his future, Johnny's aunt asks him what he'd like to be when he grows up. "Well," says Johnny, "I've decided I want to be a vitamin." "A vitamin?" exclaims his aunt. "I just got the idea today," says Johnny. "On my way home I passed the drug-store and it had a sign out front saying 'Vitamin $B_1$.' "

*Dose 2*: The Mr. Rogers joke: Ten-year-old Amanda approaches her mother giggling one evening. "Mom," Amanda says in a sweet voice, "Won't you be my neighbor?" "Sure I will, honey," her mother responds. "Good!" blurts Amanda, "Move next door!"

*Dose 3*: Jessica walks out to the elementary school playground and runs into her friend Jonina. "Jonina," Jessica announces, "Did you know your mother was pregnant?" "No way! No she's not!" retorts Jonina. "Oh no," replies Jessica. "She had you, didn't she?"

*Dose 4*: Speaking of medicine, did you hear about the man who went to see the doctor about his loss of memory? The doctor made him pay in advance.

*Dose 5*: Do you know how many psychiatrists it takes to change a light bulb? Just one, but it takes a very long time because the light bulb really has to want to change.

*Dose 6*: Friend: Joan, how much did you lose on Dr. Quick's new diet book?
Joan: About $14.95.

*Dose 7*: Medicine has become so specialized that when her cold moved from her head to her chest, she had to change doctors.

*Dose 8*: A patient walks into a doctor's office.
Patient: Doc, I'm not feeling very well.
Doctor: But your pulse is as steady as a clock.
Patient: But *Doc*, your hand is on my watch.

*Dose 9*: A man finds a conch shell on the beach, puts it to his ear, and says to his friend, "If you concentrate, you can hear the ocean."

*Dose 10*: Refill this prescription by reading a joke book or by watching a comedy. Doses 4, 5, and 7 came from *Dr. Burns' Prescription for Happiness* by comedian George Burns. *The Subtreasury of American Humor* and *The Enjoyment of Laughter* are also good sources of laughs. Norman Cousins thinks the daily dose of laughter should be ten minutes. The sound of laughter is one of the healthiest sounds in the world.

# Chapter 3

## *The Inside Story of Nutrition*

*"How did I enter the field of nutrition?" (Marilyn repeated the question she was asked.) "Nutrition kept entering into my life. I was in charge of the health of my family. I was both concerned about and responsible for the nutrition of myself, my husband, and our four children. But I hated to cook and wasn't at all sure I was making the right decisions when it came to feeding the family. I felt I needed to learn enough about nutrition so I would know what to feed my family while causing a minimum of harm.*

*"I read everything about nutrition I could get my hands on, but the books and articles made little sense. The information and advice presented in one book were often at odds with what another one said. My reading got me nowhere. At the end of it all, I still didn't know if sugar was good, bad, or okay for kids; if I should avoid foods that contain food additives; or if I was priming my husband for heart disease.*

*"Out of frustration, I enrolled in an introductory nutrition course at Syracuse University. I found the "truth" fascinating and stayed on at the university to complete a doctorate in nutrition."*

▼The sort of nutrition information available to most people comes in confusing bits and pieces—the kind that raises more questions than it answers. Should I take a calcium supplement? Do I have enough iron in my diet? What is a balanced diet, anyway? Are irradiated foods safe? Bits and pieces of information don't help much when you want answers to questions like these, so you know what action to take. For Marilyn, it meant taking a college course to get the facts. For you, it may mean "enrolling" in the crash nutrition course presented in this and the following three chapters. Unlike a college course, the contents here are condensed and there are no tuition costs, pop quizzes, or papers due. It's learning strictly because you want to learn. Take from this chapter as much, or as little, of the discussion as you need or want. Just remember, it's here if you want to look up something or to check something you read or hear.

Reading these chapters won't make you a nutrition expert (although you will probably have studied the topic more than most of your health advisers). But the information will help you make some sense out of the bits and pieces of nutrition information you get. It may help you feel comfortable about the nutrition decisions you make and the action you take.

Nutrition principles and related topics are discussed in this chapter. The principles are not controversial and change little with time; they represent the basic "truths" that serve as the core of our understanding about human nutrition, and as the foundation for growth in knowledge. These principles are fundamental to an understanding of the relationships among food, nutrition, and health.

### PRINCIPLE 1: FOOD IS A BASIC NEED OF HUMANS

This first principle is very straightforward: humans need food to live. The basic need for food must be met if humans are to achieve a fulfilling existence.

### PRINCIPLE 2: FOODS PROVIDE NUTRIENTS NEEDED FOR LIFE AND HEALTH

Our need for food is based on the body's requirement for nutrients found in food. Nutrients are chemical substances needed by the body for health and growth. There are six categories of nutrients (and no others):

Carbohydrates
Proteins
Fats
Vitamins
Minerals
Water

Carbohydrates, proteins, and fats supply calories and are called the *energy nutrients*. Although each of these three types of nutrients perform a variety of functions, they share the property of being the body's sole source of fuel. Vitamins, minerals, and water are chemicals needed for the conversion of carbohydrates, proteins, and fats into energy, and for the building and maintenance of muscles, components of blood, bones, and all other parts of the body. The major features of nutrients within these categories will be highlighted after the discussion of principles.

Each specific nutrient within the categories is a unique chemical substance; its role in the body is dictated by its specific chemical characteristics. The chemical characteristics of nutrients allow them to be used by, and become part of, living tissue. Whether nutrients are obtained preassembled from foods or are manufactured in a laboratory makes no difference to the roles they perform in the body.

There is a major advantage to getting your nutrients from foods rather than pills, however. We are not yet able to imitate nature, to obtain exactly what we get in foods through pills. Taking vitamin C supplements, for example, in no way replicates the nutrients you would get from an orange. Oranges contain vitamin C and much more—carbohydrates, B-complex vitamins, potassium, and other minerals.

### *The Nutrient Composition of Foods*

The nutrient composition of foods varies substantially by food type. The amounts and types of nutrients in foods are principally determined by genetic blueprints that dictate their nutrient composition. Without the required nutrients, plants and animals fail to stay healthy and grow. So it is assumed that food items making it to market contain nutrients that were needed for their health and growth.

The types of nutrients taken up by plants and animals that are not required for their growth or health, however, vary by growing conditions. The variety of nutrients present in soil and water, the use of fertilizers, the nutrient composition of feed, and food storage and processing methods all influence the nutrient content of foods we eat. Plants grown in soil rich in selenium or iodine contain more of these minerals than those grown in selenium- or iodine-poor soil. Although they have different nutrient contents, plants grown in both types of soil look the same (or, you can't pick out iodine-rich spinach by its appearance). Oysters harvested from the shores off the East Coast contain four times more zinc than oysters netted from the West Coast. The difference in zinc content is due to the high zinc content of Atlantic coastal waters. Beef that comes from grass-fed cattle contains more polyunsaturated fats than beef from grain-fed cattle.

### PRINCIPLE 3: SOME NUTRIENTS MUST BE PROVIDED BY THE DIET

Many nutrients are required for growth and health. Some of these can be manufactured in the body from raw materials supplied by food, while others must come assembled. Nutrients that the body cannot make, or make in sufficient quantity, are referred to as *essential* nutrients. The meaning of *essential* here is "required in the diet." Vitamin A, iron, and calcium are examples of essential nutrients.

Nutrients manufactured by the body from components of our diet are considered *nonessential*. They are not a required part of our diet. Fructose, lecithin, cholesterol, and glucose are nonessential nutrients. They may be present in food and used by the body, but are not required in our diet because we can produce them.

Both essential and nonessential nutrients are required for life and health. The difference between them is whether we need a dietary source. A dietary deficiency of an essential nutrient will cause a specific deficiency disease, but a dietary lack of a nonessential nutrient will not.

So far, forty nutrients have been identified as essential. A few more that are possibly required in extremely small amounts, such as arsenic and carnitine, may be added to the list in years to come. Nutrients now considered essential for adults include the following:

Energy Nutrients
- Carbohydrates
- Proteins (source of nine amino acids)
- Fats (source of linoleic acid)

Vitamins
- Thiamin ($B_1$)
- Riboflavin ($B_2$)
- Niacin ($B_3$)
- Pantothenic acid
- Folacin
- Biotin
- Vitamin $B_6$ (proxidine)
- Vitamin $B_{12}$
- Vitamin C (ascorbic acid)
- Vitamin A
- Vitamin E
- Vitamin D
- Vitamin K

Minerals
- Calcium
- Chloride
- Chromium
- Copper
- Fluoride
- Iodine
- Iron
- Magnesium
- Manganese
- Molybdenum
- Phosphorus
- Potassium
- Selenium
- Sodium
- Zinc
- Water

The amount of essential nutrients needed each day by humans varies a lot, from amounts measured in cups to micrograms. (A microgram is a very small measure. A grain of sugar weighs several hundred micrograms.) Generally speaking, humans need about ten cups of water from fluids and foods, nine tablespoons of protein, one-fourth teaspoon of calcium, and only one-thousandth teaspoon (a thirty-microgram speck) of vitamin $B_{12}$ each day. How much we need of a nutrient in part depends on how good the body is at conserving it. Some are lost or inactivated quickly, while others are saved and used repeatedly.

### *Individual Variation in Nutrient Need*

We all need the same nutrients, but not always in the same amounts. The amounts needed vary among people based on:

- Age
- Sex
- Growth status
- Genetic traits
- Physical activity level

They are also based on the presence of conditions such as:

- Pregnancy
- Breast-feeding
- Illnesses
- Drug use
- Exposure to environmental contaminants

Each of these factors, and others, can influence nutrient requirements. General recommendations for diets that provide all the essential nutrients usually make allowances for major factors that influence level of nutrient need, but they cannot allow for all of the factors. The Recommended Dietary Allowances (RDAs) are the most widely used standard for identifying desired intake levels of essential nutrients. This set of standards apply to healthy people and are categorized by a person's age and gender and by whether a woman is pregnant or breast-feeding.

### *The RDAs*

Recommended levels of intake have been established for nineteen essential nutrients, and "provisional" ranges of estimated safe and adequate intake have been defined for an additional seven. These levels, a very common standard used in nutrition, are listed in tables

3–5. The RDAs do not indicate the required level of nutrient intake or minimal levels of nutrient need. Rather, they represent estimates, based on the best available scientific data, of the levels of essential nutrients that would meet the needs of 95 percent of all healthy people. In calculating the RDAs, a margin of safety is added to the average nutrient-intake level required for the maintenance of the nutrient's functions. For example, the adult RDA for protein is set at a level 30 percent higher than the amount needed to maintain the normal functions of protein.[1] RDA levels are generally set well above the amounts associated with the development of deficiency diseases. Although the RDAs are widely accepted and used, they are not without controversy. The lack of agreement on what the recommended levels of nutrients such as vitamins A and C should be resulted in the failure of the release of the 1985 edition of the tables.

A major assumption underlying the RDAs is that food serves as the source of essential nutrients. Foods consumed that contain the RDA levels of nutrients are also likely to contain adequate amounts of essential nutrients for which there are no RDAs. So you can't guarantee that you'll be getting an adequate diet if you consume a "100% fortified" cereal or supplement pills.

An offshoot of the RDAs surfaced in 1971 to help consumers become informed about the nutrient value of food products. These standards are the *U.S. RDAs.*

### THE U.S. RDAs

The U.S. RDAs are nutrient levels devised by the Food and Drug Administration for the sole purpose of providing a legal standard for the nutrition labeling of foods and supplements. In general, the U.S. RDAs represent the highest level of nutrients recommended in 1968 RDA tables, excluding values for pregnant and breast-feeding women. Many of the U.S. RDAs are out of date based on current knowledge.

Prior to the introduction of U.S. RDAs, standards called Minimum Daily Requirements (MDRs) were used on food and supplement labels. They represented the minimum amount of nutrients needed to prevent deficiency diseases. The MDRs are two to six times lower than the U.S. RDAs and are no longer recognized as appropriate standards for food and supplement labeling. (You may still see the MDRs on some supplement labels, but they should not be there. The U.S. RDAs are now the legally required standard for supplement labels.)

TABLE 3. RECOMMENDED DIETARY ALLOWANCES (RDA), 1989[a]

| | | | | | FAT-SOLUBLE VITAMINS | | | | | WATER-SOLUBLE VITAMINS | | | | | | | MINERALS | | | | | | |
|---|---|---|---|---|---|---|---|---|---|---|---|---|---|---|---|---|---|---|---|---|---|---|---|
| CATEGORY | AGE (YEARS) OR CONDITION | WEIGHT[b] (LB) | HEIGHT[b] (IN) | PROTEIN (G) | VITAMIN A (μgRE)[c] | VITAMIN D (μG)[d] | VITAMIN E (MGα-TE)[e] | VITAMIN K (μG) | VITAMIN C (MG) | THIAMIN (MG) | RIBOFLAVIN (MG) | NIACIN (MG NE)[f] | VITAMIN $B_6$ (MG) | FOLATE (μG) | VITAMIN $B_{12}$ (μG) | CALCIUM (MG) | PHOSPHORUS (MG) | MAGNESIUM (MG) | IRON (MG) | ZINC (MG) | IODINE (μG) | SELENIUM (μG) |
| Infants | 0.0–0.5 | 13 | 24 | 13 | 375 | 7.5 | 3 | 5 | 30 | 0.3 | 0.4 | 5 | 0.3 | 25 | 0.3 | 400 | 300 | 40 | 6 | 5 | 40 | 10 |
| | 0.5–1.0 | 20 | 28 | 14 | 375 | 10 | 4 | 10 | 35 | 0.4 | 0.5 | 6 | 0.6 | 35 | 0.5 | 600 | 500 | 60 | 10 | 5 | 50 | 15 |
| Children | 1–3 | 29 | 35 | 16 | 400 | 10 | 6 | 15 | 40 | 0.7 | 0.8 | 9 | 1.0 | 50 | 0.7 | 800 | 800 | 80 | 10 | 10 | 70 | 20 |
| | 4–6 | 44 | 44 | 24 | 500 | 10 | 7 | 20 | 45 | 0.9 | 1.1 | 12 | 1.1 | 75 | 1.0 | 800 | 800 | 120 | 10 | 10 | 90 | 20 |
| | 7–10 | 62 | 52 | 28 | 700 | 10 | 7 | 30 | 45 | 1.0 | 1.2 | 13 | 1.4 | 100 | 1.4 | 800 | 800 | 170 | 10 | 10 | 120 | 30 |
| Males | 11–14 | 99 | 62 | 45 | 1,000 | 10 | 10 | 45 | 50 | 1.3 | 1.5 | 17 | 1.7 | 150 | 2.0 | 1,200 | 1,200 | 270 | 12 | 15 | 150 | 40 |
| | 15–18 | 145 | 69 | 59 | 1,000 | 10 | 10 | 65 | 60 | 1.5 | 1.8 | 20 | 2.0 | 200 | 2.0 | 1,200 | 1,200 | 400 | 12 | 15 | 150 | 50 |
| | 19–24 | 160 | 70 | 58 | 1,000 | 10 | 10 | 70 | 60 | 1.5 | 1.7 | 19 | 2.0 | 200 | 2.0 | 1,200 | 1,200 | 350 | 10 | 15 | 150 | 70 |
| | 25–50 | 174 | 70 | 63 | 1,000 | 5 | 10 | 80 | 60 | 1.5 | 1.7 | 19 | 2.0 | 200 | 2.0 | 800 | 800 | 350 | 10 | 15 | 150 | 70 |
| | 51 + | 170 | 68 | 63 | 1,000 | 5 | 10 | 80 | 60 | 1.2 | 1.4 | 15 | 2.0 | 200 | 2.0 | 800 | 800 | 350 | 10 | 15 | 150 | 70 |
| Females | 11–14 | 101 | 62 | 46 | 800 | 10 | 8 | 45 | 50 | 1.1 | 1.3 | 15 | 1.4 | 150 | 2.0 | 1,200 | 1,200 | 280 | 15 | 12 | 150 | 45 |
| | 15–18 | 120 | 64 | 44 | 800 | 10 | 8 | 55 | 60 | 1.1 | 1.3 | 15 | 1.5 | 180 | 2.0 | 1,200 | 1,200 | 300 | 15 | 12 | 150 | 50 |
| | 19–24 | 128 | 65 | 46 | 800 | 10 | 8 | 60 | 60 | 1.1 | 1.3 | 15 | 1.6 | 180 | 2.0 | 1,200 | 1,200 | 280 | 15 | 12 | 150 | 55 |
| | 25–50 | 138 | 64 | 50 | 800 | 5 | 8 | 65 | 60 | 1.1 | 1.3 | 15 | 1.6 | 180 | 2.0 | 800 | 800 | 280 | 15 | 12 | 150 | 55 |
| | 51 + | 143 | 63 | 50 | 800 | 5 | 8 | 65 | 60 | 1.0 | 1.2 | 13 | 1.6 | 180 | 2.0 | 800 | 800 | 280 | 10 | 12 | 150 | 55 |
| Pregnant | | | | 60 | 800 | 10 | 10 | 65 | 70 | 1.5 | 1.6 | 17 | 2.2 | 400 | 2.2 | 1,200 | 1,200 | 320 | 30 | 15 | 175 | 65 |
| Lactating | 1st 6 months | | | 65 | 1,300 | 10 | 12 | 65 | 95 | 1.6 | 1.8 | 20 | 2.1 | 280 | 2.6 | 1,200 | 1,200 | 355 | 15 | 19 | 200 | 75 |
| | 2nd 6 months | | | 62 | 1,200 | 10 | 11 | 65 | 90 | 1.6 | 1.7 | 20 | 2.1 | 260 | 2.6 | 1,200 | 1,200 | 340 | 15 | 16 | 200 | 75 |

[a] *The allowances, expressed as average daily intakes over time, are intended to provide for individual variations among most normal persons as they live in the United States under usual environmental stresses. Diets should be based on a variety of common foods to provide other nutrients for which human requirements have been less well defined.*

[b] *Weights and heights of reference adults are actual medians for the U.S. population of the designated age, as reported by NHANES II. The median weights and heights of those under 19 years of age were taken from Hamill et al. (1979). The use of these figures does not imply that the height-to-weight ratios are ideal.*

[c] *Retinol equivalents. 1 retinol equivalent* = 1 μg retinol or 6 μg β-carotene.

[d] *As cholecalciferol. 10* μg cholecalciferol = 400 IU of vitamin D.

[e] α-Tocopherol equivalents. 1 mg d-α tocopherol = 1 α-TE. See text for variation in allowances and calculation of vitamin E activity of the diet as α-tocopherol equivalents.

[f] *1 NE (niacin equivalent) is equal to 1 mg of niacin or 60 mg of dietary tryptophan.*

*Reproduced from* Recommended Dietary Allowances, *10th ed. (1989), with the permission of the National Academy of Sciences, Washington, D.C.*

TABLE 4. ESTIMATED SAFE AND ADEQUATE DAILY DIETARY INTAKES OF SELECTED VITAMINS AND MINERALS[a]

| | | VITAMINS | | TRACE ELEMENTS[b] | | | | |
|---|---|---|---|---|---|---|---|---|
| CATEGORY | AGE (YEARS) | BIOTIN (μG) | PANTO-THENIC ACID (MG) | COPPER (MG) | MAN-GANESE (MG) | FLUO-RIDE (MG) | CHRO-MIUM (μG) | MOLYB-DENUM (μG) |
| Infants | 0.0–5 | 10 | 2 | 0.4–0.6 | 0.3–0.6 | 0.1–0.5 | 10–40 | 15–30 |
| | 0.5–1 | 15 | 3 | 0.6–0.7 | 0.6–1.0 | 0.2–1.0 | 20–60 | 20–40 |
| Children and | 1–3 | 20 | 3 | 0.7–1.0 | 1.0–1.5 | 0.5–1.5 | 20–80 | 25–50 |
| adolescents | 4–6 | 25 | 3–4 | 1.0–1.5 | 1.5–2.0 | 1.0–2.5 | 30–120 | 30–75 |
| | 7–10 | 30 | 4–5 | 1.0–2.0 | 2.0–3.0 | 1.5–2.5 | 50–200 | 50–150 |
| | 11+ | 30–100 | 4–7 | 1.5–2.5 | 2.0–5.0 | 1.5–2.5 | 50–200 | 75–250 |
| Adults | | 30–100 | 4–7 | 1.5–3.0 | 2.0–5.0 | 1.5–4.0 | 50–200 | 75–250 |

[a]*Because there is less information on which to base allowances, these figures are not given in the main table of RDA and are provided here in the form of ranges of recommended intakes.*
[b]*Since the toxic levels for many trace elements may be only several times usual intakes, the upper levels for the trace elements given in this table should not be habitually exceeded.*

TABLE 5. MEAN HEIGHTS AND WEIGHTS AND RECOMMENDED ENERGY INTAKE

| CATEGORY | AGE (YEARS) | WEIGHT (KG) | WEIGHT (LB) | HEIGHT (CM) | HEIGHT (IN) | ENERGY NEEDS (KCAL) |
|---|---|---|---|---|---|---|
| Infants | 0.0–0.5 | 6 | 13 | 60 | 24 | 650 |
| | 0.5–1.0 | 9 | 20 | 71 | 28 | 850 |
| Children | 1–3 | 13 | 29 | 90 | 35 | 1,300 |
| | 4–6 | 20 | 44 | 112 | 44 | 1,800 |
| | 7–10 | 28 | 62 | 132 | 52 | 2,000 |
| Males | 11–14 | 45 | 99 | 157 | 62 | 2,500 |
| | 15–18 | 66 | 145 | 176 | 69 | 3,000 |
| | 19–24 | 70 | 154 | 177 | 70 | 2,900 |
| | 25–50 | 70 | 154 | 178 | 70 | 2,900 |
| | 51+ | 70 | 154 | 178 | 70 | 2,300 |
| Females | 11–14 | 46 | 101 | 157 | 62 | 2,200 |
| | 15–18 | 55 | 120 | 163 | 64 | 2,200 |
| | 19–22 | 55 | 120 | 163 | 64 | 2,200 |
| | 23–50 | 55 | 120 | 163 | 64 | 2,200 |
| | 51–75 | 55 | 120 | 163 | 64 | 1,900 |
| Pregnant | | | | | | +300 |
| Lactating | | | | | | +500 |

Four sets of U.S. RDAs have been developed. They consist of nutrient levels set for:

Infants
Children one to four years of age
Children four years of age and over and adults
Pregnant and breast-feeding women

The category "adults and children four years and older," most commonly used on food and supplement labels, is shown in table 6.

Providing nutrition information on food labels is voluntary in the United States, except for products that make a claim about nutrient content. Vitamin and mineral supplements, however, must be labeled with the U.S. RDAs. If a food product is labeled, the information has to include the percentage of the U.S. RDAs per serving for ten specific vitamins and minerals. The calorie, carbohydrate, and fat content of one serving must also be included on the label. Other U.S. RDA levels for vitamins and minerals *may* be listed in addition to the required ten. They *must* be listed if added to a food (such as a breakfast cereal or fruit drink), or if a claim is made about them on the package. The sodium, sucrose, fiber, and cholesterol content of the foods may also be included on the nutrition label, but they are not required unless a specific claim relating to them is made.

It is important not to confuse the U.S. RDAs used for labeling purposes with the RDAs. The U.S. RDAs generally exceed the nutrient needs of people and they may not accurately reflect variations in nutrient needs related to a person's sex and age.

Foods are often labeled with nutrition information that is primarily intended to help products sell. The meaning of some of the common

TABLE 6. THE U.S. RDAs

| FOOD LABEL COMPONENTS (PER SERVING) | U.S. RDAs FOR ADULTS AND CHILDREN (FOUR YEARS AND OLDER) |
|---|---|
| *Required components* | |
| Calories | – |
| Carbohydrates | – |
| Fats | – |
| Protein | |
| • animal protein source | 45 g |
| • vegetable protein source | 65 g |
| Vitamin A | 5,000 IU |
| Vitamin C | 60 mg |
| Thiamin (vitamin $B_1$) | 1.5 mg |
| Riboflavin (vitamin $B_2$) | 1.7 mg |
| Niacin (vitamin $B_3$) | 20 mg |
| Calcium | 1,000 mg |
| Iron | 18 mg |
| *Optional components* | |
| Vitamin D | 400 IU |
| Vitamin E | 30 IU |
| Vitamin $B_6$ | 2.0 mg |
| Folic acid (folacin) | 400 mcg |
| Vitamin $B_{12}$ | 6 mcg |
| Phosphorus | 1,000 mg |
| Iodine | 150 mcg |
| Magnesium | 400 mg |
| Zinc | 15 mg |
| Copper | 2 mg |
| Biotin | 300 mcg |
| Pantothenic acid | 10 mg |

terms used on food labels to describe the nutritional attributes of products is given below.

LABEL LINGO

**Dietetic** One or more ingredient (usually sodium or sugar) has been changed, substituted, or restricted. *Not* necessarily low in calories.

**Enriched** The replacement of selected nutrients lost in the manufacturing process. Most common is the addition of vitamins $B_1$, $B_2$, and $B_3$ and iron to refined grain.

**Fortified** The addition of nutrients to foods that did not originally contain them. The additions of vitamins A and D to milk, iodine to salt, and vitamins or minerals to cereals are examples.

**Extra Lean** No more than 5 percent fat by weight—*not* by calories.

**Lean** No more than 10 percent fat by weight—*not* by calories.

**Leaner** At least 25 percent less fat (by weight) than the original product.

**No Cholesterol** Currently, no legal definition. Remember, though, that a product labeled no or low cholesterol may still contain saturated fats that raise blood cholesterol, and that this label does not mean *no fat*. Remember also that only animal products contain cholesterol.

**Organic** Usually *implies* that no synthetic fertilizers or pesticides were used when growing, processing, or packaging the food, but this definition is not backed by federal law. In other words, there is no guarantee that organic foods are completely free from pesticides, fungicides, or fertilizers.

**Reduced Calorie** One-third fewer calories than the product it most resembles, except meat and poultry, which must contain 25 percent fewer calories than similar products.

**Low in Calories** No more than 40 calories per serving and no more than 0.4 calorie per gram.

**Sodium-Free** No more than 5 mg sodium per serving.

**Very Low Sodium** No more than 35 mg sodium per serving.

**Low Sodium** No more than 140 mg sodium per serving.

**Reduced Sodium** At least 25 percent less sodium than the original product.

**No Salt Added and Salt-Free** No salt added in processing. However, the food could have significant amounts of natural sodium, or sodium from other sources such as soy sauce or preservatives.

**Sugar-Free/Sugarless** Contains no sucrose (table sugar), but might contain corn syrup fructose, honey, sorbital, or other sweeteners. *Not* necessarily low in calories.

*Sources: Learning the Tricks of Food Labeling. Environmental Nutrition 11(5), May 1988. Hamilton, E., Whitney, E., Sizer, F.:* Nutrition: Concepts and Controversies, *3d ed., St. Paul, Minn.: West Publishing Company, 1985.*

## PRINCIPLE 4: MOST HEALTH PROBLEMS RELATED TO NUTRITION ORIGINATE WITHIN CELLS

The main employers of nutrients are cells. The processes for which nutrients are required take place within cells and the fluid that surrounds them. There are over 100 trillion (100,000,000,000,000) cells in the human body. Each is a living unit fueled and maintained by the supply of nutrients it receives.

Cells are the building blocks of tissues (such as muscles and bones), organs (kidney, heart, liver, for example), and systems (such as respiratory, reproductive, circulatory, and nervous). Cells are responsible for all of the biological processes carried out in the body. Optimal cell health and functioning are maintained when a nutritional and environmental utopia exists within and around cells. Disruptions in the availability of nutrients, or the presence of harmful substances in the cell's environment, initiate diseases and disorders that eventually affect tissues, organs, and systems. Health problems in general begin with disruptions in the normal activity of cells.

The types and amounts of foods consumed by people affect the environment of cells and their ability to function normally. Excessive and inadequate supplies of nutrients and other chemical substances produce the disruptions in cell functions that ultimately become identified as health problems. Humans are as healthy as their cells.

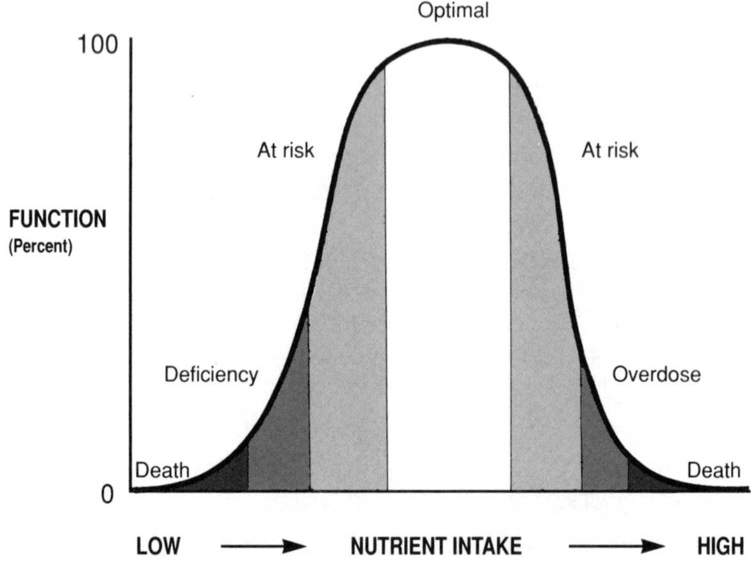


**FIGURE 2. HOW MUCH IS ENOUGH? VARIATIONS IN FUNCTION BY LEVEL OF NUTRIENT INTAKE**

*Source: Adapted from Mertz, 1981*

PRINCIPLE 5: POOR NUTRITION CAN RESULT FROM EXCESSIVE AS WELL AS INADEQUATE LEVELS OF NUTRIENT INTAKE

For each nutrient, for every individual, there is a range of optimal intake that produces the best level for cell and body functions. On either side of the optimal range are levels of intake associated with impaired functions. This concept is illustrated in figure 2. Inadequate essential nutrient intake, if prolonged, results in obvious deficiency diseases. Marginally deficient diets produce subtle changes in behavior or physical condition. If the optimal intake range is exceeded, then mild to severe changes in mental and physical functions occur, depending on the amount of the excess and the nutrient. Overt vitamin C deficiency, for example, produces bleeding gums, pain upon being touched, and a failure of bone growth. A marginal deficiency may cause delayed wound healing. On the excessive side, high intakes of vitamin C may contribute to the development of diarrhea and kidney stones.[2]

Severe consequences of deficient and excessive intake of nutrients are indeed rare in the United States. But marginally inadequate and excessive intakes of some nutrients are probably quite common.[3] Nearly all cases of vitamin and mineral overdose result from the excessive use of supplements—they are almost never caused by foods.

### *Nutrient Deficiencies Are Usually Multiple*

Most foods contain many nutrients, so inadequate diets will affect the intake levels of more than a single nutrient. Inadequate diets generally produce a spectrum of signs and symptoms related to multiple nutrient deficiencies. For example, protein, vitamin $B_{12}$, iron, and zinc are packaged together in many high-protein foods. Diets low in protein, therefore, are also likely to provide low amounts of these other nutrients.

Dietary changes also affect the intake level of many nutrients. Switching from a high-fat to a low-fat diet, for instance, generally results in a lower intake of calories, cholesterol, and vitamin E as well. So dietary changes to improve the intake level of a particular nutrient produce a ripple effect on the intake of other nutrients.

## PRINCIPLE 6: MALNUTRITION CAN BE CAUSED BY POOR DIETS AND BY DISEASE STATES

*Malnutrition* means "poor nutrition" and applies to both ends of the nutrient-intake range. You can be malnourished because you eat high amounts of nutrients as well as if you eat low amounts of them. Obesity is an example of malnutrition just as starvation is.

Malnutrition can result from poor diets as well as diseases that interfere with our body's ability to use the nutrients we consume. Diarrhea, alcoholism, cancer, and kidney disease, for example, may be responsible for the development of malnutrition in people with these disorders.

In healthy people, the amount of nutrients consumed in a diet can directly cause malnutrition in the form of deficiency and toxicity (overdose) diseases. The length of time it takes to develop nutrient deficiencies or toxicities depends on the type and amount of nutrient consumed, the extent of body-nutrient stores, and the body's need for the nutrient.

Malnutrition due to inadequate diets generally develops in the stages outlined in figure 3. After a period of deficient intake of an essential nutrient, tissue reserves become depleted. Blood levels of the nutrient then decrease because there are no reserves left to replenish the blood supply. Without an adequate supply of the nutrient in the blood, cells get shortchanged. They no longer have the nutrients needed to maintain normal function. If the deficiency is prolonged, the malfunctioning cells cause sufficient impairment to

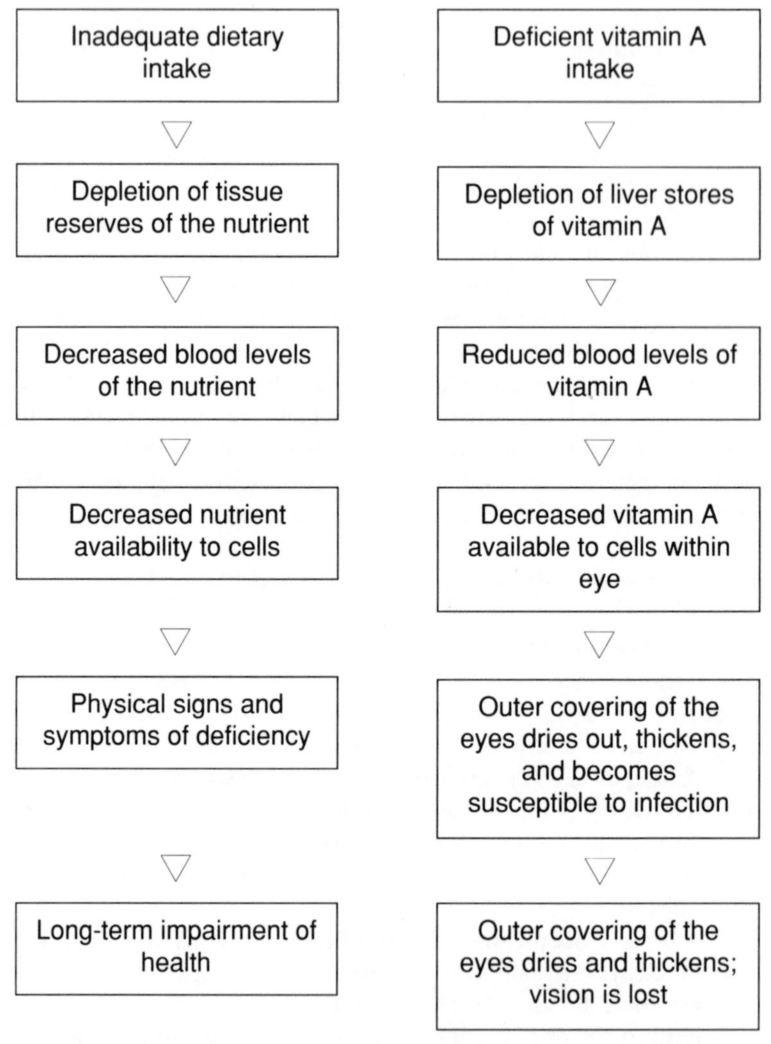


**FIGURE 3. USUAL SEQUENCE OF EVENTS IN THE DEVELOPMENT OF A NUTRIENT DEFICIENCY AND AN EXAMPLE OF HOW VITAMIN A DEFICIENCY DEVELOPS**

*Source: Adapted from Underwood, 1986, and Goodman, 1984*

produce physically obvious signs of a deficiency disease. Eventually, some of the problems produced may no longer be repairable, and permanent changes in health and function may occur. In most cases, the problems resulting from the deficiency can be reversed if the nutrient is supplied before this final stage occurs.

Excessively high intakes of some nutrients such as vitamin A and niacin produce toxicity diseases. The signs of the toxicity disease stem from increased levels of the nutrient in blood and the subsequent oversupply of the nutrient to cells. The high nutrient load upsets the balance needed for normal cell function. The changes in cell functions lead to the signs and symptoms of toxicity diseases. For both deficiency and toxicity diseases, the best time for correction of the problem is before tissue stores are adversely affected. In that case, no harmful effects on health and cell function occur—they are prevented.

### PRINCIPLE 7: SOME GROUPS OF PEOPLE ARE AT HIGHER RISK OF BECOMING INADEQUATELY NOURISHED THAN OTHERS

Every human requires the same nutrients, but not in the same amounts. Women who are pregnant or breast-feeding, growing children, and the ill and those recovering from illness have a higher requirement for nutrients than those of us who fit into none of the above categories. It is a situation that leaves those with greater nutrient needs at higher risk of becoming malnourished than other people. Their growth or health is more rapidly and seriously affected by inadequate diets than other people who require a lower level of nutrients. In cases of widespread food shortages, such as those induced by natural disasters or war, it is these nutritionally vulnerable groups whose health is compromised most by inadequate diets.

### PRINCIPLE 8: MALNUTRITION CAN INFLUENCE THE DEVELOPMENT OF CERTAIN CHRONIC DISEASES

The result of malnutrition is not always a nutrient deficiency or toxicity disease. Malnutrition can be caused by overeating, an excess consumption of fat, cholesterol, sodium, alcohol, and sugars; or the underconsumption of fiber. Faulty diets appear to play an important role in the development of heart disease, hypertension, cancer, osteoporosis, dental disease, and other disorders. The harmful effects of negative dietary practices on the development of these diseases and disorders may take years to develop.

### PRINCIPLE 9: FOODS CONTAIN MANY CHEMICAL SUBSTANCES IN ADDITION TO NUTRIENTS THAT MAY AFFECT HEALTH AND THE SAFETY OF FOODS

Nutrients come packaged in foods along with thousands of other chemical substances. Information on the health effects of these other chemical substances is far from complete, but evidence indicates that some can have either harmful or beneficial effects on health.

Chemical substances in food (other than nutrients) that may affect health can be classified into three groups:

Naturally occurring toxicants
Environmental contaminants
Intentional food additives

EXAMPLES OF NATURALLY OCCURRING TOXICANTS, ENVIRONMENTALLY CONTAMINATED FOODS, AND FOOD ADDITIVES

| SUBSTANCE | SOURCES | EFFECTS OF EXCESSIVE INTAKE |
|---|---|---|
| | *Naturally Occurring Toxicants* | |
| Allergens | Wheat gluten, cow's milk protein | Diarrhea, rash in genetically susceptible people |
| Avidin | Raw egg whites | Inhibits biotin (a B vitamin) absorption |
| Goitrogens | Cabbage, turnips, kale, brussels sprouts, rutabaga | Goiter (enlarged thyroid) |
| Oxalic acid | Spinach, Swiss chard, beet greens, rhubarb | "Oxalic-acid poisoning," which includes gastrointestinal upset and convulsions |
| Phytic acid | Whole grains | Inhibits absorption of calcium, zinc, and other minerals |
| Tryramine | Aged cheese and wine, and some chocolates | Severe hypertension and headaches among people taking certain types of antidepressants |
| Toxins in fish | Puffer fish toxins, dinoflagellates, others | Wide range; may include gastrointestinal upset, paralysis, and coma |
| | *Environmentally Contaminated Foods* | |
| Aflatoxin | Moldy grains, beans, peas, and peanuts | Liver damage |

| SUBSTANCE | SOURCES | EFFECTS OF EXCESSIVE INTAKE |
|---|---|---|
| | *Environmentally Contaminated Foods* | |
| Bacteria | Chicken, salads, honey, cheese and other foods contaminated with bacteria | Food poisoning |
| Lead | Lead-based paint flakes, car exhaust, contaminated soil | Anemia, mental retardation |
| Mercury | Industrial pollution of water and fish | Numbness, loss of coordination, visual disturbances |
| Radioactive particles | Fallout from nuclear plant accidents, leakages of stored or discarded radioactive particles | Gastrointestinal upset, cancer |
| Pesticides/herbicides | Plants | Wide range; may include rash, numbness, headaches, birth defects |

| TYPE | SUBSTANCES | FOOD SOURCES |
|---|---|---|
| | *Intentional Food Additives* | |
| Flavoring agents | Sugar, salt, herbs, fructose, saccharin, extracts, plus over 1,000 natural and artificial flavors | Soft drinks and fruit drinks, breakfast cereals, frozen desserts, cakes, candy, breads (and much more) |
| Flavor enhancers | MSG (trade names: Accent, Ajinomoto, Vestin) | Oriental foods, some processed meats (May cause "Chinese-restaurant syndrome"—temporary chest pain, headache, burning sensation, and sweating.) |

| TYPE | SUBSTANCES | FOOD SOURCES |
|---|---|---|
| | *Intentional Food Additives* | |
| Food coloring agents | Blue #1 and 2, Green #3, Red #3 and 40, Yellow #5, and six carotenes and other natural coloring agents | Margarine, soft drinks, fruit drinks, candy, bakery products, ice cream, orange skin, cheese, and many other products |
| Nutrients | Ferrous sulfate (iron), reduced iron, niacinamide (niacin $NB_3$), thiamin hydrochloride and thiamin mononitrate (thiamin or B), riboflavin ($B_3$), calcium carbonate (calcium), sodium ascorbate (vitamin C), pyridoxine hydrochloride ($B_6$), vitamin A palmitate (vitamin A), zinc oxide (zinc), trisodium phosphate (phosphorus), iodine | Refined flour and rice, bakery products, breakfast cereals, dairy products, beverages |
| Preservatives | BHA/BHT, citric acid, gamma radiation sulfites (sulfur dioxide), sodium nitrate, sodium benzoate, vitamins C and E | Breakfast cereals, bakery products, fruit drinks, soft drinks, fruits, vegetables, bacon, sausage, ham, snack foods, salad dressings |
| Texture enhancers | Mono- and diglycerides, alginates, gelatin, gums, carrogean, lecithin, starches | Margarine, ice cream and other frozen desserts, puddings, cheese spreads, gravies, bakery products |

| SUBSTANCES | FOOD SOURCES |
|---|---|
| *Unintentional Food Additives* | |
| Iodine | Milk and milk products |
| Estrogen | Meats |
| Antibiotics | Meats |
| Vitamin $B_{12}$ | Microorganisms in food |
| Lead | Calcium supplements made from crushed bone |

*Food Safety*

Virtually every chemical substance—such as water, fiber, caffeine, nitrogen, and sodium—is toxic at some level of consumption. Whether chemical substances found in foods are hazardous to health primarily depends upon our level of exposure to them. Just exposing the tongue to poisonous parts of a puffer fish, for example, is enough to cause death within hours. Oxalic acid, a chemical found in a number of dark green, leafy vegetables, must be consumed in ounces before signs of a toxic reaction occur. You can get "oxalic-acid poisoning" from eating raw rhubarb.

People are exposed to potential toxins in foods every day that they eat. Our level of exposure to toxins is rarely high enough to cause problems, though. Most overdoses of toxins in food result from consuming foods that contain strong toxins or those that have been contaminated with toxins.

*Naturally Occurring Toxicants*

Have you ever noticed a bright green area right beneath the skin of a potato or on the border of a potato chip? The greenish area contains a very small amount of *solanine*, a poisonous substance. *Phytates* are a natural part of whole grains that attach firmly to calcium, zinc, and other minerals in foods during digestion. The tightness of the bond between phytates and certain minerals causes them to be excreted rather than absorbed into the bloodstream. Perhaps the most bizarre example of a naturally occurring toxin is one contained in human tissue. *Kuru*, a degenerative disorder of the central nervous system, is believed to be transmitted by cannibalism among close relatives of the Fore tribe in New Guinea.

*Environmental Contaminants*

Toxic chemicals can enter foods as a result of environmental contamination. Aflatoxin, a substance formed by molds allowed to grow on stored beans, grains, and some other foods, causes liver damage if the contaminated foods are regularly consumed. Aflatoxin poisoning is considered a major cause of liver disease in certain developing countries where stockpiles of grain commonly become contaminated during storage.[6]

Dangerously high levels of lead, mercury, radioactive particles, and other substances can end up in foods as a result of environmental contamination. Lead poisoning usually results from the ingestion of lead-based paint flakes, air pollution from car exhaust, or the consumption of plants grown in lead-contaminated soil. Mercury poisoning has occurred among people eating fish from industrially contaminated water. Warnings of "Do not eat the fish" are generally posted by waters known to be contaminated with mercury and other toxic substances. Radioactive particles enter the atmosphere, groundwater, and soil as a result of nuclear weapon testing, nuclear power-plant accidents, and other industrial and toxic-waste storage accidents. It is generally agreed that health risks from radioactive particle contamination of food are small except in areas where significant levels of radioactive fallout have occurred. The levels of radioactive particles in the atmosphere have generally decreased since 1965, when nuclear weapon testing declined dramatically.[7]

### *Intentional Food Additives*

Chemical substances that are intentionally or inadvertently added to foods are considered *food additives.* This category includes over ten thousand different substances that affect the chemical and physical characteristics of food. Most additives are intentionally put in foods to improve the flavor, texture, color, appearance, nutrient value, and physical properties of foods. The two most common intentionally used food additives are sugar and salt. Among food additives used in smaller amounts, flavorings are by far the most common.

## FOOD IRRADIATION

*Frozen foods are antedated, ask for yours IRRADIATED.*

(Science Digest *magazine over twenty years ago)*

A different sort of food additive, one that does not fit very neatly into this group of chemical substances, but legally belongs there, is irradiation. *Irradiated* foods have been treated with a powerful stream of gamma radiation, or high-energy waves emitted by gamma particles contained in the nucleus of radioactive atoms. Gamma radiation passes completely through foods, much as microwaves pass through foods cooked in microwave ovens, so no irradiation remains in the food. The intense energy of the gamma rays destroys bacteria and other microorganisms, thus rendering the food sterile. The process substantially increases the time it takes for food to spoil. As long as irradiated foods are stored in airtight containers, they will remain unspoiled.

Irradiation has been used as a commercial method of food preservation in the United States since 1985, but only on a limited number of foods such as spices and some vegetables and fruits. Any foods that have been preserved by irradiation must state that fact on the label. The method is most widely employed in China, but by 1990 it is expected that there will be fifty commercial irradiation plants in seventeen countries.[8] Irradiation has been hailed as a major breakthrough in food preservation for developing countries where a high proportion of the available food supply spoils during storage.

Food irradiation is considered a food preservation method of the future. Although its use appears to cause no harm, the safety of the process has not been fully tested and many questions about it remain. Unless consumers are convinced that the process is safe, it is unlikely that irradiation will be much used as a food preservation technique in the United States.

ADVANTAGES AND DISADVANTAGES OF FOOD IRRADIATION

| *Advantages* | *Disadvantages* |
|---|---|
| Highly effective method for preservation | Safety not fully documented |
| Reduces food losses from spoilage | Does not destroy all types of toxins present in foods |
| Eliminates need for cold storage of foods | Destroys or chemically alters certain vitamins and fats |
| Reduces the need to use chemical preservatives | Alters the taste and texture of some foods |
| May reduce the incidence of food poisoning from spoiled food | Cannot be used on foods with low moisture content |

### WHAT ABOUT ARTIFICIAL SWEETENERS?

Both artificial and naturally occurring sweeteners are used extensively as food additives. Their attraction is their sweet taste.

Many chemicals in addition to the simple sugars impart a sweet taste to foods. Of the hundreds identified so far, saccharin and aspartame are used commercially. Saccharin is a complex, noncarbohydrate substance that has no caloric value; it cannot be broken down by the body to yield energy. The acceptability of the taste, and concerns about a possible relationship between saccharin intake and cancer, have lead to the decreased use of saccharin in foods. Aspartame is now the major type of artificial sweetener in use.

It has long been known that certain amino acids (the building blocks of proteins) have an intensely sweet taste and potential for use as low-calorie sweeteners. Developing a protein sweetener that was nontoxic, tasty, and inexpensive to produce became a priority of a number of food companies and absorbed a lot of industry time and money. The product finally identified was aspartame—a small protein containing two amino acids: aspartic acid and phenylalanine. Although these two amino acids exist in nature, they do not naturally exist together. Aspartame was developed by chemists, not Mother Nature.

Aspartame provides calories because it is made from protein. Most aspartame-sweetened products contain few calories, however, because little aspartame is needed to sweeten a product. Gram for gram, aspartame is several hundred times as sweet as sucrose. It is at the top of the list with saccharin when the relative sweetening power of all sweet substances now in use are compared. Aspartame is found in soft drinks, gelatins, whipped toppings, jellies, fruit drink mixes, cereals, puddings, and even in some medicines. Because it breaks down when heated and loses its sweetening power, aspartame is not recommended for use in cooked food products.

Although generally recognized as safe, precautions about the use of aspartame by pregnant women and young children have been issued.[9] Aspartame is fully absorbed by the body and increases blood levels of aspartic acid and phenylalanine. In laboratory animals, aspartame causes a decreased synthesis of serotonin (a chemical substance that affects mood, appetite, and other behaviors) by the brain.[10] The effect of aspartame on brain serotonin and possibly other neurotransmitter levels may be related to some of the physical signs reported among humans consuming relatively high amounts of it. Depression, headaches, increased appetite, and seizures have been reported among individuals consuming more than five cups of aspartame-sweetened beverages per day.[11] Other reports have not identified such side effects. Physical signs associated with aspartame use disappear after its use is discontinued. It appears that some people may be sensitive to aspartame and should avoid its use. Individuals with PKU (phenylketonuria)—a rare genetic disorder that causes phenylalanine to accumulate in the blood—must limit the amount of phenylalanine in their diets. PKU, if not managed adequately with a low-phenylalanine diet, produces mental retardation. Since aspartame contains phenylalanine, all products containing the sweetener must carry a warning label.

Artificially sweetened products are often touted as being good for dieters because they can help to cut down on caloric intake. As unexpected as it may sound, artificially sweetened products do not appear to help people control their weight. Two studies have shown that people who use them regularly tend to gain more weight over time than people who don't.[12,13]

### ALCOHOL SUGARS

Alcohol sugars and alcohols are chemically similar to the simple sugars. They are formed when simple sugars *ferment* (are converted to alcohol by enzymes).

Alcohol sugars are found in very small amounts in foods such as fruits. Their presence in foods is most often due to their use as sweetening agents in gums and so-called dietetic candies. Their use in such candies is a bit misleading. They provide 4 calories a gram, just as the other carbohydrates do, and may not contribute to lowering the caloric value of a food product.

The alcohol sugars have a sweet taste. Xylitol is by far the sweetest and it takes less xylitol to sweeten a product than sugar. Mannitol and sorbitol, the two other major alcohol sugars, are about half as sweet as xylitol. The extensive use of alcohol sugars as sweetening agents is limited by their tendency to cause diarrhea and other side effects.

One negative feature of simple sugars not shared by alcohol sugars is a tendency to promote tooth decay. Bacteria that cause tooth decay don't dine on the alcohol sugars.[14]

### FAKE FAT AS A FOOD ADDITIVE

The first artificial fat was discovered over twenty years ago by accident. Researchers at a large company were attempting to develop a synthetic fat that could easily be absorbed by premature infants. Instead, the product developed wasn't absorbed well at all. It had the taste and texture of fat, but since it was not broken down by digestive enzymes or absorbed, it did not provide calories. Although the researchers failed to develop the product they sought, they had opened the doors to what has become a multimillion-dollar industry.

Two types of artificial fat have been developed. Olestra™ and Simplesse™. Both look and taste like fat and contain no cholesterol, but have little else in common. Olestra is made by chemical reactions that tightly bind sucrose to fat. The resulting chemical is a "sucrose polyester." (Sounds like it should be a primary ingredient of leisure suits, right?) Olestra provides no calories, is heat-stable so it can be used in cooked, baked, or fried products, and may help lower blood cholesterol levels.

The raw ingredient for Simplesse is egg white or milk protein (both work). Simplesse is partially digested and provides 1⅓ calories per gram, or one-seventh of the calories provided by an equal amount of fat. Because it forms a gel when heated, Simplesse is not suitable for use in cooked products.

Several side effects of artificial fats have been noted in human studies. It appears their use can decrease the absorption of the fat-soluble vitamins (vitamins A and E, for example), and cause flatulence (gas), diarrhea, and other gastrointestinal upsets.

Whether artificial fats will fail the way starch blockers, liquid-protein diets, and lipase for weight loss did, or will turn out to be a revolutionary cure for overweight and the ill effects of high-fat diets, is yet to be seen. Because artificial fats are classified as foods and not drugs, there's not much information on their effects on health. Foods don't have to be rigorously tested and confirmed to be safe and effective, as drugs do.

For now, nutritionists have voiced concerns that the quality of diets may decrease if foods with artificial fat are widely consumed.[15] It's not that they are nay-sayers. It is because so little is known about the products. Are the diets and health of people improved by freely consuming foods with artificial fat? Will such products lower total fat intake? Are there side effects associated with the consumption of artificial fats that outweigh their potential benefits in saving calories? Will it turn out, as it seems to have for artificial sweeteners, that people who consume foods with artificial fat gain more weight than people who don't? How nutritious are products that will use them most of all? Would we be better off with diets lower in potato chips, salad dressings, and sauces or diets that contain these types of foods but that were made from ersatz fat? For these products, it appears that only time will tell.

### *Unintentional Food Additives*

Chemical substances that incidentally end up in foods during processing or storage are also considered food additives. Foods processed or stored in aluminum, tin, or copper containers end up absorbing a small amount of the minerals. Estrogen (a hormone), antibiotics, and other substances given to livestock to improve their growth and health may be found in trace amounts in the animal products that reach our plates. Because they can affect human health, the presence and use of unintentional and intentional food additives are regulated by the Food and Drug Administration.

Relatively few of the enormous number of food additives in current use are suspected of producing harm to health. Concerns have been raised about the safety of sulfides, monosodium glutamate (MSG), nitrates, saccharin, aspartame (NutraSweet™), and some color dyes, however.[16] Many consumers and scientists are questioning the need for certain additives, especially those used for cosmetic reasons, such as food dyes. As can be clearly observed from food labels that brightly announce "no preservatives," "no artificial colors," or "all natural flavors," there is a trend in the United States toward selecting foods made without additives.

## FOOD POISONING

A primary concern about food safety revolves around avoiding food poisoning. It is estimated that two million cases of food poisoning occur in the United States each year, and many more cases may go undiagnosed. (To be fair, some illnesses such as the flu get mislabeled as "food poisoning.") For the most part, the ingestion of food that has been contaminated with bacteria causes an upset stomach, vomiting, and/or diarrhea. The effects may be serious if food poisoning occurs in young children or adults who already have a digestive system problem or are in frail health.

One of the most effective ways to prevent foods from spoiling is to store them at, and heat them to, the right temperatures (see figure 4). Most types of bacteria don't grow at temperatures below 40° F and above 170° F. When holding foods before serving, hot foods should be kept hot, and cold foods cold. Freezing foods halts the growth of all of the main types of bacteria that contaminate foods. Once the foods are thawed, however, bacteria growth resumes and the foods may become contaminated with new bacteria while thawing.

The range of temperature that is best suited for bacterial growth is 60° to 120° F. The room temperature of homes is within this

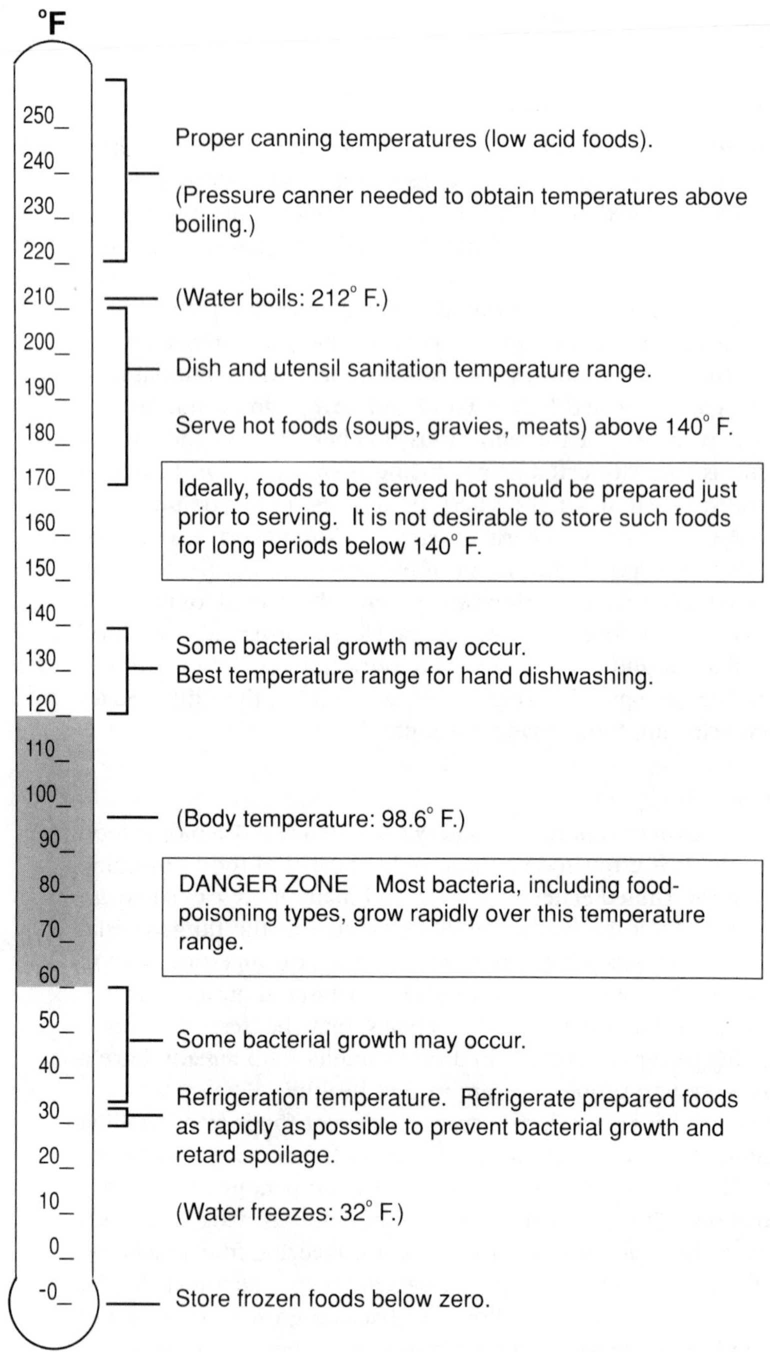


**FIGURE 4. TEMPERATURE GUIDE FOR SAFE HANDLING OF FOOD IN THE HOME**

*Source: Adapted from Minnesota Extension Service, University of Minnesota*

range and that's why foods that spoil should not be stored outside of the refrigerator or freezer for more than two hours. If a food smells or looks unusual, or if it has been improperly stored or stored past the expiration date on the label, it should not be eaten. The general rule should apply: When in doubt, throw it out.

Foods that are commercially canned are heated to the point where all bacteria are killed after the can is sealed. Consequently, the contents of canned foods are sterile and will not spoil if left on the shelf for years. The contents of canned foods may spoil if the can develops a pinhole leak or if errors made during the canning process allow bacteria to enter the food. A cardinal sign that canned foods have spoiled is a buildup of pressure inside the can. The pressure will cause the top of the can to bulge out instead of curving in. Because a buildup of pressure inside a can may result from bacteria that cause botulism, the food should be tossed.

A form of food poisoning that can lead to serious health problems is salmonella infection. It is the infection that can lead to the Memorial Day picnic-type outbreaks of food poisoning among everyone who eats the potato salad. The cause of the food poisoning can generally be traced back to the eggs that were used (and *not* the mayonnaise!). In the northeastern United States, over two thousand cases of salmonella and eleven deaths were reported in the eighteen-month period ending July 1987. Two-thirds of the outbreaks were due to the use of eggs contaminated with salmonella bacteria. Salmonella can occur on the outside of dirty eggs or may grow on the inside of eggs and the chicken if the chicken is infected with the bacteria. Washing eggs and hands after the eggs have been touched, promptly cleaning utensils and surfaces used in the preparation of eggs and chicken, and not eating raw or undercooked eggs and underdone chicken are the best ways to prevent salmonella infection. Keeping potato, macaroni, and other salads made with eggs cold prevents the bacteria from growing and ending a picnic on a sour note.

Some types of food spoil more quickly than others, so particular care needs to be taken when handling and storing them. Dairy products such as milk and cheese may spoil in about a week or sooner if contaminated with germs from the air or hands. If you hold cheese by the wrapper when you take it out of the refrigerator to cut a slice off, it will likely last longer than if you touch the cheese with your hands. Handling foods with clean hands and utensils on clean surface areas reduces the number of bacteria that come in contact with the food. The same principle applies to other foods that spoil easily. Meats, if tightly wrapped and kept clean and cold, for example, will normally stay fresh for two to three days.

The incidence of food-borne diseases in the United States is on the increase, and consumer interest in the topic has justifiably increased too.

HOW TO AVOID FOOD POISONING

1. Cook and heat foods thoroughly. Poultry should be cooked to an internal temperature of 180°–185°F. Beef should be cooked to an internal temperature of 140°F for rare, 160°F for medium, and 170°F for well done. Cook veal, lamb, and pork to an internal temperature of 170°F.
2. When reheating sauces, gravies, and soups, be sure to bring them to a rolling boil for a few minutes before serving.
3. Don't allow foods to sit out of a warm (140°F or above) oven or a cold refrigerator (40°F or below) for more than an hour or two. Freezers should be kept at 0°F or below.
4. Divide large batches of hot food into smaller containers before cooling in refrigerator so they cool quickly and thoroughly.
5. Thaw frozen foods in the refrigerator. When cooking frozen foods, allow 1½ to 2 times the amount of cooking time required for thawed food.
6. Marinate meats in the refrigerator and discard the marinade after using. Though acids such as lemon juice, wine, and vinegar in some marinades slow bacterial growth, they don't stop it.
7. Wash foods before cooking or eating. Poultry can contain salmonella, and fruits and vegetables can harbor bacteria from the dirt or soil they grow in.
8. Wash utensils and cutting boards, especially wooden ones, that have come in contact with poultry or meat. Dirty can openers are also a source of contamination. Using a diluted-bleach-and-water solution to clean these may be helpful. Keep kitchen towels and sponges clean as well.
9. Use clean lunch boxes and lunch bags. Wet or food-stained containers could harbor bacteria that, after multiplying overnight, may contaminate the next day's lunch.
10. Wash hands after going to the bathroom, diapering a baby, and blowing your nose.
11. Never use food from a bulging can.

*Source: Tracy Phelps, R.D., Health Education Unit, Minneapolis Health Department, Minneapolis, Minn.*

### PRINCIPLE 10: HUMANS HAVE ADAPTIVE MECHANISMS FOR MANAGING FLUCTUATIONS IN DIETARY INTAKE

Healthy humans come equipped with a number of adaptive mechanisms that partially protect the body from malnutrition due to fluctuations in diet. In the context of nutrition, adaptive mechanisms act to conserve nutrients when dietary supply is low, and to eliminate them if present in excessively high amounts. For some nutrients, dietary surpluses are stored within tissues for later use. For others, however, the body has no storage facilities and excesses must be quickly eliminated to prevent damage to cell functions.

Here are some examples of how the body adapts to changes in dietary intake:

> When caloric intake is reduced by fasting, starvation, or dieting, the body adapts to the decreased supply by lowering energy expenditure. Declines in body temperature and the capacity to do physical work act to decrease the body's need for calories. When caloric intake exceeds the body's need for energy, the excess is stored as fat for energy needs in the future.
>
> The ability of the gastrointestinal tract to absorb dietary iron increases when the body's stores of iron are low. The mechanisms that facilitate iron absorption in times of need rapidly shut down when enough iron has been absorbed, to prevent iron overload.
>
> The body has no absorption barriers for some vitamins, so the amount absorbed is directly related to the amount consumed. To avoid the toxic effects of high blood levels of these vitamins, excessive levels in the blood are rapidly cleared by the kidneys and excreted in the urine.

Although these built-in mechanisms do not protect humans from all the consequences of poor diets, they do provide an important buffer against the development of malnutrition.

### PRINCIPLE 11: BALANCE AND VARIETY ARE KEY CHARACTERISTICS OF A HEALTHY DIET

All of the nutrients humans need for health are available from foods, and many different combinations of foods can lead to a healthy or balanced diet. A balanced diet contains a variety of foods that together provide calories, nutrients, and other substances in amounts that promote health. As the name implies, balanced diets are balanced in both directions. They provide neither too few nor too many calories, and healthy proportions of carbohydrate, protein, fat, vitamins, minerals, water, and other substances such as alcohol and fiber. Balanced diets, regardless of what specific foods go into them, all have one property in common: they include a variety of foods.

Balanced diets require a variety of foods because no one food, with the exception of breast milk for young infants, provides all the nutrients humans need. Most foods do not even come close. It matters little what specific foods go into a balanced diet; it could include ants, snails, and raw sea cucumbers. What matters is whether the calorie and nutrient composition of the foods complement each other and add up to a healthy diet.

### *Nutrient Density*

Balanced diets are most easily achieved if they are composed of foods that are good sources of a number of nutrients while not being packed with calories. Foods that provide multiple nutrients in appreciable amounts relative to calories are considered ***nutrient dense.*** Those that provide calories but few nutrients are spoken of as ***empty-calorie foods.*** It is obviously easier to build a balanced diet around nutrient-dense foods such as fruits, vegetables, breads, cereals, lean meats, and milk than around a varied assortment of soft drinks, candy, pastries, chips, and alcoholic beverages. Variety by itself is not enough to ensure a balanced diet, however. It develops from a foundation of nutrient-dense foods.

A number of guides have been developed to help people choose an appropriate assortment of foods that will make up a balanced diet. Given today's food supply, our habit of consuming a high-fat diet and "eating on the run," and an attraction by many Americans to fast-food restaurants, putting a balanced diet together takes some planning.

# Chapter 4

## *Healthy Eating: Achieving the Balance between What Tastes Good and What Is Good for You*

*Before you get into this chapter, I'd like you to relax. To start, take a deep breath. Now release any tense muscles. Relaxed? Okay. For a moment, wrap your complete attention around the following statements:*

*A plump, golden peach. It's so ripe that juice spurts from it and drips down your chin when you take a bite.*

*A Thanksgiving turkey. It's still in the oven roasting, and the wonderful smell fills the whole kitchen.*

*A steaming loaf of golden-brown homemade bread that has just been set out to cool.*

*A perfectly ripe, just-picked tomato that melts in your mouth.*

*If your mouth is watering and you're ready to go out and buy some ripe peaches, you have found the balance between what tastes good and what's good for you.*

▼ Eating right has to mean eating foods you enjoy. If it doesn't, if it's too much of a struggle, good diets don't last. Healthy diets are those that people can live with and enjoy for a lifetime. The trick to getting one going that will last is planning. In return for up-front planning, you can end up eating right with foods and meals you like that don't take long to prepare.

For most of us, it isn't a dislike of good-for-you foods that keeps us from a healthy diet. It's a lack of time to shop for food and prepare meals, as well as a concern about calories and weight. This chapter focuses on the needs of adults who have little time to prepare meals and who don't want high-calorie diets. It does, however, call for taking some time to plan grocery shopping so you have the right foods on hand when it's time to zip a meal on the table or a lunch in a bag. Because about half of all meals are eaten outside the home, attention is also paid to eating right while eating out.

## EATING RIGHT DEFINED

*Eating right* means consuming a diet that promotes health and helps prevent disease. Such a diet provides adequate amounts of vitamins, minerals, and fiber, and a balanced supply of carbohydrates, proteins, and fat. In addition, healthy diets are built around basic foods that are naturally low in salt and sugar. The concept of *balance* is key to the definition of eating right. The American diet has gotten way out of balance. Too much of the U.S. diet is made up of fried or fat-rich foods and salted and sugared processed foods. On the low end of the balance are dietary fiber and complex carbohydrates from whole grain products, fruits and vegetables, and low-fat milk and milk products. How well-balanced diets are depends on the variety of foods that go into them. And most people like enough of the different types of foods that go into balanced diets to achieve one.

## BUILDING BALANCED DIETS

A balanced diet is not formed food by food. It is made up of the collection of foods we eat over the course of a day or several days. It's the sum of the contributions made by components of our usual food intake that produces a diet that either balances or doesn't.

How do you select the combination of foods that adds up to a balanced diet? One easy and straightforward way is to build diets around the recommended number of servings from the basic food groups.

(Food groups. I bet this term rings a bell. We all memorized them in health or home economics class, didn't we? As a matter of fact, you can almost tell a person's age by finding out what number of basic food groups she or he studied in school. Since 1916, food guides have been based on four, five, seven, eleven, and even sixteen food groups. The author had to learn the "Basic seven.")

The basic food groups, although boring to memorize, are nifty. They have worn well and continue to be used as a cornerstone of nutrition education in this country and many others. The food-group approach to selecting balanced diets has endured over the years because it focuses on foods (which people eat) and not nutrients (which people don't eat), because it allows leeway for personal choices within each group, and because foods selected according to the plan generally produce a healthy diet. The list of food groups that go into a balanced diet are shown in table 7.

TABLE 7. FOOD GROUPS THAT SERVE AS THE FOUNDATION OF A BALANCED DIET

| | RECOMMENDED MINIMUM NUMBER OF SERVINGS | | | |
|---|---|---|---|---|
| FOOD GROUP | CHILDREN | TEENAGERS | ADULTS[a] | VEGETARIANS |
| BREAD AND CEREALS | 4 | 4 | 4 | 6 |
| Whole grain and enriched bread, 1 slice or 1 ounce | | | | |
| English muffin, ½ | | | | |
| Roll, biscuit, muffin, 1 | | | | |
| Bagel, ½ | | | | |
| Tortilla, 1 | | | | |
| Noodles, macaroni, ½ cup | | | | |
| Rice, ½ cup | | | | |
| Ready-to-eat cereal, 1 cup or 1 ounce | | | | |
| Cooked cereal, ½ cup | | | | |
| Crackers, 4 squares | | | | |
| Pancake, 5" × ½" | | | | |
| Waffle, 4" × 4" × ½" | | | | |
| VEGETABLES AND FRUITS | 4 | 4 | 4 | 4 |
| (Includes at least one serving from each category) | | | | |
| *Vitamin-A-Rich* | | | | |
| Broccoli, ½ cup | | | | |
| Carrots, ½ cup | | | | |
| Collards, ½ cup | | | | |
| Spinach, ½ cup | | | | |
| Green peppers, ½ cup | | | | |
| Sweet potatoes, ½ cup | | | | |
| Winter squash, ½ cup | | | | |
| Apricots, 3 | | | | |
| *Vitamin-C-Rich* | | | | |
| Cantaloupe, ¼ whole | | | | |
| Orange/juice, 1 or 6 ounces | | | | |
| Grapefruit/juice, ½ or 6 ounces | | | | |
| Tomato/juice, 1 or 1 cup | | | | |
| Strawberries, ⅔ cup | | | | |
| Cabbage, raw, 1 cup | | | | |
| Brussels sprouts, ½ cup | | | | |

TABLE 7. CONTINUED

| FOOD GROUP | RECOMMENDED MINIMUM NUMBER OF SERVINGS | | | |
|---|---|---|---|---|
| | CHILDREN | TEENAGERS | ADULTS[a] | VEGETARIANS |
| VEGETABLES AND FRUITS (continued) | 4 | 4 | 4 | 4 |
| (Includes at least one serving from each category)<br>*Other*<br>Potatoes, 1<br>Corn, ½ cup<br>Peas, ½ cup<br>Green beans, ½ cup<br>Beets, ½ cup<br>Banana, 1<br>Apple/juice, 1 or 6 ounces<br>Pear, 1<br>Peach, 1<br>Grape/juice, 1 cup or 6 ounces<br>Watermelon, 1 cup | | | | |
| MILK AND MILK PRODUCTS (includes low-fat products) | 3 | 4 | 2 | 2 |
| Milk, 1 cup<br>Fortified soy milk, 1 cup<br>Yogurt, 1 cup<br>Cheese, 1½ ounces<br>Cottage cheese, 1 cup<br>Pudding, 1 cup<br>Ice cream, 2 cups<br>Ice milk, 1 cup | | | | |
| MEAT AND MEAT ALTERNATES (includes lean meats) | 2 | 2 | 2 | 3 |
| Beef, fish, poultry, pork, and other meats, 3 ounces or ½ cup diced<br>Eggs, 2<br>*(Vegetable protein sources)*[b]<br>Dried beans, cooked, 1 cup<br>Peanut butter, 4 tablespoons<br>Nuts, seeds, ½ cup<br>Tofu, ½ cup | | | | |
| MISCELLANEOUS | Based on caloric need | | | |
| Fats (butter, margarine, oil, mayonnaise), 1 teaspoon | | | | |

TABLE 7. CONTINUED

| FOOD GROUP | RECOMMENDED MINIMUM NUMBER OF SERVINGS | | | |
|---|---|---|---|---|
| | CHILDREN | TEENAGERS | ADULTS[a] | VEGETARIANS |
| MISCELLANEOUS (continued) | Based on caloric need | | | |
| Cream, whipped toppings, 2 tablespoons | | | | |
| Salad dressing, 2 tablespoons | | | | |
| Gravy, sauces, cup | | | | |
| Bacon, sausage, 1 ounce | | | | |
| Sweets (candy, sugar, soft drinks, fruit drinks, etc.), 1 ounce solids, 8 ounces beverages | | | | |
| Alcoholic beverages (if any) | | | | |

[a]*Pregnant and breast-feeding women should consume two additional servings from the milk and milk products group and one more serving from the meat and meat alternates group. Women beyond the age of fifty may benefit from more than two daily servings of low-fat milk and milk products.*
[b]*Vegetable protein sources should be consumed along with grains.*

KEY NUTRIENTS PROVIDED BY THE FOOD GROUPS

| *Food Group* | *Key Nutrients* | |
|---|---|---|
| Breads and cereals | Thiamin ($B_1$) | Iron |
| | Riboflavin ($B_2$) | Fiber |
| | Niacin ($B_3$) | |
| Vegetables and fruits | Vitamin A | Carbohydrates |
| | Vitamin C | Fiber |
| Milk and milk products | Calcium | Protein |
| | Riboflavin ($B_2$) | |
| Meat and meat alternates | Protein | Niacin ($B_3$) |
| | Iron | |
| Miscellaneous (other) | Fats | Sodium |
| | Sugars | Alcohol |

Foods included in the basic food groups are organized by their content of key nutrients. In other words, foods within a group are good sources of the same set of nutrients. Diets that contain at least

TEMPLATE FOR PLANNING BALANCED DIETS BASED ON THE FOOD GROUPS
*(Include one or more servings of foods from each group listed.)*

*Meal One*

- Vitamin-C-rich fruit
- Breads and cereals
- Milk and milk products

*Meal Two*

- Vegetables and fruits
- Breads and cereals
- Meat and meat alternates
- Milk and milk products
- Miscellaneous (1 serving)

*Meal Three*

- Vitamin-A-rich vegetables
- Other vegetable or fruit
- Meat and meat alternates
- Breads and cereals
- Milk and milk products
- Miscellaneous (1 serving)

*Snack*

- Breads and cereals,
- Vegetables and fruits, or
- Milk and milk products

the minimum number of servings recommended from each group tend to provide 80 percent or more of the RDAs for nutrients. The caloric level of diets that just meet the minimum recommended number of servings, however, is generally on the low side—1,000 to 1,400 calories. Calories can be increased to meet needs by eating more than the minimum number of servings.

A balanced diet is a bit easier for some people to plan if they have a framework with which to work. Although dietary patterns vary a lot, you can pull together a balanced diet using an approach that places foods from the different food groups into three meals and a snack. For guidance, see the basic template for designing meals and snacks that correspond with the assortment of foods prescribed in the food groups.

The basic food groups can be used for practical applications such as planning grocery lists, meals, and ordering from a restaurant menu. Of these, organizing grocery shopping by the food groups is one of the most useful applications.

*Guide for Grocery Shopping*

Eating right usually starts in the grocery store. Buying the right foods means they will be available when you need them. You can use the basic food groups to make up a big part of your grocery list, or to make sure what you plan to buy includes the right variety of foods. To make this easier to accomplish, follow the Shopping for a Balanced Diet guide, Appendix C, page 325. This checklist includes a wide variety of foods from each of the food groups so you can see the choices and decide which ones you want to buy. If you follow the plan as you shop, you'll probably find it takes less time to prepare meals and snacks. You won't have to fish around or run to the store to get the healthy assortment of foods you need when it's time to prepare them.

*Okay Snacks and Desserts*

Snacks and desserts are important parts of many diets and they, too, can fit into a balanced diet. A healthy diet doesn't have to omit all sweets and high-calorie snacks, but it does require limiting them to reasonable amounts. Diets that are based on the food groups usually have room for a serving or two a day of foods you eat mostly for fun. Children, because of their high need for energy, may need more of the calories provided by fun snacks or desserts. The problem comes when sweet or high-calorie snacks replace basic foods in the diet, and when weight becomes a problem because too many empty-calorie foods are consumed. Some types of snacks and desserts have more to offer nutritionally than others. See the list of "good snacks" and "okay desserts" to get an idea of the types of snacks and desserts that tend to be lower in calories and higher in nutrients than alternatives such as pies, cakes, candy, and chips.

GOOD SNACKS AND OKAY DESSERTS

| *Good Snacks* | *Okay Desserts* |
|---|---|
| Banana bread | Angel food cake |
| Carrots | Applesauce |
| Celery | Frozen yogurt |
| Cheese and crackers | Fruit |
| Cottage cheese | Fruit and cheese |
| Cucumbers | Ginger bread |
| Fruit, fruit juice | Ginger snaps |
| Fruit roll-ups | Ice milk |
| Graham crackers | Milk chocolate |
| Milk | Oatmeal cookies |
| Muffins | Peanut butter cookies |
| Nuts | Pudding |
| Peanut butter and crackers | Yogurt with fruit |
| Popcorn | |
| Rice wafers | |
| Yogurt | |

*Recipes for Good and Quick Meals*

Diets based on the food groups can take the form of delicious (and nutritious) beverages, appetizers, entrees, side dishes, and desserts. We have placed a healthy cookbook in chapter 13 so you can find the dinner menus and recipes when you want them. Most of the recipes provided take less than thirty minutes to prepare. They are nearly all low in fat and come with an analysis of their caloric and nutrient content.

*Eating Right while Eating Out*

For many women and men who organize meals, the question about what to eat often boils down to choosing a restaurant. The average American spends more than 43 percent of his or her food dollar on meals eaten out or ordered in. Ordering foods that fit into a balanced diet has become as important a skill as planning and preparing meals at home. With some forethought, eating out doesn't have to mean tipping the balance in your diet.

The goal of eating right while eating out has become easier to reach over the last few years because many restaurants have improved their menus. A recent survey by the National Restaurant Association showed that 23 percent of restaurants featured health and nutrition promotions in their menus. The special dishes are called everything from "Diet Plates" to "Fitness Foods" to "Light and Healthy." You can often order foods that are "spa" cooked—prepared without fat or salt. Restaurants frequently give customers the choice of fried or broiled fish, poultry, and beef, and will leave out the sauces and gravies upon request.

The general trend in restaurant offerings is very encouraging. But obviously not only nutritionists and dietitians are making up these "healthy" menus. Sometimes, they appear to have been designed by a marketing department more interested in making the items sound low calorie and healthy than being that way. Many "diet plates" aren't at all low in calories. For example, steak and cottage cheese, two relatively high-calorie foods, are often featured on diet plates. But potatoes and bread, two lower calorie foods, aren't because they're thought of as "too fattening." Salads and salad bars convey a "nonfattening, good-for-you" message, until you remember about the salad dressing. . . .

Outlined below are two types of "diet" meals and a popular fast-food meal. Which provides the fewest calories?

*Diet Plate*
6 ounces cooked beef pattie
1 cup cottage cheese
2 slices whole wheat bread
1/2 cup canned peaches

*Fast–Food Meal*
Big Mac
Regular order of french fries

*Salad Bar*
2 cups lettuce
1 ounce ham
1 ounce turkey
1 ounce American cheese
1/2 hard–boiled egg
1/2 tomato
2 ounces Italian dressing

The diet plate option weighs in at around 940 calories, similar to the 980 calories provided by the fast-food meal. Neither is very "diet-friendly" for a person interested in low-calorie balanced meals. The salad bar meal shown has the fewest calories, approximately 630, most of which come from the salad dressing. If you doubled the amount of salad dressing (from two to four ounces), you would increase the caloric content of the meal to 970—right up there with the diet plate.

It helps to stay on track if you decide what to eat before you look over a restaurant's menu. That may mean deciding *before* you enter the restaurant to order soup and a salad (with dressing on the side), seafood that is not fried, a half-portion, or no dessert. If you eat on planes frequently, you may want to give your travel agent a standing order for a vegetarian meal (they are generally low calorie, nutrient rich, and fiber rich) or a low-fat meal. If you're going to a party or business event where food will be served, decide before you go what types of food you'll eat, and what you will drink. If all you are presented with are high-calorie foods, plan on taking a small portion and stopping there. Impulse ordering and spur-of-the-moment food choices are two big environmental hazards that can whack diets out of balance.

The crash course continues in the next chapter with a closer look at the nutrients that provide energy. You'll find out what carbohydrates, proteins, and fats are, why we need enough but not too much of each of them, and what they do for us.

# Chapter 5

## A Look at Carbohydrates, Proteins, and Fats

*One of the very nicest things about life is the way we must regularly stop whatever we are doing and devote our attention to eating.*

*Luciano Pavarotti,* Pavarotti My Own Story

▼ Food is one of the greatest pleasures of humankind. It provides relief from hunger and a feeling of comfort and security, and it makes the taste buds smile. The pleasure and relief provided by food are strong incentives for eating. The body has developed these "eating reward systems" for one main purpose. It is only through eating that the body has a chance of getting the energy and nutrients it needs to stay alive and well.

The first and foremost need of the body is for energy, or the *calories* supplied in food. Calories are a unit of measure for food energy, just like *watts* of a light bulb or the *horsepower* of a car. The number of calories of energy in a food equals the amount of fuel it supplies to the body. Without a constant supply of energy, body processes would fail quickly. Without energy, we cannot use the proteins, vitamins, and minerals in foods to build and maintain healthy tissues or to fight off and recover from illness.

When we consume more calories from food than our body needs, the excess is converted to fat and stored for later use. When fewer calories are taken in than needed, we draw on the energy stores and reduce them and our body weight.

Because the body can form energy from carbohydrates, proteins, and fats in foods, those elements are called *energy nutrients.* Both carbohydrates and proteins supply 4 calories per gram, while fat provides over twice that much—9 calories per gram. (Does it help to know there are about 28 grams in 1 ounce? Or 1 ounce in

2 tablespoons of liquid?) If you have observed the flames produced by dripping fat from a steak or hamburger on a grill, you have seen the powerhouse of energy stored in fat. The carbohydrate and protein contents of grilled foods don't burn with nearly the same intensity. They have less energy to give.

## CHARACTERISTICS OF THE ENERGY NUTRIENTS

Shortly after the energy nutrients were discovered in the late 1800s, it was recognized that protein did more than supply energy. It also provided the building blocks for the construction and repair of body tissues. Because only protein can perform those essential functions, the body "spares" protein from use as an energy source if carbohydrates and fats are available. When the supply of carbohydrates and fats is limited, protein will be used to form energy, making less protein available for tissue formation and repair. So protein can only be used for its unique functions if enough carbohydrates and fats are available to meet the body's need for energy.

Of the energy nutrients, the body's favorite source of fuel is carbohydrates. They can be most readily converted into energy and, unlike protein and fat, can be directly used as a source of fuel by all cells in the body.

As dictated by the first law of thermodynamics, energy can neither be created nor destroyed, but it can change forms. The energy stored in the carbohydrates, proteins, and fats we consume in foods can be used for physical movement, digestion, and so on, or it can be changed to a storage form of energy. If the foods we consume supply more energy than we need at the time, the excess is largely converted to fat and stored for later use. The body can make fat out of excess amounts of *any* of the energy nutrients—carbohydrates, fat, *and* protein. When our food intake supplies less energy than we need, stored fat is called upon to make up the deficit.

Carbohydrates can also be stored by the body in the form of glycogen. But glycogen stores are much smaller than fat stores. People are usually limited to about an 1,800-calorie supply of glycogen stored in muscles and the liver. On the other hand, the body can store extraordinary amounts of fats—on average, 140,000 calories in adults (figure 5).

In general, foods have substantially more carbohydrates, proteins, and fats than vitamins or minerals, which reflects our larger need for those energy nutrients. They rarely are the sole nutrients provided by foods. With the exception of sugar and alcohol, foods that supply the energy nutrients also add vitamins, minerals, water, and other substances to our diets.

Alcohol also provides calories. It is chemically similar to carbohydrates and supplies 7 calories per gram. The relatively high energy content of alcohol makes cherries jubilee and other flambeaus possible.

Carbohydrates, proteins, and fats do more for the body than serve as energy sources. Next, a look is taken at the special features of each, and their effects on health.

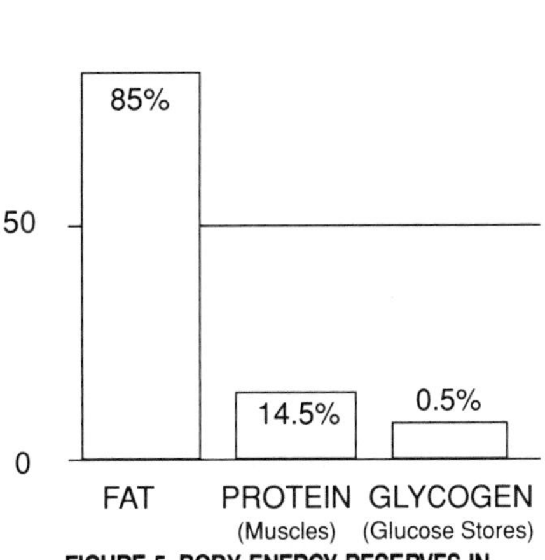


**FIGURE 5. BODY ENERGY RESERVES IN HEALTHY HUMANS**

## CARBOHYDRATES

Carbohydrates are the body's leading source of fuel. Foods that are rich in carbohydrates—some examples are rice, potatoes, beans, millet, cassava, pasta, and breads—are the main ingredients in the diets of people throughout most of the world. The diets of people who live in the United States and several other economically developed countries stand out in that carbohydrates take a backseat to foods rich in protein and fat.

Carbohydrates serve one major body function: they are a source of energy. The cells of the central nervous system, certain cells in the kidneys, and red blood cells must use carbohydrates for energy formation. Carbohydrates can be completely used to form energy—there are no waste products that the body must take care of, as when energy is formed from protein or fats.

### *The Types of Carbohydrates in Foods*

Carbohydrates are a diverse group of substances that range from the simple sugars to the complex and indigestible dietary fibers. They are usually grouped into two basic classes, *simple sugars* and *complex carbohydrates*. Because alcohol is a close chemical relative of the carbohydrates, it will be discussed in this section. You will find a listing of the carbohydrate content of common foods in table 8. To make it easier to picture the carbohydrate value of the foods listed, the percentage of total calories in the food that is contributed by carbohydrates is also given in the table.

TABLE 8. CARBOHYDRATE CONTENT OF COMMON FOODS
*(Recommended intake of carbohydrates: 58% of total caloric intake)*

| | CARBOHYDRATE CONTENT | | |
|---|---|---|---|
| FOOD | AMOUNT | GRAMS | % OF CALORIES PROVIDED BY CARBO-HYDRATES |
| *Sugars and Sweeteners* | | | |
| Sugar | 1 tsp. | 4 | 100 |
| Honey | 1 tsp. | 6 | 100 |
| Maple syrup | 1 tsp. | 4 | 100 |
| Corn syrup | 1 tsp. | 5 | 100 |
| *Grains and Grain Products* | | | |
| Corn starch | 1 tsp. | 3 | 100 |
| Apple Jacks | 1 cup | 26 | 94 |
| Cornflakes | 1 cup | 15 | 84 |
| Noodles | ½ cup | 27 | 84 |
| White rice | ½ cup | 25 | 84 |
| Whole wheat bread | 1 slice | 12 | 74 |
| Oatmeal | 1½ cups | 12 | 74 |
| Cheerios | 1 cup | 8 | 73 |
| *Legumes* | | | |
| Lima beans | ½ cup | 17 | 72 |
| White beans | ½ cup | 21 | 71 |
| Kidney beans | ½ cup | 20 | 67 |
| *Fruits* | | | |
| Apple | 1 medium | 20 | 92 |
| Banana | 1 medium | 25 | 93 |
| Pear | 1 medium | 25 | 90 |
| Peach | 1 medium | 10 | 93 |
| Orange | 1 medium | 18 | 90 |
| *Vegetables* | | | |
| Carrot | 1 medium | 7 | 93 |
| Potato | 1 medium | 35 | 89 |
| Corn | ½ cup | 15 | 86 |
| Broccoli | ½ cup | 4 | 80 |
| *Beverages* | | | |
| Cola | 12 oz. | 40 | 100 |
| Mountain Dew | 12 oz. | 43 | 100 |
| Fruit drink | 1 cup | 29 | 98 |
| Grapefruit juice | 6 oz. | 25 | 95 |
| Orange juice (sweetened) | 6 oz. | 18 | 90 |
| Whole milk | 1 cup | 11 | 28 |

### *The Simple Sugars*

There are three major simple sugars that are as simple as carbohydrates come in foods: *glucose* (blood sugar), *fructose* (fruit sugar), and *galactose*—which has no nickname. The body rapidly converts nearly all of the fructose and galactose consumed in foods into glucose, the only form of sugar the body can use to produce energy.

Simple sugars also come in packages of two units of glucose, fructose, and/or galactose. *Maltose* (malt sugar) consists of two units of glucose, whereas *sucrose*, or table sugar, and honey are formed from glucose and fructose. The milk sugar *lactose* contains glucose plus galactose.

Most of the simple sugars have a very distinct sweet taste, which is why many people love to eat them. In addition to our normal dentition, Mother Nature has given us a special, sweet-seeking tooth.

#### THE HUMAN SWEET TOOTH

Humans, like most mammals, are born with a preference for a sweet taste. Even before birth, a fetus will react positively (or move toward) the source of sweetness if a sucrose solution is injected into the womb. It will withdraw from bitter and sour fluids. After birth, infants will select sweet fluids over solutions with other tastes. The preference for the strength of sweet solutions may decline with age, but a preference for a sweet taste is a human trait from womb to tomb.[1]

#### SUGAR SOURCES

There are more than a hundred sweet substances that can be correctly described as sugars. Sucrose, or table sugar, is the most common. It is manufactured by a refining process that converts cane or beet sugar to molasses, then to brown sugar, then to "raw" sugar, and finally to white sugar. Per person consumption of sucrose in the United States averages 5.4 ounces per day (3/4 cup) or around 123 pounds per year.[2] On average, almost 30 percent of the total calorie intake of Americans is from sugar.

Most of the sugar in the U.S. diet is added to foods before purchase. Of the total amount of sugar produced, 65 percent is used by the food and beverage industry in the manufacture of soft drinks, beer, wine, bakery products, cereals, candy, and processed foods.[3] One 12-ounce cola, for example, contains about ten teaspoons of sugar. Some presweetened cereals have 4 teaspoons of added sugar per serving. Added sugars can make up as much as 45 percent, or

TABLE 9. SUGAR CONTENT OF BREAKFAST CEREALS

| CEREAL | SUCROSE (GRAMS) | % OF CALORIES PROVIDED BY SUCROSE | TOTAL CALORIES |
|---|---|---|---|
| Raisin bran | 9 | 45 | 80 |
| Frosted Flakes | 11 | 40 | 110 |
| Ice Cream Cone Cereal | 11 | 37 | 120 |
| All-Bran | 5 | 29 | 70 |
| Frosted MiniWheats | 6 | 24 | 100 |
| Bran Flakes | 5 | 22 | 90 |
| Life | 6 | 20 | 120 |
| 100% Natural | 6 | 17 | 140 |
| Grape-Nuts | 3 | 11 | 110 |
| Product 19 | 3 | 11 | 110 |
| Special K | 3 | 11 | 110 |
| Wheaties | 3 | 11 | 110 |
| Wheat Chex | 2 | 8 | 100 |
| Cornflakes | 2 | 7 | 110 |
| Cheerios | 1 | 4 | 110 |
| Shredded Wheat | 0 | 0 | 110 |

*Source: Nutrition Information Labeling on Breakfast Cereal Packages, 1988.*

as little as 0 percent of the total calories in a breakfast cereal. The sugar content of several brands of cereal is given in table 9.

You can get a rough estimate of the sugar content of breakfast cereals by noting on what shelf they are displayed in the grocery store. The cereals on the lower shelves, those that are about eye level to the six-year-old shopper, are often the sweetest.

Do you know what *levulose, dextrose*, and *sorghum* are? They are three names for different types of sugars. If you spend time reading nutrition information labels on food packages, you have probably seen them before. There is a wide array of simple sugars added to foods, and many have names that don't mean "oh, this is a sugar" to most people. Do you find any surprises in this list of sugars?

| | | |
|---|---|---|
| Corn syrup | Glucose | Xylitol |
| Dextrose | Mannitol | Lactose |
| High-fructose corn syrup | Sorbitol | Levulose |
| Honey | Sorghum syrup | Maltose |
| Fructose | Sucrose | Maltodextrin |

A relative newcomer to the sweetener scene is a product called "high-fructose corn syrup." Food companies have known about its remarkable sweetening powers for some time, but it wasn't widely used in foods because it was too expensive to make. New technology has made it inexpensive to manufacture, and high-fructose corn syrup is taking over a good chunk of the sweetener market. Made from corn starch, high-fructose corn syrup can contain up to 90 percent fructose, which makes it a very sweet fluid. It is used in candy, soft drinks, bakery products, cereals, and "sucrose-free" seltzers. (A close look at the label of these seltzers reveals that they are indeed sucrose-free, but they are by no means sugar-free. Many are loaded with fructose and it has 4 calories per gram, just like the other sugars.)

Our inborn preference for a sweet taste and the wide availability of sugary foods can put us at odds with what we think we ought to be eating. Although they please the taste buds, sweet foods are generally thought of as "being bad for you." Some people (with a tendency to draw and publicize unfounded conclusions) have even suggested that excessive sugar intake is the root of mental illness and violent and criminal behavior. In addition, it has been claimed that sugar depletes nutrients from our bodies. None of these purported relationships hold any scientific water. However, there is one established relationship between sugar and health that is beyond question—the relationship between sugar intake and tooth decay. There are two other potential relationships that are matters of heated scientific debate. One concerns sugar intake by children and hyperactivity, and the other the role of sugar intake in contributing to diabetes. In a well-designed study by the National Institute of Mental Health, children aged two to six years who were said to be "sugar responsive" by their parents tended to be more physically active after consuming around 8 teaspoons of sugar than after they ingested aspartame (NutraSweet™) or saccharin.[4] The differences in activity level were not large, and not all of the children tested showed increased activity after the sugar.

Although there is no direct proof that sugar intake is related to the development of diabetes, there is evidence to suggest the two may be related. Diabetes is considered a "disease of civilization"; its incidence increases as a population becomes urbanized. Diabetes is a relatively rare condition in developing nations, where traditional diets are similar to those consumed by our early ancestors and where few people are obese. However, when traditional diets move toward being high in calories and simple sugars, the incidence of diabetes in the adult population tends to increase.[5]

### SUGARS AND TOOTH DECAY

The suspicion that diet may be related to tooth decay was expressed as long ago as 350 B.C., when Aristotle posed the question: "Why do figs when they are soft and sweet produce damage to the teeth?"[6]

Sugar intake is strongly related to the development of tooth decay. However, enough is known about diet and tooth decay to give sound and practical guidance on how to prevent it.

Tooth decay is the leading dental health problem in the world. It has been a bothersome problem to humankind for thousands of years, but only became a widespread problem late in the 17th century, when great quantities of sucrose began to be imported from the New World. Sugar consumption is so closely linked to the development of tooth decay that periods of sugar shortage, such as occurred during World Wars I and II, corresponded to decreased rates of tooth decay in the United States and Europe.[7]

Eating sugary foods and drinking sweetened beverages between meals is more hazardous to dental health than is eating or drinking them with meals.[8] People who drink coffee or tea sweetened with sugar throughout the day tend to have more decayed teeth than people who only drink them with meals.[9] Candy, cookies, crackers, and syrups eaten between meals are much more likely to promote decay than when the same foods are mixed with a meal.[8] Chewing as few as two sticks of gum made with sugar daily has also been found to increase tooth decay significantly.[10]

Some foods have been identified that actually protect teeth from developing tooth decay.

Tooth decay, although still one of the most important, preventable health problems of our time, is on the decline in the United States and many other developed countries. Decreased rates of tooth decay are strongly associated with declining consumption of sugary foods between meals and the increased availability of fluoridated drinking water and mouth rinses.[12]

A growing body of expert opinion indicates that many people in the United States would benefit from lower sugar intake. The reason is not only that sugars promote tooth decay, but also because sugars and most sugary foods provide *empty calories*. They take up space in a diet that would be better occupied by fresh fruits, vegetables, grains, and other sources of *replete* calories. Foods high in sugar are often high in fat, so that fat intake increases along with sugar intake. Cutting down on sugar may well result in a bonus reduction in fat intake.

| Foods that DO NOT PROMOTE Tooth Decay | Foods that DO PROMOTE Tooth Decay |
|---|---|
| Milk | Sugars |
| Ice cream | Fruit drinks and juices |
| Cheese | Soft drinks |
| Yogurt | Candy |
| Eggs | Crackers |
| Meat | Milk chocolate |
| Fruit | Cookies |
| Nuts | Cereals |
| Artificial sweeteners | Chocolate milk |
| Artifically sweetened gum | Pastries |
| Peanut butter | Raisins |
| Fats and oils | Regular gum |
| Coffee, tea | Jelly, jam |
| Club soda | Syrups |

*Source: Reference 11*

*The Complex Carbohydrates*

The complex carbohydrates consist of *starches* and *dietary fiber*, or "bulk," as our mothers used to say. (Or perhaps your mother said "roughage"?) Complex carbohydrates come from plants and they lack the sweet taste of the simple sugars.

Starches differ from simple sugars in that it takes the body longer to digest them and they generally don't cause a "rush" in blood-sugar levels. Complete digestion of starch yields glucose—a simple sugar. Potatoes, corn, dried beans, rice, cereals, bread, and pastas are leading food sources of the complex carbohydrates. Dietary fiber, or the bulk just mentioned, differs from starches in that it is not digested at all by human digestive enzymes.

DIETARY CARBOHYDRATES: HOW MUCH?

*I never met a carbohydrate I didn't like.*

*Boynton cartoon, 1979*

Recommendations for diets that promote health indicate that about 58 percent of the total calories in a person's diet should come from carbohydrates—particularly the complex, starchy sources such as potatoes, pastas, breads, and cereals.[13] Most people in the United

States get too few calories from complex carbohydrates and too many from simple sugars and fat.

### DIETARY FIBER

Dietary fiber comes in two basic types: the fibrous components of plant cells, particularly plant cell walls, and nonfibrous components of plant cells, found primarily inside cells. Many foods, such as dried beans, potatoes, and corn, hide their fiber content very well. They are not crunchy and don't look a bit fibrous, yet they are among our best sources of fiber. The bottom line is that you can't tell a plant's fiber content by its looks or crunch value. Table 10 shows the dietary fiber content of foods and reveals the hidden truths.

Fibrous sources of dietary fiber, such as the bran that covers wheat, rice, and some other whole grains, do not dissolve in water. However, they do hold water and will swell up when combined with water. Nonfibrous dietary fibers form a gel-like solution when combined with water. Primary sources of the gel-like fibers are the pulp parts of fruits, vegetables, dried beans, and oat bran.

Although humans do not produce the types of digestive enzymes needed to break down dietary fiber, certain bacteria that dwell in our large intestine do. Bacteria that consume dietary fibers as food don't completely break them down. They excrete fragments of fats and gases as their end products of dietary fiber ingestion. The gases produced by the bacteria can sometimes cause discomfort after a meal when an unusually high amount of dietary fiber has been consumed, particularly if the fiber comes from dried beans, which contain several types of fiber that bacteria feast upon.

### THE SPECIAL EFFECTS OF DIETARY FIBER

Dietary fibers, even though they are not absorbed into the body proper, have a number of effects on the body. The type of effect varies according to the type of dietary fiber eaten. Cellulose, a fibrous component of bran and plant cell walls, makes food move along the digestive tract more quickly than when it is not present. Gel-forming, nonfibrous fibers such as contained in the pulp of fruit have a less pronounced effect. Fibrous forms of dietary fiber such as wheat bran tend to bind with zinc, magnesium, and other minerals during digestion and decrease their absorption. Some types of fibers appear to decrease glucose and cholesterol absorption, features that make gel-forming fibers such as guar gum, psyllium (pronounced "silly-um"), and other fibers found in dried

TABLE 10. FOOD SOURCES OF DIETARY FIBER
*Recommended Intake for Adults: 25–35 grams*

| FOOD | AMOUNT | DIETARY FIBER (GRAMS) |
|---|---|---|
| *Grains* | | |
| All-Bran | ¾ cup | 11.2 |
| Grape-Nuts | ¾ cup | 5.9 |
| Shredded wheat | 1 biscuit | 2.7 |
| Oatmeal | ¾ cup | 2.1 |
| Cornflakes | ¾ cup | 2.1 |
| Whole wheat bread | 1 slice | 2.0 |
| Bran | 1 T. | 1.8 |
| Rice Krispies | ¾ cup | 0.9 |
| White bread | 1 slice | 0.6 |
| *Fruits*[a] | | |
| Apple (with skin) | 1 medium | 2.4 |
| Peach (with skin) | 1 medium | 2.3 |
| Strawberries | 10 large | 2.1 |
| Pear (with skin) | 1 medium | 2.1 |
| Banana | 6" long | 1.8 |
| Grapefruit, canned | ½ cup | 0.5 |
| *Legumes*[b] | | |
| Kidney or navy beans | ⅓ cup | 6.2 |
| Peas | ½ cup | 5.7 |
| Peanuts | 3 T. | 2.5 |
| Peanut butter | 2 T. | 2.3 |
| *Nuts* | | |
| Brazil | ¼ cup | 2.7 |
| *Vegetables* | | |
| Corn, canned | ½ cup | 4.7 |
| Potato (with skin) | 1 medium (2¼") | 3.5 |
| Broccoli | ½ cup | 3.4 |
| Carrots, boiled | ½ cup | 2.8 |
| Green beans | ½ cup | 2.7 |
| Brussels sprouts | ½ cup | 2.0 |
| Cauliflower | ½ cup | 1.4 |
| Tomato, fresh | 1 small | 1.4 |
| Potato chips | 1 oz. | 0.9 |
| Lettuce, iceberg | ½ cup | 0.8 |

[a] *Where are the prunes? You may notice that prunes are not among the sources of dietary fiber listed. The distinct effect of prunes on the intestinal tract is primarily related to their content of a naturally occurring laxative.*

[b] *Legumes: Dried seeds or their pods that will "split down the middle"; includes beans (such as kidney, pinto, black, and red), split peas, lentils, and yes—peanuts.*

beans and oat bran a lot more popular than they used to be.[14,15] It is also possible that an increased-fiber diet may help people lose weight. In one study, women who increased their fiber intake by 23 grams decreased their caloric intake by 115 to 153 calories per day.[16]

The intake of dietary fiber by most people in the United States is in the order of 10 to 20 grams per day.[17] An intake of 25 to 35 grams per day is thought to represent a desired intake level.[18] If you are thinking about increasing the fiber content of your diet, try following these three suggestions:

Eat a high-bran cereal for breakfast or for a snack each day. Or, add 1 tablespoon of oat or wheat bran to your hot or cold breakfast cereal. (If you're trying to lower your cholesterol level, choose the oat bran.)

Eat more than four servings of fruits and vegetables every day.

Use whole grain breads with added bran.

Remember, you probably need to increase your fluid intake when you add fiber to your diet. (Fiber can be constipating if your fluid intake is too low.) You may need to add 2 to 3 cups of water to your diet each day to help the fiber work.

Newcomers to increased-fiber diets often experience diarrhea, cramping, bloating, and gas for the first several days (or more) of increased fiber use. Because the intestines and their bacterial colonies take awhile to adjust to the larger supply of fiber, it should be added to the diet gradually.

If diarrhea and the other symptoms continue beyond a few days, there is likely too much fiber in the diet and you should cut back. How much dietary fiber is needed to promote peak intestinal performance varies substantially among individuals. Some people develop diarrhea on relatively small amounts of fiber; others need a lot to prevent constipation. Perhaps the best level of dietary fiber intake is one that produces neither diarrhea nor constipation. You've got the amount right when stools are well formed but soft, and float.

### *Alcohol*

Alcohol enters our diets through beverages such as beer, wine, and whiskey. Data for the United States indicates that for every person over the age of fourteen years, fourteen cases of beer, twelve fifths of wine, and twelve fifths of distilled spirits are sold each year.

However, about 80 percent of the alcohol consumed in the United States is by the 30 percent of adults who consume it regularly.[19]

Alcohol-containing beverages are classic examples of empty-calorie foods. You can see the caloric value of various alcoholic beverages in table 11.

TABLE 11. CALORIC VALUES OF VARIOUS ALCOHOLIC BEVERAGES

| ALCOHOL-CONTAINING BEVERAGE | AMOUNT | CALORIES |
|---|---|---|
| Beer | | |
| Regular | 12 oz. | 150 |
| Light | 12 oz. | 95 |
| Liquor (86 proof) | | |
| Gin, rum, vodka, whiskey | 1½ oz. | 105 |
| Wine | | |
| Sweet | 3½ oz. | 200 |
| Dry, red | 3½ oz. | 110 |
| Dry, white | 3½ oz. | 115 |
| Cordials and liqueurs (80 proof) | 1½ oz. | 145 |

Alcohol-containing beverages, if consumed in moderation by nonpregnant adults, appear to cause no harm and may decrease the risk of developing heart disease.[20] A moderate amount of alcohol is considered to be two or fewer standard-size drinks per day. Heavy drinking (usually defined as six or more drinks per day) puts people at high risk of developing a variety of social, economic, and health problems. Among health problems common in heavy drinkers are malnutrition, hypoglycemia, ulcers, heart disease, hypertension, certain types of cancer, and cirrhosis.[21] Cirrhosis of the liver is the eighth leading cause of death in U.S. males, and over 90 percent of the cases are associated with heavy drinking.[19] Far fewer women drink excessively than men.[19]

## PROTEIN

*Protein*. The word conjures up the thought "good for you." It gets a much more positive reaction than other terms of the trade such as *diet*, *calories*, and *fat*. You don't have to talk about the importance of protein; people are already convinced of it. Protein is an essential structural component of all living matter that is involved in most every human biological process.

Protein's primary role is to provide building materials for body tissue. (It is also used for energy.) Muscles, connective tissue (ligaments and cartilage, for example), hemoglobin, enzymes, many hormones, and antibodies are derived from protein.

Protein consists of units of amino acids linked together in chemical chains. It is really the amino acids, not protein per se, that are needed for health. It's just that we get the amino acids we need by eating food sources of protein (table 12).

Twenty amino acids serve as the building blocks for the thousands of proteins formed by the body. Of these, nine are *essential*,

TABLE 12. FOOD SOURCES OF PROTEIN
*(Adult RDA for women = 50 g)*

| | | PROTEIN CONTENT | |
|---|---|---|---|
| FOOD | AMOUNT | GRAMS | % OF CALORIES PROVIDED BY PROTEIN |
| *Animal products* | | | |
| Shrimp | 3 oz. | 11 | 84 |
| Low-fat cottage cheese | 1 cup | 38 | 74 |
| Chicken (no skin) | 3 oz. | 20 | 70 |
| Pork chop (lean) | 3 oz. | 20 | 59 |
| Tuna | 3 oz. | 24 | 56 |
| Beef liver | 3 oz. | 20 | 46 |
| Beef steak (lean) | 3 oz. | 24 | 44 |
| Beef roast (lean) | 3 oz. | 25 | 41 |
| Skim milk | 1 cup | 9 | 40 |
| Fish (haddock) | 3 oz. | 19 | 38 |
| Leg of lamb | 3 oz. | 22 | 37 |
| Hamburger (regular) | 3 oz. | 21 | 34 |
| Sausage (pork links) | 3 oz. | 17 | 28 |
| Swiss cheese | 1 oz. | 8 | 30 |
| Egg | 1 medium | 6 | 30 |
| Cheddar cheese | 1 oz. | 7 | 27 |
| Low-fat yogurt | 1 cup | 8 | 27 |
| Whole milk | 1 cup | 9 | 23 |
| Hot dog | 1 | 6 | 15 |
| *Legumes and nuts* | | | |
| Soybeans (cooked) | 1 cup | 20 | 33 |
| Split peas (cooked) | 1 cup | 9 | 31 |
| Lima beans (cooked) | 1 cup | 12 | 27 |
| Dried beans (cooked) | 1 cup | 15 | 26 |
| Peanuts | ¼ cup | 9 | 17 |
| Peanut butter | 1 T. | 4 | 17 |
| Walnuts | ¼ cup | 7 | 14 |
| Almonds | ¼ cup | 7 | 13 |
| *Grains* | | | |
| Corn | 1 cup | 5 | 29 |
| Egg noodles | 1 cup | 7 | 25 |
| Oatmeal | 1 cup | 5 | 15 |
| Whole wheat bread | 1 slice | 2.5 | 15 |
| Macaroni | 1 cup | 5 | 13 |
| White bread | 1 slice | 2.2 | 13 |
| Rice | 1 cup | 4 | 11 |

or must be obtained from the diet, and eleven are considered *nonessential* because they can be manufactured by the body. (They still perform essential roles in the body, however, and are as important to health as the essential amino acids. They are not considered an essential part of our *diet* because we don't have to obtain them from foods.) The two essential amino acids we hear the most about are *tryptophan* and *tryosine.* (You'll hear more about them in an upcoming section on amino acids and neurotransmitters.)

Proteins are classified by their ability to support protein tissue construction in the body. Not all sources of protein do this equally well; it depends on their content of essential amino acids. How well dietary proteins support protein synthesis in the body is captured by tests of the protein's "quality." The quality of dietary sources of protein is an especially important issue in countries where too few high-quality protein foods are available, and among people who consume vegetarian diets.

### *Protein Quality*

High-quality proteins contain all of the essential amino acids in the amounts needed to support protein tissue formation by the body. If any of the essential amino acids is missing in the dietary protein source, protein synthesis does not take place—even for those proteins that could be synthesized from available amino acids. It may appear inefficient for the body to shut off all protein synthesis for want of an amino acid or two. But if all protein synthesis did not cease, cells would end up with an imbalanced assortment of protein that would seriously affect cell functions. Without the needed levels of each essential amino acid, proteins consumed can only be used to form energy. Because the body does not store amino acids, we need to make them available for the body's use all at once. This means we need to consume some high-quality protein at every meal to get the essential amino acids needed for protein synthesis.

Food sources of protein that contain all of the essential amino acids in the amount needed to support protein synthesis are called *complete proteins*, and include those found in animal products such as meat, milk, and eggs. *Incomplete proteins* are deficient in one or more essential amino acids. Proteins found in plants are incomplete; however, you can complement the essential amino acid composition of plant sources of protein by combining them to form a complete source of protein.

### *Combining Proteins*

Which combinations of plant proteins complement each other depends on which essential amino acids are missing, or present in low amounts, in the individual plants. The essential amino acid that is missing or found in the lowest amount is referred to as the *limiting amino acid*. The goal of combining plant sources of protein to form a complete source of protein is the selection of foods that complement each other's amino acid content—or the selection of *complementary proteins*. The three most common limiting amino acids in plant foods are lysine, methionine, and tryptophan. Wheat, rice, nuts, and seeds, for example, contain a good amount of methionine but limited amounts of lysine. Legumes, except for peanuts, contain a high amount of lysine, but a low amount of methionine. So combining a grain, such as rice, with a legume like dried beans provides a source of complete protein. In general, complementary proteins are obtained from plants by combining:

Rice and dried beans
Rice and green peas
Bulgur (wheat) and dried beans
Barley and dried beans
Corn and dried beans
Corn and lima beans (succotash)
Soybeans and seeds
Peanuts and rice and dried beans
Seeds and green peas

### *The Diets and Health of Vegetarians*

About 3 percent of the U.S. population practice some form of vegetarianism, and the percentage appears to be increasing.[22] Individuals choose vegetarian diets for health, religious, or philosophical reasons. Vegetarian diets have been practiced by people in some religious groups for centuries, bearing testimony to the general safety of well-established vegetarian eating patterns.[23]

The most common categories of vegetarian diets are semivegetarian (a relatively new type that excludes only red meats), lacto-ovo vegetarian, and vegan. *Lacto-* refers to milk and *ovo-* to eggs. Less common vegetarian diets include macrobiotic and fruitarian regimes. These two types of vegetarian diets exclude many types of foods and are generally inadequate in many nutrients.[23]

Vegetarian diets that are nutritionally inadequate generally violate the principle that a wide variety of foods are needed for a

VEGETARIAN MEAL PLAN FOR ADULTS

| *Basic food group* | | *Minimum number of servings per day* |
|---|---|---|
| PROTEIN FOODS | | 2 |
| 1½ cups cooked dried beans | ½ cup nuts | |
| 8 oz. tofu | 4 T. peanut butter | |
| 2 cups fortified soy milk | 2 cups yogurt | |
| | 2 oz. cheese | |
| | 2 eggs | |
| WHOLE GRAINS | | 6 |
| 1 slice bread | ½ cup cooked cereal | |
| 1 muffin | ½ cup brown rice | |
| ¼ cup seeds | ½ cup pasta | |
| VEGETABLES | | 2 |
| VITAMIN-A-RICH EXAMPLES: | OTHER EXAMPLES: | |
| ½ cup broccoli brussels sprouts collards, squash | ½ cup "other" vegetables: potatoes, green beans, corn, lettuce | |
| FRUITS | | 2 |
| VITAMIN-C-RICH EXAMPLES: | OTHER EXAMPLES: | |
| ¾ cup berries | 1 apple | |
| ¼ cup cantaloupe | 1 banana | |
| 1 orange | 1 pear | |
| ½ grapefruit | 1 peach | |
| ½ cup orange juice | ½ cup grapes | |
| FATS | | 0–4 |
| 1 tsp. margarine | 2 tsp. mayonnaise | (depends on caloric need) |
| 1 tsp. butter | 1 T. cream cheese | |
| 1 tsp. oil | | |

healthy diet. They become more restrictive as they move from semi-vegetarian to vegan. With careful food selection, it is possible to obtain complete nutrition from vegetarian diets.[23] In fact, well-balanced vegetarian diets have some advantages over diets of many omnivores, or people who eat both plant and animal foods. Vegetarian diets usually contain over twice as much dietary fiber, lower levels of saturated fat and cholesterol, and fewer calories than the diets of meat eaters. Vegetarians following established dietary practices tend to have lower levels of blood cholesterol and are less likely to be overweight than omnivores. They are less likely than their nonvegetarian counterparts to develop heart disease, diabetes, and cancer of the colon.[23,24]

Excessively restrictive or poorly planned vegetarian diets, especially when consumed by people with high protein needs, such as women who are pregnant and children, can compromise health. Dietary deficiencies of protein, iron, zinc, calcium, riboflavin, and vitamins $B_{12}$ and D are commonly found in vegetarians consuming an imbalanced assortment of foods.[25] Iron, zinc; and calcium in plants are poorly absorbed due to the presence of phytates, oxalates, and dietary fiber.[26] Although intake of those nutrients may be adequate in a vegetarian diet, they are incompletely absorbed and deficiencies may develop. Vegetarian diets that exclude milk, or appropriately fortified soy milk, may contain inadequate amounts of calcium, riboflavin, and vitamin D. Vitamin $B_{12}$ is only found in appreciable amounts in animal and fermented products. Vegetarians who don't eat any type of meat or fermented food products are at high risk of becoming deficient.[23] Poor growth and a higher incidence of osteoporosis are common consequences of inadequate vegetarian diets.[23,25]

Nutritional deficiencies may be very common among lifelong vegans. A study of 138 vegans from birth identified deficiencies of vitamin $B_{12}$ in 69 percent, iron in 63 percent, vitamin D in 14 percent, and folic acid deficiency in 3 percent.[27] Among the common vegetarian diets, those of vegans are the most difficult to balance.

### *Amino Acids and Neurotransmitters*

Neurotransmitters act as chemical messengers within the body's network of over 100 billion nerve and brain cells. They influence functions such as memory, mood, appetite, and muscular coordination. Known neurotransmitters number around thirty-five and primarily include substances formed from one or two amino acids.

Three major neurotransmitters are serotonin, dopamine, and norepinephrine. Serotonin is derived from the essential amino acid tryptophan, whereas dopamine and norepinephrine are made from the nonessential amino acid tyrosine. The level of activity of each of these neurotransmitters can be influenced by diet composition.[28] That makes them unusual, because diet composition doesn't generally affect production of the body's chemical messengers. This area turns out to be such a fascinating one that we'll take a close look at one example of the influence of diet on neurotransmitter synthesis and discuss how it may affect behavior. The neurotransmitter we'll discuss is serotonin, and the behavior, food intake.

#### MOOD FOODS?

The level of serotonin in the brain is influenced by dietary carbohydrate and tryptophan intake. When a high-carbohydrate diet is consumed, tryptophan in the blood is selectively transported into the brain. The high level of tryptophan in the brain leads to an increased production of serotonin. Elevated serotonin levels increase the feeling of well-being, decrease appetite, and may reduce depression. The increased serotonin levels following a high-carbohydrate meal may serve as a form of self-medication that perpetuates a desire for carbohydrates. This notion fits the observation that some people "crave carbohydrates" and could help explain why it happens. Carbohydrates have been shown to have mild antidepressing effects in some people. The mood-associated urge to eat carbohydrate-rich foods may also hinder prolonged weight-reduction efforts and account for the higher prevalence of more carbohydrate cravers among overweight than normal-weight adults.[29]

#### SLEEP DISORDERS

Tryptophan and tryosine also affect sleep through their actions as neurotransmitters. Tryptophan tends to induce sleep, whereas tyrosine tends to prevent it. Both have been used to treat sleep disorders but this practice is no longer recommended. The sale of tryptophan supplements was banned in the United States in 1990 because the habitual use of this amino acid was found to cause a serious form of paralysis. Amino acid supplements should only be taken under close medical supervision.

### *Protein: How Much?*

How much protein a person requires is affected by the quality of the protein consumed (complete or incomplete), total caloric intake (are energy needs being met?), body size, illness, pregnancy, and growth. The amount of protein needed is less when dietary sources of complete protein are consumed. For example, people consuming animal products require less protein to obtain sufficient amounts of the essential amino acids than do vegans. The adult RDA for protein is 50 grams for women and 63 grams for men. The recommended level assumes that people are consuming a mix of animal and plant sources of protein.

The usual diet in the United States is high in protein, a feature that has not been associated with health benefits. The major, negative side effect of high-protein diets is that they are generally rich in fat. Most meats and dairy products that are good sources of protein are also loaded with fat. Many people think that lean hamburger is a rich source of protein and not high in fat—after all, it's labeled "lean." But the truth is that hamburger labeled as "90 percent lean" provides 48 percent of its total calories as fat. Low-fat meats and dairy products do help lower our total fat intake, but they don't always reduce it as much as is hoped.

You'll find out why everybody needs some fat in their diet, what fat does for us, and why the U.S. diet is getting a bad reputation as an artery-clogging one in the next section.

## FATS

Dietary fat. Body fat. Cholesterol. Blood lipids. Saturated fats. Polyunsaturated fats. Fish oils, corn oil, safflower oil. Sound familiar? Most of us have quite a "fat" vocabulary. Hardly a day passes when we don't hear something about the latest research on dietary fat and clogged arteries or new diet-drug therapies that unclog them. TV commercials for margarines and oils keep us informed about the specific types of vegetable oils available and tell us why one type of margarine or oil is better than others for our hearts. The latest weight-loss book lets us know how we can get rid of that ugly, excess body fat. The word *fat* means a lot more than "energy nutrient" to most people. In this section, we'll discuss the functions, categories, and food sources of dietary fat and why there are so many health issues that surround them.

Fats consist of a group of substances found in food that have one major property in common: they dissolve in fat and not in water. If you have ever tried to get vinegar and oil to mix before you poured it over a salad, you have observed firsthand the principle of water and fat solubility.

Fats are actually a subcategory of the fat-soluble substances known as *lipids*. Lipids include all types of fats and oils. Fats are often distinguished from oils by their property of being solid at room temperature. Butter, margarine, lard, shortening, and animal fat belong in this group because they don't melt if left on a shelf. Oils, on the other hand, are liquid at room temperature. The physical difference between fats and oils is due to their chemical structures. You can, however, change a liquid oil to a solid fat by adding hydrogen, or *hydrogenating* the oil.

Fats in foods not only supply energy, but also fat-soluble nutrients. Fats "carry" the essential fatty acid, linoleic acid, and fat-soluble vitamins A, D, E, and K. So part of the reason that we need fats in our diet is to get a supply of the essential nutrients they carry. They also increase the flavor and palatability of foods. Although "pure" fats by themselves are tasteless, they absorb and retain the flavor of substances that surround them. Because fats in meats and other foods exist in different "flavor environments," the characteristic taste of foods containing fat is due to the flavors picked up and incorporated into the fat. That is why butter, if placed next to the garlic in the refrigerator, ends up tasting like garlic.

Fats in foods contribute to the sensation of feeling full (as they should at 9 calories per gram!). Fats stay in the stomach longer than carbohydrates or proteins, and are absorbed over a longer period of time. Foods with fat "stick to your ribs."

A crucial role of fat is to serve as a component of cell membranes. To an extent, the type of fat found in our cell membranes reflects the type of fat we consume in our diets, and that may influence how susceptible cells are to certain disease processes. For example, cell membranes that contain a high proportion of polyunsaturated fats may break down more easily than cell membranes that contain fewer.

The body has two sources of fats: those consumed in the diet and those produced from carbohydrates and proteins. Humans eat only a few times a day, but energy is needed throughout the day. To ensure a constant supply of energy, the body converts carbohydrates and proteins not used to meet immediate needs to storage forms of energy. Although glycogen, the storage form of glucose, makes up some energy stores, excess carbohydrates and protein are mostly converted to fat.

Fats found in the body are not only skin deep. Fat is also located around organs such as the kidneys and heart. It's there to cushion and protect the organs, and to keep them insulated. (Fat is a great insulation material; everybody needs some body fat to help keep them warm on the inside.)

### *The Types of Fat*

There are many types of fat and fatlike substances in food and our bodies. Of primary importance are triglycerides, saturated and unsaturated fats, cholesterol, and omega fatty acids. The subject of fats is introduced here. It is extensively covered in chapter 7 under the topics of diet and heart disease and cancer.

The type of fat that makes up 98 percent of our dietary fat intake and the vast majority of our body's fat stores are ***triglycerides***. They consist of one glycerol unit and three fatty acids. Triglycerides are also found in the blood, where their job is to transport fat to fat stores and to cells where it is needed for energy formation.

As far as health is concerned, the glycerol component of fat is relatively unimportant. It's the fatty acids that influence what the body does with the fat we eat and, in part, how fat influences health. There are many different types of fatty acids and you've heard of the major ones: ***saturated*** and ***unsaturated*** fatty acids.

### *Saturated and Unsaturated Fats*

Whether a fat is saturated or not depends on the type of fatty acids that are attached to glycerol. Saturated fatty acids are saturated with hydrogens. The chemical bonds that hold the atoms of the fatty acid together are linked to as many hydrogens as possible. Unsaturated fatty acids have fewer hydrogens than they can hold. So the whole business about saturated and unsaturated fats boils down to the hydrogen content of fatty acids.

Triglycerides that contain saturated fatty acids are called saturated fats. If one or more of their three fatty acids are two hydrogens short, the fat is called *monounsaturated*. Triglycerides that have fatty acids with four or more absent hydrogens are considered *polyunsaturated fats*. Although plants and animals contain both types of fats, plants tend to be richer sources of unsaturated fats than animal products.

### *Food Sources of Fat*

Three types of food provide around 90 percent of the fat consumed in the United States: fats and oils (43 percent), beef, poultry, and fish (36 percent), and dairy products (12 percent).[30] The most concentrated sources of fats in our diets are foods like butter, margarine, and oils. Many fast foods, such as hamburgers, fried chicken, french fries, potato and taco chips, soft ice cream, and shakes, are high in fat. Most vegetables are naturally low in fat—at least they are before we add margarine or sauces to them. You won't find much fat in fruits other than avocados, either. Food sources of fat, and the percentage of total calories in the foods that are supplied by fat, are shown in table 13.

You can't always tell the fat content of a food by looking at its cover. Bacon and sausage look fatty and they are, but what about nuts, milk chocolate, and cheese? They are also high in fat, but we

TABLE 13. FOOD SOURCES OF FAT[a]
*(Recommended intake of fat for adults: 30% or less of total caloric intake)*

| FOOD | AMOUNT | FAT CONTENT: GRAMS | FAT CONTENT: % OF CALORIES PROVIDED BY FAT |
|---|---|---|---|
| *Fats and oils* | | | |
| Butter | 1 tsp. | 4 | 100 |
| Margarine | 1 tsp. | 4 | 100 |
| Oil | 1 tsp. | 4.7 | 100 |
| Mayonnaise | 1 T. | 11 | 99 |
| Heavy cream | 1 T. | 5.5 | 93 |
| Salad dressing | 1 T. | 6 | 83 |
| Gravy | ¼ cup | 14 | 77 |
| Salad dressing, low-cal | 1 T. | 1 | 45 |
| *Animal meats, egg* | | | |
| Hot dog | 1 (2 oz.) | 17 | 83 |
| Bologna | 1 oz. | 8 | 80 |
| Sausage | 4 links | 18 | 77 |
| Bacon | 3 pieces | 9 | 74 |
| Salami | 2 oz. | 11 | 68 |
| Egg | 1 | 6 | 68 |
| Pork, beef, or veal with fat | 3 oz. | 18 | 62 |
| Hamburger, regular (20% fat) | 3 oz. | 16.5 | 62 |
| Chicken, fried with skin | 3 oz. | 14 | 53 |
| Big Mac | 6.6 oz. | 31.4 | 52 |
| Quarter Pounder with cheese | 6.8 oz. | 28.6 | 50 |
| Whopper | 8.9 oz. | 32 | 48 |
| Hamburger, lean (10% fat) | 3 oz. | 9.5 | 45 |
| TV dinner, pork | 11 oz. | 21.9 | 43 |
| Pork, beef, or veal, lean | 3 oz. | 8 | 39 |
| Tuna in oil, drained | 3 oz. | 7 | 38 |
| Flounder, baked | 3 oz. | 1 | 13 |
| Chicken, baked without skin | 3 oz. | 4 | 25 |
| Shrimp, boiled | 3 oz. | 1 | 74 |
| Tuna in water | 3 oz. | 1 | 7 |
| *Dairy products* | | | |
| Cheddar cheese | 1 oz. | 9.5 | 74 |
| Whole milk | 1 cup | 8.5 | 49 |
| 2% milk | 1 cup | 5.0 | 32 |
| 1% milk | 1 cup | 2.7 | 24 |
| Skim milk | 1 cup | 0.4 | 4 |
| *Other* | | | |
| Avocado | ½ | 15 | 84 |
| Sunflower seeds | ¼ cup | 17 | 77 |
| Peanut butter | 1 T. | 8 | 76 |

TABLE 13. CONTINUED

| FOOD | AMOUNT | FAT CONTENT | |
|---|---|---|---|
| | | GRAMS | % OF CALORIES PROVIDED BY FAT |
| *Other* | | | |
| Peanuts | ¼ cup | 17.5 | 75 |
| Potato chips | 1 oz. (13 chips) | 11 | 61 |
| Chocolate chip cookies | 4 | 11 | 54 |
| French fries | 20 fries | 20 | 49 |
| Taco chips | 1 oz. (10 chips) | 6.2 | 41 |
| Mashed potatoes | ½ cup | 4.5 | 41 |
| Baked potato | 1 | 0.2 | 1 |

[a]*Diets providing less than 30% of total caloric intake as fat would include less than 34 grams of fat per 1,000 calories or, for most adults, less than 78 grams of fat per day.*

just can't see it. Dry roasted nuts don't have the oily shine that other roasted peanuts have, but if you crush a dry roasted nut between two paper towels, you'll see that it makes quite a grease spot. Dry roasting doesn't take the fat out of nuts. Most of the fat that we consume in food is invisible to the eye.

The type of fat present in foods is as important a consideration as the total amount of fat. Sources of fat classified by the primary type of fat present are shown below. More detailed information about food sources of saturated, monounsaturated, and polyunsaturated fats is provided in chapter 7.

### *Cholesterol*

Cholesterol is a close chemical relative of fat. It is invisible to the naked eye and distributed in both the fat and lean portions of animal products. Consequently, you can't assume that only the fat portion of meats and other animal products is high in cholesterol. Liver and eggs are two of the richest sources of cholesterol, yet neither food is very high in fat. Beef is a moderate source of cholesterol, but is generally high in fat. Whole milk and bacon both contain a good deal of fat, but not cholesterol. Beyond the fact that cholesterol is only found in animal products, it is hard to make generalizations about its food sources. You have to refer to a table if you want to check out the cholesterol content of foods (table 14), or read the nutrition information provided on the packaging of some meat and dairy products. Most of the cholesterol consumed by people in the

FOOD SOURCES OF SATURATED AND UNSATURATED FAT*

| *Saturated fats* | *Monounsaturated fats* | *Polyunsaturated fats* |
|---|---|---|
| American cheese | Eggs | Corn oil |
| Brick cheese | Corn oil margaine | Soybean oil |
| Cheddar cheese | Olive oil | Sunflower oil |
| Cottage cheese | Peanut oil | Sunflower seeds |
| Milk (whole) | Soybean oil margarine | |
| Butter | Chicken | |
| Beef | Pork | |
| Bacon | Cashews | |
| Sausage | Macadamia nuts | |
| Coconut oil | Peanuts | |
| Palm oil | Peanut butter | |

**The most abundant type of fat found in a food has been used as the criterion for placing it in one of the three categories listed.*
*Source: USDA Handbook No. 8, Volumes 1, 4, and 5, Washington, D.C. 1980–85.*

United States comes from eggs and meat, with far less contributed by dairy products and animal fats such as butter and lard.

A rather absurd trend has recently developed in the cholesterol labeling of foods. Fruits, breads and cereals, and other nonanimal products have been labeled "contains no cholesterol." Why would they? Only animal products contain cholesterol. Such labeling practices only confuse the issue about food sources of cholesterol. In addition, because saturated fat intake is more strongly associated with elevated blood cholesterol than is cholesterol intake, what consumers really need to know is the saturated-fat content of foods. That information is rarely, if ever, listed on food packages.

The rest of the story about cholesterol and heart disease is located in chapter 7.

### *The Omega Fatty Acids*

Recently, a long-established but rarely used classification system for unsaturated fatty acids has come into vogue. The *omega* system classifies unsaturated fatty acids by the location of their missing hydrogens; the fish diets of some Eskimos have made the system famous. This type of fatty acid is highly unsaturated and also appears to have exceptional effects on health. We'll get to these effects and the food sources of omega fatty acids in chapter 7 as well.

TABLE 14. FOOD SOURCES OF CHOLESTEROL
*(Recommended intake for adults: 300 mg or less)*

| FOOD | AMOUNT | CHOLESTEROL MG |
|---|---|---|
| *Animal products* | | |
| Brain | 3 oz. | >2,000 |
| Liver | 3 oz. | 470 |
| Egg | 1 | 210 |
| Shrimp | 3 oz. | 119 |
| Prime rib | 3 oz. | 80 |
| Baked chicken (no skin) | 3 oz. | 75 |
| Hamburger, regular | 3 oz. | 64 |
| Pork chop, lean | 3 oz. | 60 |
| Fish, baked (haddock, flounder) | 3 oz. | 58 |
| Ice cream | 1 cup | 56 |
| Sausage | 3 oz. | 55 |
| Hamburger, lean | 3 oz. | 50 |
| Whole milk | 1 cup | 34 |
| Crab, boiled | 3 oz. | 33 |
| Lobster | 3 oz. | 29 |
| Cheese (cheddar) | 1 oz. | 26 |
| 2% fat milk | 1 cup | 22 |
| Yogurt, low-fat | 1 cup | 17 |
| 1% fat milk | 1 cup | 14 |
| Skim milk | 1 cup | 7 |
| Margarines | 1 tsp. | 0 |

# Chapter 6

## *Basic Truths about Vitamins and Minerals*

*The decade was the 1920s. Horse-drawn carriages competed with cars for space on the road, and "My Blue Heaven" was a hit tune. Industries, cities, and the population of the United States were rapidly expanding. It was a boom period that produced both prosperity and poverty. It was also a period when thousands of people in this country suffered from vitamin and mineral deficiency diseases. Pellagra, the niacin deficiency disease, and rickets due to a lack of vitamin D were common problems. Thousands of people died from pellagra and many children's hospitals were filled with victims of rickets.*

*Those days are gone now, but the consequences of vitamin and mineral deficiency diseases have not been forgotten. Their importance to health is a fact firmly implanted in our minds.*

▼ Vitamins and minerals are referred to as *trace nutrients*. It is true that they are needed by humans in very small amounts, but the title *trace* may convey the wrong impression. Very small amounts of these essential substances have profound effects on body functions. The amount of vitamins and minerals we need is way out of proportion with the magnitude of their effects on body processes.

Today, concerns about vitamin and mineral intake center on marginal deficiencies and toxicity diseases. Habitually low intake of certain vitamins and minerals has been related to cancer, osteoporosis, depression, poor growth, and other disorders. The overuse of supplements by Jane S. Public and John Q. Citizen has greatly increased our knowledge about the hazards of overdosing on vitamins and minerals. Toxicity diseases, which lie at the opposite end of the spectrum from deficiency diseases, are becoming increasingly common in the United States. Most overt vitamin and mineral deficiency diseases, on the other hand, now occur so infrequently that they are apt to be diagnosed incorrectly, or accurately only after many other disease possibilities have been ruled out.

## AN OVERVIEW OF VITAMINS AND MINERALS

Each essential vitamin and mineral performs unique roles in the body, roles that cannot be replaced by any other chemical substance. Given an inadequate or excessive intake of any of the essential vitamins or minerals, specific deficiency or overdose symptoms result that can be traced back to their unique functions.

Vitamins and minerals enable the body to use carbohydrates, proteins, and fats to build and maintain muscles, bones, blood, and all other tissues in our body. They do that for the most part by their work with enzymes. Enzymes are protein substances that greatly increase the rate at which chemical changes take place in the body. Every function the body performs, from breathing to sleeping, depends on enzymes and their ability to speed up the body's chemical assembly lines. Nearly all of the vitamins, and most minerals, perform the major role of activating enzymes so they can get to work on keeping our bodies alive and well.

Can you accelerate enzyme activity by loading up with extra vitamins and minerals? Well, actually, no. High levels of vitamins and minerals do not improve or accelerate enzyme functions because they do not cause an increase in enzyme levels. So, even with an excess intake of vitamins and minerals, you can't speed up your enzymes. To come back to a point made earlier for nutrients, "Enough is as good as a feast."

The notion that extra vitamins and minerals can wake up lazy enzymes, no matter how unfounded, has been used by peddlers of nutrition nonsense as a pitch for supplement sales. But the nonsense doesn't stop there. Enzymes are added to some vitamin and mineral supplements to boost your supply. The truth is, however, that, taken orally, enzymes are digested and their activity is destroyed in the intestines. They never make it into our bloodstream to do their work.

### *Will the Real Vitamins Please Stand Up?*

Thirteen vitamins are known to be essential for health. Nine are water soluble, or completely dissolve in water, and four dissolve only in fats. These vitamins are:

| **WATER-SOLUBLE VITAMINS** | **FAT-SOLUBLE VITAMINS** |
|---|---|
| B-complex vitamins | Vitamin A (retinol) |
| Thiamin ($B_1$) | Vitamin E (tocopherol) |
| Riboflavin ($B_2$) | Vitamin D (1,25-dihydroxycolicalciferol) |
| Niacin ($B_3$) | Vitamin K (phylloquinone, menaquinone) |
| Vitamin $B_6$ (pyridoxine) | |
| Folacin (folic acid) | |
| Vitamin $B_{12}$ (Cyanocobalamin) | |
| Biotin | |
| Pantothenic acid (pantothenate) | |
| Vitamin C (ascorbic acid, ascorbate) | |

These are the "real" vitamins. But there are a number of bogus ones too. Vitamins are "fake" either because they are produced in the body and therefore aren't required in the diet or because they have no special role to play in the body. Here is a list of some popular nonvitamins that are added to supplements, skin care creams, hair care products, and other items.

**NONVITAMINS**

| | |
|---|---|
| Bioflavonoids (vitamin P) | Lipoic acid |
| Choline | Nucleic acids |
| Gerovital H-3 | Pangamic acid (vitamin $B_{15}$) |
| Hesperidin | Para-aminobenzoic acid (PABA) |
| Inositol | Provitamin $B_5$ complex |
| Laetrile (vitamin $B_{17}$) | Rutin |
| Lecithin | |

Deficiency diseases do not result from low intake of these substances, nor has extra intake been shown to be beneficial. Nonetheless, the benefits of vitamin imposters are extolled: inositol is promoted for preventing hair loss, gerovital H-3 for slowing down the aging process, and lecithin for burning away excess body fat. Laetrile, a cyanide-containing component of apricot pits, has been illegally and ineffectively used to treat cancer. In an attempt to circumvent regulations controlling the sale of drugs, laetrile was labeled as a vitamin by enterprising quacks. Some of the nonvitamins do, however, have a contribution to make. Although nutritionists are at a loss for identifying an essential function of PABA, it does make a fine sunscreen.

### *What You Eat May Not Be What You Get*

Just because you consume your RDA level of iron, vitamin C, or calcium doesn't mean you actually end up with the amount you need in your body. Many factors can affect the level of vitamins and minerals that become available for service to the body. The amount of the zinc in our diet that ends up in the body proper, for example, can vary from 0 to 100 percent. People who eat lots of whole grains may develop zinc deficiency because so little of the zinc in the grains can be absorbed into the bloodstream. Although adequate levels of zinc are present in the whole grains, only a small amount can be absorbed because the zinc is tightly bound to phytic acid, a natural component of whole grains.[1] Another example is the interaction between tea and iron. Drinking tea with a meal can decrease iron absorption by 50 percent or more. In the intestines, iron combines with the tannic acid in tea and forms a compound that cannot be absorbed.[2]

Not all vitamin and mineral interactions with other substances reduce their absorption. Vitamin C and alcohol, for example, increase iron absorption. The amount of vitamin C in a half cup of orange juice will nearly quadruple the amount of iron that can be absorbed from plant foods.[2] In days gone by, people would put iron nails in oranges or apples, let them sit for a while, and then drink the juice as an iron tonic. (Knowledge of tetanus has ended the practice.) Iron overdose has occurred among people who drink alcoholic beverages brewed in iron vats.

The availability of vitamins and minerals in food is one important issue for those concerned about getting full value out of foods eaten. A parallel concern is whether vitamins and minerals originally present in foods are being lost en route to their destination—your plate.

### *Preserving the Vitamin and Mineral Content of Foods*

Food storage and preparation techniques can influence the vitamin and mineral content of food. Vitamins, however, are much more vulnerable to processing, storage, and cooking losses than are minerals. Unlike the vitamins, minerals are indestructible. Minerals are lost by soaking or boiling foods, and through fluids that drip out of foods during the cooking process.

RELATIVE STABILITY OF VITAMINS DURING FOOD STORAGE AND PREPARATION

| *Stable* | *Unstable* | *Very unstable* |
|---|---|---|
| Niacin | Vitamin $B_6$ | Vitamin C |
| Vitamin K | Riboflavin | Thiamin |
| Vitamin $B_{12}$ | Pantothenic acid | Folic acid |
| Vitamin D | Vitamin A | |
| | Beta-carotene (a provitamin) | |
| | Vitamin E | |

Vitamins and minerals may also be removed from foods during processing. The process of refining flour, for example, removes the whole wheat grain from the germ and outer coverings, both of which are good sources of a variety of vitamins and minerals. Freeze drying of raw foods causes the least loss of vitamins and minerals. Freezing foods causes less loss than canning, and steaming or microwaving preserves the vitamin and mineral content of cooked foods the best.[3]

The list below categorizes vitamins by their stability during food storage and preparation. As you can see, vitamin C, thiamin, and folic acid are the most fragile vitamins.

Vitamins in food can be broken down or depleted by exposure to light, acidic or basic conditions, air, heat, and moisture. Until the early 1960s, milk was bottled in clear glass containers. However, it was discovered that the exposure of milk to sunlight reduced the milk's vitamin content. That finding led to the use of colored glass, fogged plastic, and cardboard milk containers. Vitamin C is highly stable in acid solutions like orange and tomato juice, but breaks down in low-acidity solutions, such as apple juice. Consequently, vitamin-C-fortified apple juice doesn't really provide much vitamin C.

Major losses of vitamins often occur during the final preparation of food. Overcooking, holding cooked foods on a warmer or steam table, cooking foods in lots of water, and tossing out the water that foods are cooked in all result in vitamin losses. (Overcooking vegetables is a nutritional misdemeanor—in addition to causing vitamin losses, it tends to make people dislike them.) Green beans and peas, if held hot for three hours before serving, lose over half of their content of thiamin, riboflavin, and vitamin C.[4] Approximately one-third of the vitamin content of boiled vegetables is tossed out with the cooking water.[5] On the other hand, foods may

FOOD STORAGE AND PREPARATION METHODS FOR PRESERVING VITAMINS AND MINERALS

*Storing Foods*

Store foods for the shortest amount of time possible.

Choose fresh, freeze-dried, and frozen products over heavily processed and canned products.

Store vegetables and fruits not needing refrigeration in a cool, dry, and clean place.

Store leftover, perishable foods tightly wrapped in a refrigerator set just above 32 °F.

Avoid the freeze-thaw-freeze cycle. Foods defrosted, heated, and then refrozen show major losses in vitamin content.

*Preparing Foods*

Don't overcook foods, especially vegetables. Cook vegetables to the point where they are still a bit crunchy.

Microwave, stir fry, steam, or broil foods. Use just enough water to prevent scorching.

Serve foods right after they have been prepared (or be the first one in the cafeteria line). Time food preparation so that the foods served are all ready at the same time.

gain vitamins and minerals during processing. How that happens is the subject of this next section.

*Enriching and Fortifying Foods*

Enrichment and fortification are two procedures used to increase the nutrient content of certain foods. Both processes were started over forty years ago to help prevent then-widespread vitamin and mineral deficiency diseases. *Enrichment* refers to replacing particular vitamins and a mineral lost during the refining of grains. For example, bread that is made from refined flour is enriched. *Fortification* means simply the addition of nutrients to foods whether they were originally present in the food or not. Many foods, from breakfast cereals to cupcakes, are fortified with vitamins and minerals. Only refined grains can be labeled as enriched, but any food can be fortified.

Refining comes with a cost to the nutrient content of grains. Lost along with the outer bran covering is much of the whole grain's content of dietary fiber, calcium, phosphorus, magnesium, zinc, vitamin $B_6$, pantothenic acid, and folic acid. Some of the thiamin, riboflavin, niacin, and iron content of grains is also lost due to refining, but these four nutrients (and only these four) are replaced by enrichment. The term *replaced* here is key. Enriched nutrients are added back at levels that approximately equal the amount lost due to refining.

Enrichment does not add back all of the nutrients lost during the refinement of grains, nor does it guarantee that they won't be lost during food preparation. Rice, for example, is often enriched by spraying the four nutrients on the grains. They wash off if you rinse rice with water before you cook it.

Now to individualized discussion of the genuine items, starting with the water-soluble B-complex vitamins and vitamin C.

TABLE 15. FOOD SOURCES OF THIAMIN
*(RDA for women = 1.1 mg per day)*

| FOOD | AMOUNT | THIAMIN MG |
|---|---|---|
| *Meat* | | |
| Pork roast | 3 oz. | 0.8 |
| Beef | 3 oz. | 0.4 |
| Ham | 3 oz. | 0.4 |
| Liver | 3 oz. | 0.2 |
| *Nuts and seeds* | | |
| Sunflower seeds | ¼ cup | 0.7 |
| Peanuts | ¼ cup | 0.1 |
| Almonds | ¼ cup | 0.1 |
| *Grains* | | |
| Bran flakes | 1 cup | 0.6 |
| Macaroni | 1 cup | 0.2 |
| Rice | 1 cup | 0.2 |
| Bread | 1 slice | 0.1 |
| *Vegetables* | | |
| Peas | ½ cup | 0.3 |
| Lima beans | ½ cup | 0.2 |
| Corn | ½ cup | 0.1 |
| Broccoli | ½ cup | 0.1 |
| Potato | 1 | 0.1 |
| *Fruit* | | |
| Orange juice | 1 cup | 0.2 |
| Orange | 1 | 0.1 |
| Avocado | ½ | 0.1 |

## A CLOSER LOOK AT VITAMINS

### *Thiamin (Vitamin $B_1$)*

Thiamin was neither the first vitamin discovered nor is it any more important than the other vitamins; it was simply first in line when the B-complex vitamins were announced.

Thiamin is needed to activate enzymes that convert glucose to energy. It is found in a wide variety of foods and most people in the United States have more than enough thiamin in their diets. Only milk and milk products fail to qualify for table 15, the list of good food sources of thiamin.

The thiamin deficiency disease is ***beriberi***. The disease is still found among people in developing countries who consume refined, unenriched grain products such as white rice or flour products as staple foods.[6] It is rarely identified in the United States

TABLE 16. FOOD SOURCES OF RIBOFLAVIN
*(RDA for women = 1.3 mg per day)*

| FOOD | AMOUNT | RIBOFLAVIN MG |
|---|---|---|
| *Milk and milk products* | | |
| Milk | 1 cup | 0.5 |
| 2% milk | 1 cup | 0.5 |
| Low-fat yogurt | 1 cup | 0.5 |
| Skim milk | 1 cup | 0.4 |
| Yogurt | 1 cup | 0.1 |
| American cheese | 1 oz. | 0.1 |
| Cheddar cheese | 1 oz. | 0.1 |
| *Meat* | | |
| Liver | 3 oz. | 3.6 |
| Pork chop | 3 oz. | 0.3 |
| Beef | 3 oz. | 0.2 |
| Tuna | ½ cup | 0.1 |
| *Vegetables* | | |
| Collard greens | ½ cup | 0.3 |
| Broccoli | ½ cup | 0.2 |
| Spinach, cooked | ½ cup | 0.1 |
| *Eggs* | | |
| Egg | 1 | 0.2 |
| *Grains* | | |
| Macaroni | 1 cup | 0.1 |
| Bread | 1 slice | 0.1 |

because nearly all the refined grain products we consume are enriched with thiamin.

Thiamin appears to be one of the safest vitamins as far as overdoses are concerned. There are no reports (at least yet) of thiamin overdose due to supplements.

*Riboflavin (Vitamin $B_2$)*

Riboflavin is everywhere in the body. It is a key activator of enzymes involved in the release of energy from glucose, proteins, and fats. Dairy products are the leading source of riboflavin in our diet. You can see its presence in skim milk, as a matter of fact; riboflavin gives skim milk its fluorescent yellowish-blue color. Specific foods that are considered good sources of riboflavin are shown in table 16.

Riboflavin deficiency occurs throughout many parts of the world.[6] People in the United States are generally spared because we consume enough dairy products, meats, and grain products to meet our need for riboflavin. However, it does occur from time to time among vegans, people with alcoholism, and long-term users of certain tranquilizers and antidepressants.

Even when taken in high-dosage supplements, riboflavin appears to be nontoxic because it is rapidly excreted by the body.

*Niacin (Vitamin $B_3$)*

*In 1914, the bacteriologist Joseph Goldberger of the U.S. Public Health Service was dispatched to the southern United States. His mission was to discover the cause of pellagra, a common and horrible disease that would be shown to be due to niacin deficiency over twenty years later. At the time Goldberger started his studies, however, it was fully expected that he would identify a bacterial cause of what was thought to be an infectious disease.*

*Goldberger observed that pellagra was most likely to occur among poor people and children in orphanages, and that it was not spread by contact. Dramatic differences in diets were noted between the poor and well off, with the diets of people with pellagra primarily consisting of cornmeal, grits, fatback, molasses, and little meat or milk. People with higher incomes ate more milk, meat, and vegetables. The observation that children in orphanages who did not develop the disease were the same ones who had habitually raided the milk and meat supplies at night provided a strong clue that the disease was due to diet.*

*In dramatic fashion, Goldberger disproved the notion that pellagra was an infectious disease. He, his wife, and fourteen volunteers were injected with the blood of people with pellagra. No volunteer developed pellagra, and the search for the dietary cause of the disease intensified. It took until 1937 before niacin deficiency was identified as the culprit. The prevalence of pellagra declined rapidly in the United States as dietary intake improved.*[6]

Niacin has one of the most interesting histories of any of the vitamins. It is also interesting in another respect: our bodies can make niacin out of the essential amino acid *tryptophan*. If you consume the same sort of high-protein diet that most people in the United States do, about three-fourths of the niacin in your diet comes from tryptophan.[7] The list of food sources of niacin shown in table 17 includes foods high in tryptophan.

The major roles of niacin are in energy formation and the activation of enzymes used to form certain types of fat in the body. This role is related to the experimental use of niacin as a cholesterol-lowering agent. Niacin diverts fats from forming cholesterol and consequently acts to lower cholesterol levels. Unfortunately, very high doses of niacin (3 to 6 grams) are needed to do the trick and that level produces signs of niacin toxicity.[8]

Niacin overdose can have rather alarming effects on body processes. Nausea, low blood pressure, a rapid heart rate, flushing, weakness, and hypoglycemia can develop quickly in response to one-time niacin intakes of around 3 grams.[9] Some of these signs of niacin overdose also appear when around 50 mg is taken regularly for a period of months.[10] Although the symptoms of niacin toxicity subside when supplements are stopped, people experiencing the reactions often feel their life is on the line and may seek medical attention immediately.

*Vitamin $B_6$ (Pyridoxine)*

Vitamin $B_6$ has caught the attention of many women because of its potential association with depression and components of premen-

TABLE 17. FOOD SOURCES OF NIACIN
*(RDA for women = 15 mg per day)*

| FOOD | AMOUNT | NIACIN MG |
|---|---|---|
| *Meats* | | |
| Liver | 3 oz. | 14.0 |
| Tuna | ½ cup | 10.3 |
| Turkey | 3 oz. | 9.5 |
| Chicken | 3 oz. | 7.9 |
| Salmon | 3 oz. | 6.9 |
| Veal | 3 oz. | 5.2 |
| Beef (round steak) | 3 oz. | 5.1 |
| Pork | 3 oz. | 4.5 |
| Haddock | 3 oz. | 2.7 |
| Scallops | 3 oz. | 1.1 |
| *Nuts and seeds* | | |
| Peanuts | 1 oz. | 4.9 |
| *Vegetables* | | |
| Asparagus | ½ cup | 1.5 |
| *Grains* | | |
| Wheat germ | 1 oz. | 1.5 |
| Brown rice | ½ cup | 1.2 |
| Noodles (enriched) | ½ cup | 1.0 |
| Rice (white, enriched) | ½ cup | 1.0 |
| Bread (enriched) | 1 slice | 0.7 |
| *Milk and milk products* | | |
| Milk | 1 cup | 1.9 |
| Cottage cheese | ½ cup | 2.6 |

strual syndrome (PMS). (We'll get back to these important topics in chapter 10.) Vitamin $B_6$ is directly involved in the set of chemical reactions that convert tryptophan to serotonin, a neurotransmitter that has a lot to do with mood, appetite, and sense of well-being. It also activates enzymes that form a variety of other proteins from amino acids.

The RDA for women is 2 mg of vitamin $B_6$ per day. That amount is at the upper limit of usual vitamin $B_6$ intake by women; most intakes fall somewhat below the RDA. Women who use oral contraceptive pills for more than two to three years, adolescent girls, and pregnant women are at highest risk of developing $B_6$ deficiency because marginal intake may be topped by an increased need for the vitamin during these times.[9] Mental changes, including depression and confusion, are the earliest signs of $B_6$ deficiency in adults.

TABLE 18. FOOD SOURCES OF VITAMIN $B_6$
*(RDA for women = 1.6 mg per day)*

| FOOD | AMOUNT | VITAMIN $B_6$ MG |
|---|---|---|
| *Meats* | | |
| Liver | 3 oz. | 0.8 |
| Salmon | 3 oz. | 0.7 |
| Other fish | 3 oz. | 0.6 |
| Chicken | 3 oz. | 0.4 |
| Ham | 3 oz. | 0.4 |
| Hamburger | 3 oz. | 0.4 |
| Veal | 3 oz. | 0.4 |
| Pork | 3 oz. | 0.3 |
| Beef | 3 oz. | 0.2 |
| *Eggs* | | |
| Egg | 1 | 0.3 |
| *Legumes* | | |
| Split peas | ½ cup | 0.6 |
| Dried beans (cooked) | ½ cup | 0.4 |
| *Fruits* | | |
| Banana | 1 | 0.6 |
| Avocado | ½ | 0.4 |
| Watermelon | 1 cup | 0.3 |
| *Vegetables* | | |
| Turnip greens | ½ cup | 0.7 |
| Brussels sprouts | ½ cup | 0.4 |
| Potato | 1 | 0.2 |
| Sweet potato | ½ cup | 0.2 |
| Carrots | ½ cup | 0.2 |
| Peas | ½ cup | 0.1 |

Vitamin $B_6$ is found in a rather odd assortment of foods. It is not found across the range of foods within a food group like many other vitamins, but is scattered among specific foods from a number of the food groups. Take a look at table 18 and ask yourself: "How often do I eat these foods and how much $B_6$ are they contributing to my diet?" If your diet is similar to that of most Americans, you are probably getting the majority of your vitamin $B_6$ from meats. The dried beans, fruits, and vegetables listed would be good components of a vitamin-$B_6$-bolstered diet.

Vitamin $B_6$ was considered to be nontoxic until a few years ago. Now that some women are taking large doses of the vitamin in the hope that it helps with PMS, the effects of overdoses are being seen.

Daily intake of twenty-five times the RDA (50 mg or more) is associated with the development of burning, shooting, and tingling pains in the arms and legs, clumsiness, or numbness.[11] Vitamin $B_6$ is no longer thought of as a harmless vitamin supplement.

### *Folacin (Folic Acid)*

Folacin was originally identified in *foliage* (or leaves), and dark green vegetables are still recognized as its leading source. The body heavily depends on folacin to activate many enzymes involved in DNA replication and protein tissue construction. It is a particularly important vitamin to growing children and pregnant women. Sources of folacin are listed in table 19.

The average folacin intake of people in the United States is about 600 mcg a day, or 200 mcg above the RDA of 400 mcg. Folacin intake is often as high as 1,000 to 2,000 mcg a day among people who consume six or more servings of fruit and vegetables a day.[12]

Females are at much higher risk of developing folacin deficiency than males. Adolescent girls and pregnant women are at risk because they have a high need for the vitamin for growth and often don't eat enough vegetables and fruits. It has been estimated that perhaps one-third of all pregnant women in the world develop folic acid deficiency.[13]

Folacin deficiency usually produces behavioral signs such as irritability and paranoid behavior, and will lead to abnormal changes in blood and other cells if allowed to progress. The large, irregularly shaped red blood cells seen in advanced cases of folic acid deficiency are the primary sign of the arrival of *megaloblastic anemia*. Folacin deficiency rarely advances to the stage of megaloblastic anemia in U.S. women, but marginal deficiencies are relatively common in pregnant women.[14] It's the reason why folacin supplements are recommended for pregnant women.

Dose levels of folacin for over-the-counter sale are limited to 400 mcg, making it difficult to consume a massive amount. Dose levels are limited because supplemental folacin may cover up signs of a vitamin $B_{12}$ deficiency and lead to failure to diagnose and treat $B_{12}$ deficiency.

Experimentally induced folacin toxicity has been produced with doses of 15 mg per day, or levels that are about thirty-eight times higher than the RDA for women. Symptoms of overdose do not represent serious problems, but include such aggravations as diarrhea, sleep disturbances, and irritability. Very high doses, 3 grams per day or more, can produce fever, body pain, and other ill effects.[15]

TABLE 19. FOOD SOURCES OF FOLACIN
*(RDA for women = 180 mcg (or 0.18 mg) per day)*

| FOODS | AMOUNT | FOLACIN MCG |
|---|---|---|
| *Vegetables* | | |
| Asparagus | ½ cup | 120 |
| Brussels sprouts | ½ cup | 116 |
| Black-eyed peas | ½ cup | 102 |
| Spinach, cooked | ½ cup | 99 |
| Romaine lettuce | 1 cup | 86 |
| Lima beans | ½ cup | 71 |
| Peas | ½ cup | 70 |
| Collard greens (cooked) | ½ cup | 56 |
| Sweet potato | ½ cup | 43 |
| Broccoli | ½ cup | 43 |
| *Fruits* | | |
| Cantaloupe | ¼ whole | 100 |
| Orange juice | 1 cup | 87 |
| Orange | 1 | 59 |
| *Grains* | | |
| Oatmeal | ½ cup | 97 |
| Wheat germ | ¼ cup | 80 |
| Wild rice | ½ cup | 37 |

*Vitamin $B_{12}$ (Cyanocobalamin)*

Vitamin $B_{12}$ is brought to you by bacteria, yeast, mold, and other microorganisms we think of as unsavory. Animals obtain vitamin $B_{12}$ by ingesting microorganisms or foods previously supplied with $B_{12}$ by microorganisms. Plants neither require nor produce vitamin $B_{12}$. That means our only food sources of vitamin $B_{12}$ are meats and microorganisms such as yeast and bacteria (see table 20).

Vitamin $B_{12}$ stands out from other vitamins in two other ways. It contains a mineral (cobalt) and requires a carrier found in the stomach called *intrinsic factor* for absorption into the bloodstream. Intrinsic factor binds with vitamin $B_{12}$ in the stomach and escorts the vitamin to sites in the intestines where $B_{12}$ is absorbed. People can become vitamin $B_{12}$ deficient either because diets are inadequate, or because they fail to produce intrinsic factor.

The enzymes $B_{12}$ activates are involved with the formation and maintenance of nerve, blood, and other cells. Its functions are closely related to those of folacin, and a deficiency of vitamin $B_{12}$ looks a lot like a folacin deficiency. Folacin, when mistakenly given for a $B_{12}$ deficiency, causes some improvement in health but fails to

TABLE 20. FOOD SOURCES OF VITAMIN $B_{12}$
*(RDA for Women = 2 mcg)*

| FOOD | AMOUNT | VITAMIN $B_{12}$ MCG |
|---|---|---|
| *Meats* | | |
| Liver | 3 oz. | 6.8 |
| Trout | 3 oz. | 3.6 |
| Beef | 3 oz. | 2.2 |
| Clams | ½ cup | 2.0 |
| Crab | 3 oz. | 1.8 |
| Lamb | 3 oz. | 1.8 |
| Tuna | ½ cup | 1.8 |
| Veal | 3 oz. | 1.7 |
| Hamburger, regular | 3 oz. | 1.5 |
| *Milk and milk products* | | |
| Skim milk | 1 cup | 1.0 |
| Milk | 1 cup | 0.9 |
| Yogurt | 1 cup | 0.8 |
| Cottage cheese | ½ cup | 0.7 |
| American cheese | 1 oz. | 0.2 |
| Cheddar cheese | 1 oz. | 0.2 |
| *Eggs* | | |
| Egg | 1 | 0.6 |

stop the invisible nerve damage that vitamin $B_{12}$ deficiency causes. The hideous nature of a vitamin $B_{12}$ deficiency is captured in the name of the anemia it produces: *pernicious* anemia. During the early stage of vitamin $B_{12}$ deficiency victims experience numbness and tingling in the hands and feet, moodiness, confusion, depression, and delusions.

Vegans, people who have had part of their stomach removed or stapled off, and people who genetically lack the ability to produce intrinsic factor are at highest risk of developing vitamin $B_{12}$ deficiency. Vitamin $B_{12}$ deficiency takes a while to develop from inadequate diets. The body can store enough $B_{12}$ to last three to five years. Diets that regularly contain meat of any sort generally provide an adequate amount of vitamin $B_{12}$. Adequate levels of vitamin $B_{12}$ in people who have had stomach surgery or who lack intrinsic factor can be achieved by periodic injections of the vitamin. (Vitamin $B_{12}$ injections used to be given to some seniors for an energy lift. Because benefits of $B_{12}$ shots could not be scientifically shown, health insurers decided not to cover them and the practice abruptly ended.)

Overdosing on vitamin $B_{12}$ supplements does not appear to be a problem. The body has built-in safeguards that reduce $B_{12}$ absorption when it enters the intestines in high amounts.

### *Biotin and Pantothenic Acid*

These are the two remaining vitamins of the B-complex family. Both are hard to avoid in foods, and their deficiency and toxicity diseases are very uncommon. Although biotin and pantothenic acid come in supplements, there is no evidence that they do anything special for stress, fatigue, or other conditions they are promoted to cure.

### *Vitamin C*

Why humans, unlike most animals, require a dietary source of vitamin C is one of the great unsolved mysteries of science. Except for primates like humans, chimpanzees and monkeys, pigs, the fruit-eating bat, and a couple of other species, animals manufacture vitamin C simply from glucose. Humans and other animals requiring the vitamin for some reason lack the enzyme needed to convert glucose to vitamin C.

Vitamin C was not discovered until sixty years ago, but its deficiency disease—scurvy—has been a problem for humans for thousands of years. Most cases of scurvy stem from a dietary lack of fruits and vegetables. Ocean voyagers, explorers, and soldiers were among those most likely to develop scurvy in the past. So devastating were the effects of the disease that the lack of vitamin C is thought to have influenced the course of history. Many military campaigns were abruptly ended by outbreaks of scurvy among soldiers who had run out of their supply of fruits and vegetables.[15] The lack of fruits and vegetables during winter months and periods of famine also precipitated epidemics of scurvy. Scurvy was rampant among soldiers in the Civil War, and was a life-threatening and taxing problem for sailors until the early part of the twentieth century.

Vitamin C functions in protein formation, it increases iron absorption, and it serves as an *antioxidant*. Antioxidants prevent or repair damage caused to cells by oxygen and other highly reactive chemicals. As part of its role as an antioxidant, vitamin C blocks the formation of nitrosamine from nitrates. Nitrates are often added to smoked and cured meats to protect them against spoilage and to enhance their flavor. In the absence of vitamin C, nitrates tend to combine with amino acids present in the intestine and form nitrosamines. Exposure of the gastrointestinal tract to nitrosamines has been associated with the development of certain types of cancer, but nitrates appear to be harmless.[16] Recently, producers have begun fortifying bacon, sausage, and other nitrate-containing meat products with vitamin C to protect against nitrosamine formation.

#### VITAMIN C AS THERAPY

Several therapeutic applications have been proposed for supplemental vitamin C. It has been used to:

- prevent colds and aid in their treatment,
- increase iron absorption among people with iron deficiency anemia, and
- "acidify" urine for the prevention of certain types of kidney and bladder infections among people susceptible to them.

The most effective applications are the use of vitamin C for increasing iron absorption and acidifying urine for the prevention of urinary tract infections.[10] High intakes of vitamin C produce druglike effects that may reduce the frequency and severity of colds. But the beneficial effects are mild, and may not provide enough benefit to justify taking high amounts of vitamin C routinely.[9]

#### VITAMIN C: WHERE TO FIND IT

Vitamin C is found in abundant quantities in certain fruits and vegetables (see table 21). Single servings or less of oranges, orange juice, cantaloupe, grapefruit, green pepper, cauliflower, broccoli, and brussels sprouts contain a day's supply of vitamin C for adults. Although citrus fruits are the best-known sources, they by no means have the corner on the vitamin C market.

Relatively poor sources of vitamin C, such as potatoes and cabbage, can make a big dent in the vitamin C requirement if eaten often. During the early part of this century, potatoes supplied more than one-third of the vitamin C consumed by Americans. Potatoes now supply less than one-sixth of our total vitamin C intake.[17]

#### HOW MUCH VITAMIN C DO YOU NEED?

The RDA of vitamin C for women is 60 mg per day. But there are a number of factors that affect how much vitamin C a person needs, so the figure of 60 mg isn't right for many people. The need for vitamin C is increased by smoking, oral contraceptive use, and emotional and physical stress.[9] Of these, emotional and physical stress

TABLE 21. FOOD SOURCES OF VITAMIN C
*(RDA for women = 60 mg)*

| FOOD | AMOUNT | VITAMIN C MG |
|---|---|---|
| *Fruits* | | |
| Kiwi fruit | 1 or ½ cup | 108 |
| Orange juice | 6 oz. | 87 |
| Orange | 1 | 85 |
| Cantaloupe | ¼ whole | 63 |
| Grapefruit juice | 6 oz. | 57 |
| Cranberry juice | ½ cup | 54 |
| Grapefruit | ½ cup | 51 |
| Strawberries | ½ cup | 48 |
| Watermelon | 1 cup | 31 |
| Grape juice | ½ cup | 29 |
| Raspberries | ½ cup | 18 |
| *Vegetables* | | |
| Green peppers | ½ cup | 95 |
| Cauliflower, raw | ½ cup | 75 |
| Broccoli | ½ cup | 70 |
| Brussels sprouts | ½ cup | 65 |
| Collard greens | ½ cup | 48 |
| Cauliflower, cooked. | ½ cup | 30 |
| Potato | 1 | 29 |
| Tomato | ½ | 23 |

increases our need for vitamin C the most—by as much as three to four times the normal amount.[18]

Signs of vitamin C deficiency develop within two to three months after a deficient diet has begun. The most obvious signs are black-and-blue marks that result from slight bumps to the surface of the skin. Gums bleed easily and are tender and sore, and teeth become loose. The year-round availability of fruits and vegetables in the United States has made scurvy, the vitamin C deficiency disease, a rare event.

#### VITAMIN C: HOW MUCH IS TOO MUCH?

Although often viewed as no more than minor distractions by ardent vitamin C users, daily doses that exceed 2 grams produce diarrhea, nausea, and cramping. This amount of vitamin C may also contribute to the development of kidney stones and precipitate abortion in pregnant women.[15] The results of blood and urine tests for glucose may be muddled by supplemental vitamin C. Glucose and vitamin C are very similar chemicals, and the two may not be distinguished by analyses for glucose.

Although it may sound odd, infants can develop scurvy if their mothers took a gram or more of vitamin C daily during pregnancy.[15] The baby adjusts to the high level of vitamin C it receives while in the womb by excreting large amounts of the excess. The baby continues to excrete high levels after birth, even though she or he no longer receives an excess supply of vitamin C. Infants recover from scurvy nicely if given gradually decreasing doses of supplemental vitamin C.

### *Vitamin A (Retinol)*

The discussion of the fat-soluble vitamins begins with vitamin A. It holds the distinction of being the first vitamin discovered. To date, over fifteen hundred vitamin-A-like chemical substances have been produced by scientists, and they are manufactured by the ton for use in supplements, animal feeds, fortified foods, and drugs to treat everything from acne and wrinkles to psoriasis.

Vitamin A is needed for the formation and maintenance and cells that form the outermost layer of skin and eyes, and the lining of the respiratory, reproductive, and gastrointestinal tracts. These cells are subjected to a good deal of wear and tear, and have to be replaced frequently. Vitamin A also influences bone growth and makes it possible to see in a room that is only dimly lit.

Vitamin A has what is known as a *provitamin*. Provitamins can be converted to vitamins by the body. Carotenes act as provitamins for vitamin A and they are the leading source of vitamin A in our diets. At least ten types of carotenes can be converted to vitamin A by the body. Of these, the most important is beta-carotene. It is the most common type of carotene found in foods, and yields far more vitamin A per unit weight than do any of the other carotenes. Although it was long thought that only vitamin A was used by the body, new knowledge reveals a potentially important role of beta-carotene in the prevention of cancer. (We'll talk more about vitamin A, beta-carotene, and cancer in chapter 7.)

#### VITAMIN A FOR THE TREATMENT OF SKIN CONDITIONS

The similarity between the pimplelike bumps produced by both vitamin A deficiency and acne led to the testing of vitamin A for the treatment of acne. Large amounts of the vitamin proved to be an effective treatment for cystic acne, a common, severe form of the disorder.[19]

Very high doses of vitamin A, sixty to one hundred times the RDA, are needed to treat acne. These dose levels, however, produce vitamin A toxicity. To avoid the symptoms of vitamin A toxicity, less toxic forms of vitamin A were developed and tested. Retinoic acid emerged as the form of vitamin A that best cured acne without producing vitamin A toxicity. Even though retinoic acid is less toxic in high amounts than other forms of vitamin A, it still causes problems. Malformations have occurred among newborns of women who took retinoic acid for acne shortly before and during pregnancy. Women should not take vitamin A or any of its derivatives for the treatment of acne shortly before or during pregnancy. Sexually active women should use contraception while being treated with retinoic acid for acne.

Vitamin A derivatives are also used in the treatment of psoriasis and dermatitis, and to lessen wrinkles. (Yes, there really is a "vanishing" cream.) Their use is accompanied by a risk of developing vitamin A overdose because the dose levels used are very high (100,000 IU or more). The vitamin-A-based medications are also expensive and are available on a prescription basis only. These substances, however, represent major breakthroughs in the treatment of acne and wrinkles.

#### VITAMIN A: WHERE TO GET IT

Are you getting the vitamin A you need each day? Are you eating your carrots like your mom and dad said? (If guilt helps change food intake for the better, then it's a teaching tool.) You can check it out by referring to table 22. Vitamin A and beta-carotene are found in relatively few foods; many of the best sources are listed in the table. Between 80 and 90 percent of our total intake comes from only fifty foods, and the most important sources are the beta-carotene-rich vegetables. One-half cup of carrots, sweet potatoes, or spinach supplies more than enough beta-carotene to meet our daily need for vitamin A.

#### VITAMIN A DEFICIENCY

*Night blindness* is an early sign of vitamin A deficiency. The condition exists when a person cannot adjust his or her vision to see in dim light. The effect is most striking when a person moves from a bright to a dark room. Most people can adjust to the dim light within a second or two. The person with night blindness doesn't adapt and cannot see well at all in dim light.

TABLE 22. FOOD SOURCES OF BETA-CAROTENE AND VITAMIN A
*(RDA for women = 4,000 IU [800 mcg RE])*

| FOOD | AMOUNT | VITAMIN A IU |
|---|---|---|
| | *Sources of beta-carotene* | |
| *Vegetables* | | |
| Carrots, raw | 1 medium | 7,900 |
| Sweet potato | ½ cup | 7,850 |
| Pumpkin | ½ cup | 7,840 |
| Spinach, cooked | ½ cup | 7,300 |
| Collard greens, cooked | ½ cup | 6,030 |
| Winter squash | ½ cup | 4,200 |
| Ripe peppers | ½ cup | 2,225 |
| Broccoli | ½ cup | 1,900 |
| *Fruits* | | |
| Cantaloupe | ¼ whole | 5,400 |
| Apricots, canned | ½ cup | 2,260 |
| Papaya | ½ cup | 1,595 |
| Watermelon | 2 cups | 1,265 |
| Peaches, canned | ½ cup | 1,115 |
| Nectarines | 1 | 1,001 |
| | *Sources of vitamin A (Retinol)* | |
| *Meats* | | |
| Liver | 3 oz. | 45,400 |
| Crab | ½ cup | 1,680 |
| *Eggs* | | |
| Egg | 1 medium | 590 |
| *Milk and Cheese* | | |
| Whole milk | 1 cup | 330 |
| Skim milk, fortified | 1 cup | 330 |
| 2% milk | 1 cup | 210 |
| American cheese | 1 oz. | 330 |
| Swiss cheese | 1 oz. | 320 |
| *Fats* | | |
| Butter | 1 tsp. | 160 |
| Margarine, fortified | 1 tsp. | 160 |

Vitamin A deficiency also causes the cells covering the eye to become dry and thick and susceptible to infection. Vision is partially or totally lost when this happens. Vitamin A deficiency is the leading cause of blindness in some developing countries. An estimated half million children are blinded every year and many more experience infectious diseases and stunted growth because of the deficiency.[20] The amount of vitamin A needed to meet a child's yearly need costs less than a quarter. Unfortunately, the complexities of distributing the vitamin to high-risk children in developing countries has prevented the worldwide elimination of vitamin A deficiency.

### HOW MUCH IS TOO MUCH?

Vitamin A, but not beta-carotene, is highly toxic if taken in large amounts. In children, 18,000 IU (3,600 RE) taken daily for a period of months can cause vitamin A toxicity. Adults are more resistant than children to vitamin A toxicity. Daily intakes of 20,000 to 40,000 IU (or 4,000 to 5,000 RE) are needed to produce signs of vitamin A toxicity. Doses of vitamin A in excess of 1,000,000 IU produce hypervitaminosis A in a matter of days.[10] Vitamin A toxicity has been identified among people treating themselves for acne.

People with vitamin A toxicity have blurred vision, pain in the bones and joints, headaches, dry skin, and a poor appetite. The symptoms of advanced vitamin A toxicity convincingly mimic those of a brain tumor. At least one person was transported all the way to surgery before it was discovered he was suffering from vitamin A overdose and not a brain tumor.

Excessively high intake of carrots, sweet potatoes, and beta-carotene supplements do not cause vitamin A toxicity, but a condition known as carotenemia. The major effect of carotenemia is that it turns your skin yellow. This feature of carotene overdose has led to its use in tanning pills. The yellow-colored skin produced by carotenemia is very similar to that occurring with jaundice. In cases of carotenemia, however, the whites of the eyes do not become yellow. Skin coloration returns to normal within two to six weeks after discontinued use of carotene-rich foods.

The dose level of beta-carotene from carrots or supplements that produce a yellowing of the skin was reported recently.[21] Thirty men were given 0, 12, or 30 mg of beta-carotene, or four carrots providing 38 mg of the provitamin. At the 30 mg per day dose of beta-carotene, skin became yellow in all of the men within four to six weeks. On the 12 mg dose, 80 percent of the men appeared yellow within the same time frame. The yellow color lasted for two weeks or more after the beta-carotene supplements were discontinued. Ingesting the carrots produced the carrotlike color in 60 percent of the men within a six-week period.

Carotenemia is generally not regarded as being hazardous to health. Recently, however, carotenemia has been found to produce temporary infertility in women.[22]

### *Vitamin D*

What do you get when you combine a cholesterol-like compound with ultraviolet light from the sun? Nothing less than the "sunshine" vitamin. Vitamin D is formed in the skin when its provitamin absorbs energy from ultraviolet light emitted by the sun.

Very few foods contain measurable amounts of vitamin D, and many people don't get enough exposure to sunlight to produce the level needed. To prevent vitamin D deficiency, especially among populations who get little direct exposure to sunlight, certain foods have been fortified with vitamin D. Milk has been selected as the vitamin-D-fortified food in the United States. Elsewhere, such as in England and the Scandinavian countries, margarine has been fortified. The importance of vitamin D in human nutrition lies in its role of making calcium and phosphorus available for use by the body. It does this in two ways: by increasing the absorption of calcium and phosphorus, and by promoting the incorporation of calcium and phosphorus into bones.

The list of food sources of vitamin D is the shortest one you may ever come across for an essential nutrient. As shown in table 23, liver, eggs, and butter contain some vitamin D. Nonfortified milk contains very little. By law, all milk sold in the United States must be fortified with 400 IU of vitamin D per quart. Cheese, yogurt, ice cream, and other dairy products are usually not fortified with vitamin D.

#### THE SUN AS A SOURCE OF VITAMIN D

You can obtain your RDA for vitamin D by exposing your skin to the sun. How much exposure does it take? The answer depends upon how darkly colored your skin is, and how much skin is exposed. Adults with light skin can get their RDA for vitamin D by exposing their hands, arms, and face to sunlight for ten to fifteen minutes two or three times per week. About 10,000 IU of vitamin D can be produced by sunbathing on a beach up to the point where a mild sunburn begins. People with dark skin require a longer period of exposure to the sun because less ultraviolet light is able to penetrate dark than light skin.[23] Sunlight that comes through a window doesn't promote vitamin D production in the skin because

TABLE 23. FOOD SOURCES OF VITAMIN D
*(RDA for women = 200 IU)*

| FOOD | AMOUNT | VITAMIN D IU |
|---|---|---|
| *Milk* | | |
| Whole, low-fat, or skim | 1 cup | 100 |
| *Fish and seafoods* | | |
| Salmon | 3 oz. | 340 |
| Tuna | 3 oz. | 150 |
| Shrimp | 3 oz. | 127 |
| *Organ meats* | | |
| Beef liver | 3 oz. | 42 |
| Chicken liver | 3 oz. | 40 |
| *Eggs* | | |
| Egg yolk | 1 | 27 |

the glass blocks the ultraviolet light. Tanning lights work, but other types of lights do not.

The production of vitamin D in the skin comes to a halt when 15 to 20 percent of the original provitamin stores in the skin has been converted. Consequently, you cannot receive an overdose of vitamin D by getting too much sun. (You can, however, overdose on sun and increase your risk of skin cancer.)

#### VITAMIN D DEFICIENCY

Vitamin D deficiency is generally caused by a lack of skin exposure to sunlight, a low dietary intake of vitamin D, or a combination of both. Before the fortification of milk with vitamin D, *rickets*, the deficiency disease in children, was widely prevented by a periodic dose of cod-liver oil. (Many of us who grew up in the first sixty years of this century can recall the routine of taking a spoonful of the awful-tasting stuff from time to time.)

Vitamin D deficiency contributes to the development of osteoporosis. Osteoporosis, however, is more often associated with a long-term deficiency of calcium, rather than just vitamin D.

Rickets still emerges occasionally in the United States. Between 1974 and 1978, twenty-four cases were diagnosed in Philadelphia.[24] Children affected ate vegetarian diets and wore long garments with hoods, consistent with the practices of their religious faith. A low dietary intake of vitamin D combined with low exposure to sunlight led to the development of rickets in these children.

#### OVERDOSES OF VITAMIN D

Vitamin D is the most toxic of all vitamins. Supplements that contain two times the RDA for children and ten times the RDA for adults can produce vitamin D toxicity. Excess vitamin D in the blood causes calcium to be deposited in organs such as the heart, kidney, and brain. Seizures, disorientation, joint pain, and many other problems are caused by overdoses of vitamin D. Early experiments with vitamin D supplements in children were quickly stopped when it was observed that high doses of vitamin D lead to permanent mental retardation.

### *Vitamin E*

After the discovery of vitamin E in 1922, animal studies showing its beneficial effects on reproduction, muscle development, and aging led many to believe that vitamin E held strong promise for curing a number of diseases of humankind. It became the "sex vitamin" shortly after its deficiency was shown to cause reproductive failures in rats. Research attempting to identify a direct relationship between vitamin E and human reproduction has not borne fruitful results. Few of the spectacular effects of vitamin E in laboratory animals have been shown to occur in humans. Nonetheless, vitamin E is still an intriguing vitamin. There exists a nagging suspicion among scientists that there are important applications for the vitamin in human nutrition and health, but that we are just not smart enough to figure them all out! Scientists working with vitamin E have called it the "illusive vitamin" and one that is "in search of a disease." In many respects, vitamin E is still the mysterious vitamin it was decades ago.

Vitamin E is found wherever unsaturated fatty acids are present—in vegetable oils, nuts and other oily foods, in the body's fat stores, and in the fat contained in cell membranes. It is there to protect the fragile unsaturated fatty acids from attack by oxygen and the destruction that results. Vitamin E is a powerful antioxidant.

#### VITAMIN E AND AIR POLLUTION

Vitamin E contained in cells lining the lungs provides an important barrier against the harmful effects of some types of air pollutants. Ozone and nitrogen dioxide are common air pollutants that cause damage to lung cells. Vitamin E is the body's first line of defense against cell damage due to these oxidizers that may be present in polluted air.

Low intake of vitamin E may contribute to the development of respiratory diseases due to air pollution. People who live in cities where air pollution is a problem may benefit from a higher-than-average intake of vitamin-E-rich food.[25]

#### VITAMIN E: WHERE TO GET IT

Vitamin E accompanies unsaturated fatty acids in foods, making vegetable oils and products made from them particularly rich sources. Vegetable oils, margarine, and salad dressings contribute over 70 percent of the vitamin E consumed in the United States.[17] Other foods containing unsaturated fatty acids, and therefore vitamin E, are nuts, seeds, whole grains, and seafoods. Table 24 shows examples of good food sources of this vitamin. One food you will not see on the list is oysters. Although considered by some people to be a potent source of vitamin E, oysters contain only 0.1 mg vitamin E per half cup.

#### VITAMIN E DEFICIENCY AND TOXICITY

Vitamin E deficiency is rarely seen except in premature infants. Its toxicity disease is a rare event too. You have to take over 1,000 IU of vitamin E per day to develop excessive bleeding, impaired wound healing, depression, and other signs of vitamin E toxicity.[26]

### *Vitamin K*

Vitamin K is the "coagulation" vitamin. It helps blood clot and therefore helps to control bleeding.

Vitamin K has so far escaped popular use as a supplement. That's a good thing, because there's no reason for healthy people to take it. Vitamin K is produced by bacteria in our intestines and we get it from green, leafy vegetables and meat. Diets in the United States tend to provide much more vitamin K than is required.

Only newborns and people using antibiotics for months at a time are at risk of developing vitamin K deficiency. One study showed that 31 percent of patients with gastrointestinal disorders that required long-term use of antibiotics developed vitamin K deficiency.[27] Antibiotics kill the bacteria in our intestines that produce vitamin K, and we lose that source of it. People with vitamin K deficiency bruise easily and bleed excessively if injured. Vitamin K deficiency is not related to hemophilia.

TABLE 24. FOOD SOURCES OF VITAMIN E
*(RDA for women = 12 IU)*

| FOOD | AMOUNT | VITAMIN E IU |
|---|---|---|
| *Oils* | | |
| Oil | 1 T. | 6.7 |
| Mayonnaise | 1 T. | 3.4 |
| Margarine | 1 T. | 2.7 |
| Salad dressing | 1 T. | 2.2 |
| *Nuts and seeds* | | |
| Sunflower seeds | ¼ cup | 27.1 |
| Almonds | ¼ cup | 12.7 |
| Peanuts | ¼ cup | 4.9 |
| Cashews | ¼ cup | 0.7 |
| *Vegetables* | | |
| Sweet potato | ½ cup | 6.9 |
| Collard greens | ½ cup | 3.1 |
| Asparagus | ½ cup | 2.1 |
| Spinach, raw | 1 cup | 1.5 |
| *Grains* | | |
| Wheat germ | 2 T. | 4.2 |
| Whole wheat bread | 1 slice | 2.5 |
| White bread | 1 slice | 1.2 |
| *Seafood* | | |
| Crab | 3 oz. | 4.5 |
| Shrimp | 3 oz. | 3.7 |
| Fish | 3 oz. | 2.4 |

## MINERALS

Humans require a substantially higher amount of minerals than vitamins in their diets, and foods generally contain much higher levels of the minerals. If you add up all the RDAs for one day for the fifteen minerals assigned RDAs, the total amount would fill a tablespoon. Minerals are needed in higher amounts because, unlike vitamins, they are a component part of body structures such as bones and teeth, and they are found in relatively large amounts in blood and other body fluids.

We'll start the discussion of minerals with a most interesting one: calcium.

### *Calcium*

The calcium craze hit America in the early 1980s, when the consensus of scientific opinion changed from viewing osteoporosis as an inevitable problem of aging to one strongly related to calcium intake. Lifelong adequate intakes of calcium, plus exercise, are seen as the keys to preventing osteoporosis.[28]

Concern about osteoporosis is changing the supplement- and food-buying practices of people in the United States. In the mid-1980s, sales of calcium supplements were increasing by 333 percent a year, and were expected to exceed $270 million in yearly sales by 1990.[29] Average consumption of low-fat milk and dairy products is on the way up in the United States, and the availability of calcium-fortified products is sharply increasing. Food manufacturers have responded to consumer demand for high-calcium foods by adding the mineral to an array of products—from diet soft drinks to flour.

Calcium also performs functions that keep the body alive and well from second to second. Calcium is needed to stimulate nerve impulses, muscle contractions, and blood clotting. About 99 percent of the three pounds of calcium contained in the adult body is located in bone, but the remaining 1 percent is used to perform these other important functions.

#### CALCIUM: WHERE TO GET IT

Most of the calcium supplied in American diets comes from milk and milk products. Milk, cheese, yogurt, and other products made from milk, such as ice cream and pudding, are all good sources of calcium. (That *includes* chocolate milk.) Only a few nonmilk products are good sources of calcium—spinach, collard greens, and tofu are among the best of these few sources (see table 25). However, calcium in many vegetable sources is not nearly as well absorbed as in the calcium found in milk products. Although they appear to be good sources of calcium, spinach, collard greens, and other dark, leafy vegetables tend to supply the body with only low amounts of calcium.

Most U.S. women consume about half of their RDA for calcium.[30] The gap between the recommended and actual intake is wider still for postmenopausal women. It is estimated that postmenopausal women need 1,200–1,500 mg of calcium per day but only consume an average of 475 mg.[31] The bottom line is that most women and many men in the United States do not consume enough calcium to prevent gradual losses in bone-calcium content.[32]

TABLE 25. FOOD SOURCES OF CALCIUM[a]
*(RDA for women = 800 mg)*

| FOOD | AMOUNT | CALCIUM MG |
|---|---|---|
| *Milk and milk products* | | |
| Low-fat yogurt | 1 cup | 415 |
| Low-fat yogurt with fruit | 1 cup | 315 |
| Skim milk | 1 cup | 300 |
| 1% milk | 1 cup | 300 |
| 2% milk | 1 cup | 298 |
| 3.25% milk (whole) | 1 cup | 288 |
| Swiss cheese | 1 oz. | 270 |
| Cheddar cheese | 1 oz. | 205 |
| Frozen yogurt | 1 cup | 200 |
| Cream soup | 1 cup | 186 |
| Pudding | ½ cup | 185 |
| Ice cream | 1 cup | 180 |
| Ice milk | 1 cup | 180 |
| American cheese | 1 oz. | 175 |
| Custard | ½ cup | 150 |
| Cottage cheese | ½ cup | 70 |
| Low-fat cottage cheese | ½ cup | 69 |
| *Vegetables* | | |
| Collard greens, cooked | ½ cup | 110 |
| Spinach, cooked | ½ cup | 90 |
| Broccoli | ½ cup | 70 |
| *Legumes* | | |
| Tofu | ½ cup | 155 |
| Dried beans, cooked | ½ cup | 50 |
| Lima beans | ½ cup | 40 |

[a]*Actually, the richest source of calcium is alligator meat. Three ounces contain about 1,231 mg of calcium, but just try to find it on your grocer's shelf!*

THE CONCERN ABOUT THE CALORIES IN MILK

Why is calcium intake among adult women so far below the recommended levels? One major reason is that women often give up milk after the teen years. Although most women continue to like milk, it is often viewed as fattening. After the teen years, women increasingly prefer coffee and tea, and milk loses its monopoly as their mealtime beverage choice.

Milk and other dairy products can be relatively high-calorie sources of calcium, depending on the type of product selected. The more fat in the dairy product, the higher the caloric cost of the calcium obtained. The key to getting calcium at a reasonable caloric cost is to choose low-fat milk and dairy products. Skim milk and low-fat yogurt are calorie bargains. You can get around 900 mg of calcium from 3 cups of skim milk for 270 calories. That's a 56 percent saving in calories over a similar amount of whole milk. A small container of low-fat yogurt (¾ cup or 6 ounces) has the same calorie level as a cup of corn flakes, but provides nearly one-third of the RDA for calcium for adult women. Pudding, ice cream, and cottage cheese are good, but are calorically expensive sources of calcium. The section on osteoporosis in chapter 7 includes a table with the caloric content of various food sources of calcium.

#### OTHER NOTES ABOUT CALCIUM DEFICIENCY

Dietary calcium deficiency is selective in its effects on calcium functions. Bone formation and maintenance are affected most, and the critical roles of calcium in maintaining normal nerve impulses, muscle contractions, and blood clotting are affected least by calcium deficiency. A deficiency of calcium for these latter three functions would immediately threaten life, but it takes years before a loss of calcium from bones jeopardizes health. The body ensures that the calcium needed for nerve impulses, muscle contractions, and blood coagulation is available by tightly controlling blood-calcium levels. Neither low nor high intakes of calcium make much difference in blood-calcium levels. When dietary intake is inadequate, the body uses the calcium in bones to maintain normal blood levels.

Does having and breast-feeding babies deplete calcium stores and increase a woman's chance of developing osteoporosis? For the majority of women in the United States, the answer appears to be a qualified no. A study conducted on 355 women in Washington found that those who gave birth four or more times or who breastfed more than two years were no more likely to develop osteoporosis during their postmenopausal years than women who never had babies.[33] It does appear, however, that low-calcium diets plus breastfeeding may interfere with the establishment of high, peak bone densities in adolescents.[34]

#### CALCIUM OVERDOSE

Calcium intakes near 2 grams per day do not appear to cause toxicity symptoms. However, the high levels of unabsorbed calcium in the gut that result from such an intake tend to increase bacterial production of gas and cause gut distress.[35] Although the amount of calcium absorbed decreases as calcium intake increases, a higher-than-normal level of calcium absorption can be forced by an overly generous dietary supply of vitamin D. High levels of blood calcium have been identified in people taking 2 or more grams of calcium along with 1,000 IU of vitamin D per day on a regular basis. Some people respond to high doses of calcium and vitamin D by forming calcium stones in the kidneys.

*Phosphorus*

Phosphorus is a very common ingredient in food, although it is perhaps best known for its use in friction matches (and the odor they produce when lit). We carry around about 2 pounds of phosphorus, 85 percent of it in our bones. The rest is distributed throughout the body. In addition to being a structural component of bone, phosphorus is a component of the genetic material DNA and is a key element on energy production.

Only fruits tend to be poor sources of phosphorus. It is so widely distributed in foods (table 26) that a dietary lack almost never occurs. There is some concern that people may be getting too much phosphorus due to the wide use of phosphoric acid (also called "phosphate") as a preservative. If you're a label reader, the term may be familiar. Phosphoric acid is used in diet and regular soft drinks, breakfast cereals, bakery products, and other processed foods. It has been suggested that people who drink a lot of soft drinks may be compromising their bone health by consuming far more phosphorus than calcium. Whether this is the case is not clear.

Not too long ago, nutrition textbooks and other sources of nutrition information warned against consuming diets that contained more phosphorus than calcium. An ideal ratio of dietary calcium to phosphorus was thought to be 2:1, or twice as much calcium as phosphorus. It was reasoned that since bones contain twice as much calcium as phosphorus, and because high phosphorus intake reduces calcium absorption, you needed more dietary calcium than phosphorus to achieve the proper balance for bone health.

Research results accumulating over the past decade indicate that an emphasis on maintaining a 2:1 calcium-to-phosphorus ratio is misplaced. Bone formation and maintenance appear to proceed normally with dietary calcium-to-phosphorus ratios of between 2:1 and 1:2. Current calcium-to-phosphorus intake ratios in the United States are between 1:1.4 and 1:1.8, levels that fall within the acceptable range.[30]

TABLE 26. FOOD SOURCES OF PHOSPHORUS
*(RDA for women = 800 mg)*

| FOOD | AMOUNT | PHOSPHORUS MG |
|---|---|---|
| *Milk and milk products* | | |
| Yogurt | 1 cup | 327 |
| Skim milk | 1 cup | 250 |
| Whole milk | 1 cup | 250 |
| Cottage cheese | ½ cup | 150 |
| American cheese | 1 oz. | 130 |
| *Meats* | | |
| Pork | 3 oz. | 275 |
| Hamburger | 3 oz. | 165 |
| Tuna | 3 oz. | 162 |
| Lobster | 3 oz. | 125 |
| Chicken | 3 oz. | 120 |
| *Nuts and seeds* | | |
| Sunflower seeds | ¼ cup | 319 |
| Peanuts | ¼ cup | 141 |
| Pine nuts | ¼ cup | 106 |
| Peanut butter | 1 T. | 61 |
| *Grains* | | |
| Bran flakes | 1 cup | 180 |
| Shredded wheat | 2 large biscuits | 81 |
| Whole wheat bread | 1 slice | 52 |
| Noodles | ½ cup | 47 |
| Rice | ½ cup | 29 |
| White bread | 1 slice | 24 |
| *Vegetables* | | |
| Potato | 1 medium | 101 |
| Corn | ½ cup | 73 |
| Peas | ½ cup | 70 |
| French fries | ½ cup | 61 |
| Broccoli | ½ cup | 54 |
| *Other* | | |
| Milk chocolate | 1 oz. | 66 |
| Cola | 12 oz. | 51 |
| Diet cola | 12 oz. | 45 |

### PHOSPHORUS DEFICIENCY AND OVERDOSE

Phosphorus deficiency and toxicity diseases are very unusual. Adults appear to have no problem tolerating up to 2 grams of phosphorus per day.[36] Very few people use phosphorus supplements (as should be the case) and consequently few cases of phosphorus overdose have been observed.

### *Magnesium*

Humans only contain about an ounce of magnesium, but it's a very busy ounce. Magnesium is a component of bone and is needed for the production of energy and protein; it also helps the body use calcium to form bones and to transmit impulses along networks of nerve and muscle cells.

Magnesium is found in grains, dried beans, nuts, and certain vegetables. It is more abundant in plant than animal products because chlorophyll-containing plants require magnesium for energy formation from carbon dioxide, sun, and water. (Takes you back to junior high science class, doesn't it?) Good food sources of magnesium are listed in table 27.

#### MAGNESIUM DEFICIENCY

Most people in the United States consume less than their RDA for magnesium, but enough to prevent a deficiency.[37] Cases of magnesium deficiency usually result from excessive alcohol or drugs and diseases that reduce magnesium absorption or increase its excretion. Magnesium deficiency occurs quite commonly among people who are very ill. One report indicated that 20 percent of all patients admitted to an intensive care unit were deficient in magnesium.[38] Marginal deficiencies of magnesium may be relatively common and may possibly be related to hypertension, osteoporosis, and personality changes. The diverse signs of magnesium deficiency include confusion, muscle spasms, irregular heart beat, and convulsions. Since a deficiency of magnesium interferes with the ability of calcium to form bones and transmit nerve impulses, people with this deficiency show signs of calcium deficiency too. So you get a "double deficiency" when you run out of magnesium.

#### MAGNESIUM OVERDOSE

Magnesium supplements are not very toxic to healthy people. The body protects itself from an overdose by decreasing magnesium absorption if intake is high and by excreting excess amounts in the urine. The RDA for magnesium is 300 mg per day, and it makes no sense to take more than that amount in a supplement (if one is taken at all).

TABLE 27. FOOD SOURCES OF MAGNESIUM
*(RDA for women = 280 mg)*

| FOOD | AMOUNT | MAGNESIUM MG |
|---|---|---|
| *Legumes* | | |
| Lentils, cooked | ½ cup | 134 |
| Split peas, cooked | ½ cup | 134 |
| Tofu | ½ cup | 130 |
| *Nuts* | | |
| Peanuts | ¼ cup | 247 |
| Cashews | ¼ cup | 93 |
| Almonds | ¼ cup | 80 |
| *Grains* | | |
| Bran buds | 1 cup | 240 |
| Wild rice, cooked | ½ cup | 119 |
| Fortified breakfast cereal | 1 cup | 85 |
| Wheat germ | 2 T. | 45 |
| *Vegetables* | | |
| Bean sprouts | ½ cup | 98 |
| Black-eyed peas | ½ cup | 58 |
| Spinach, cooked | ½ cup | 48 |
| Lima beans | ½ cup | 32 |
| *Milk and milk products* | | |
| Milk | 1 cup | 30 |
| Cheddar cheese | 1 oz. | 8 |
| American cheese | 1 oz. | 6 |
| *Meats* | | |
| Chicken | 3 oz. | 25 |
| Beef | 3 oz. | 20 |
| Pork | 3 oz. | 20 |

*Iron*

This mineral brings us to a very important topic, for women in particular: iron deficiency. It is the most common deficiency disease in the United States. Up to 70 percent of young women have absent or scanty iron stores. As many as 20 percent of pregnant women, 14 percent of teenage girls, and 9 percent of children in the United States are iron deficient.[39] It is estimated that 50 percent of women worldwide have iron deficiency.[40]

Iron performs its service to the body from its location in hemoglobin—the primary component of red blood cells—and myoglobin—a major protein found in muscle cells. The function of iron in these proteins is to deliver oxygen to cells and take carbon dioxide away from them. Hemoglobin, when it is loaded with oxygen, is bright red. When it returns from cells, the carbon dioxide it carries makes blood dark red.

A small amount of iron works with certain enzymes involved in energy formation. Altogether, the body's content of iron adds up to about 4 grams—or the weight of a penny.

#### IRON: WHERE TO GET IT

Nearly all foods contain iron, but not very much of it. With the exception of a limited number of foods such as liver, fortified cereals, and prune juice, the good food sources of iron provide only 10 to 20 percent of a woman's RDA per serving (see table 28). Because iron is found in small amounts in many foods, diets containing few good iron sources still provide about 6 mg of iron per 1,000 calories consumed. This situation helps men get the 10 mg of iron recommended each day, but leaves most women out. The 15 mg of iron recommended for women is difficult to obtain from the low level of calories most women consume.

The low amount of iron contained in foods and the common problem of iron deficiency have led to the addition of iron to cereals through enrichment and fortification. As a result, grain products have become a leading source of iron in the U.S. diet. About one-third of our total supply of iron comes from grain products, a third from meats, and the remaining third from a broad variety of foods.[17]

There is a pretty nifty way to increase the iron content of your diet. The tip is courtesy of the U.S. Department of Defense. Cook in iron pans. Here's the story behind the statement.

*About 30 years ago, a group of nutrition experts were brought together by the Department of Defense to study the adequacy of diets of military personnel. One component of the dietary assessment specifically addressed the adequacy of iron intake. Samples of food from different military bases were brought to a central laboratory for preparation and analysis of iron content. To the surprise of the experts, the amount of iron identified in certain foods from some of the bases was substantially higher than the same foods prepared at other bases. The reason for this unexpected result became clear when it was discovered that foods prepared in cast-iron rather than glass pans contained the unusually high levels of iron. It was further noted that acidic foods extracted a good deal more iron from the pans during the cooking process than nonacidic foods. The iron content of spaghetti sauce was twenty-nine times higher, applesauce one hundred six times higher, and beef hash, scrambled eggs, and fried potatoes over three times higher than the same foods cooked in glass pans.*[41]

Cast-iron pans are not used as much as they used to be, so their contribution to iron intake has declined in the United States. The problem is that cast-iron pans are heavy and will rust if not seasoned. You can season cast iron by lightly coating the inside of the pan with vegetable oil and then heating the pan for a few minutes on the stove. This process may have to be repeated several times to season a pan to the point where foods don't stick to it. Iron pans have to be seasoned after each washing with dish soap.

#### IRON IS NOT EASILY ABSORBED

Iron has to go through a number of hoops before it is absorbed into the bloodstream. It is perhaps the most difficult of all nutrients for humans to absorb. Several factors influence how much of the iron we consume is absorbed. They include the source of the iron (whether it is from meats or plants), what else is in our meal, and how much storage iron we have.

Iron found in meats is more easily absorbed than iron in plants. For example, both a 3-ounce hamburger and a cup of asparagus contain around 3 mg of iron. But because of differences in the availability of iron, twenty times more iron can be absorbed from the hamburger than from the asparagus. Iron in iron-fortified cereals is in the form of poorly absorbed iron. The availability of iron added to fortified cereals is about the same as it is for iron that naturally occurs in the cereal.[42] So only about 1 percent of iron added to rice or corn and around 4 percent of the iron added to wheat products are available for absorption. In general, 10 to 20 percent of iron consumed in meats are absorbed, whereas only 1 to 8 percent of the iron in plants is.[42]

The absorption of iron can be increased by consuming vitamin-C-rich food along with plant sources of iron. Because vitamin C is such a potent enhancer of iron absorption, it is thought that inadequate vitamin C intake may contribute substantially to the develop-

TABLE 28. FOOD SOURCES OF IRON
*(RDA for women = 15 mg)*

| FOOD | AMOUNT | IRON MG |
|---|---|---|
| *Meat and meat alternates* | | |
| Liver | 3 oz. | 7.5 |
| Round steak | 3 oz. | 3.0 |
| Hamburger, lean | 3 oz. | 3.0 |
| Baked beans | ½ cup | 3.0 |
| Pork | 3 oz. | 2.7 |
| White beans | ½ cup | 2.7 |
| Soybeans | ½ cup | 2.5 |
| Pork and beans | ½ cup | 2.3 |
| Fish | 3 oz. | 1.0 |
| Chicken | 3 oz. | 1.0 |
| *Grains* | | |
| Iron-fortified breakfast cereals | 1 cup | 8.0 (4–18) |
| Oatmeal (fortified) | 1 cup | 8.0 |
| Bagel | 1 | 1.7 |
| English muffin | 1 | 1.6 |
| Rye bread | 1 slice | 1.0 |
| Whole wheat bread | 1 slice | 0.8 |
| White bread | 1 slice | 0.6 |
| *Fruit* | | |
| Prune juice | 6 oz. | 7.0 |
| Dried apricots | ½ cup | 2.5 |
| Prunes | 5 medium | 2.0 |
| Raisins | ¼ cup | 1.3 |
| Plums | 3 medium | 1.1 |
| *Vegetables* | | |
| Spinach (cooked) | ½ cup | 2.3 |
| Lima beans | ½ cup | 2.2 |
| Black-eyed peas | ½ cup | 1.7 |
| Peas | ½ cup | 1.6 |
| Asparagus | ½ cup | 1.5 |

ment of iron deficiency.[43] In general, a good level of iron absorption can be expected if daily diets contain meats, or provide 75 mg of vitamin C if meats aren't consumed.[43]

How much iron is absorbed from foods and supplements depends heavily on how much of it we need. Humans cannot excrete high levels of absorbed iron as they can many vitamins and minerals. Iron becomes very toxic if allowed to pile up in blood and tissues. The body partially protects itself from the harmful effects of high iron levels by limiting the amount of iron absorbed. It also protects your health by allowing more iron to be absorbed when iron stores are low. The amount of iron absorbed from foods and supplements can increase from 2 percent when you have high iron stores to 30 percent if your stores are low or missing.[44] Although these adaptations are helpful, they do not provide complete protection against iron deficiency or overload.

#### IRON DEFICIENCY

Problems stemming from a lack of iron occur in two stages: *iron deficiency* and *iron deficiency anemia*. Iron deficiency is diagnosed when iron stores are absent and the body does not have quite as much iron as it needs to function normally. Effects of iron deficiency include reduced resistance to infection, physical sluggishness, poor appetite, and shortened attention span. Iron deficiency anemia occurs when not enough iron is available for normal hemoglobin production. Without iron, red blood cells become pale and small, and contain little hemoglobin. People with iron deficiency anemia aren't getting enough oxygen delivered to their cells. They look pale, feel tired and weak, and their heart beats rapidly in an attempt to supply more oxygen to cells.

The diagnosis of iron deficiency is often based on measurements of the amount of hemoglobin in red blood cells. Hemoglobin values of less than 12 grams per 100 ml of blood in women and less than 13 grams in men are generally used to diagnose iron deficiency.[45]

#### OTHER CAUSES OF IRON DEFICIENCY

Iron deficiency and its anemia also develop from losses in blood due to injury or disease. Hemorrhage caused by an injury and the slow but persistent losses of blood that occur with bleeding ulcers are well known to produce anemia. People who donate blood too often (over five times a year) or those who have conditions that require frequent blood tests are at risk of losing enough blood to eventually develop anemia.[46]

#### IRON OVERLOAD

The toxicity disease related to iron overload is commonly referred to as "iron poisoning." It can occur when iron intakes are habitually high (over 75 mg per day for a year or more) among people who regularly take iron pills plus vitamin C supplements or other enhancers of iron absorption.[46] Iron poisoning can also develop if large amounts of iron supplements are taken in a short period of time. Single doses of over 12 grams of iron in women, and over 17 grams in men, produce iron poisoning.[47] Acute iron overload can lead to death, and it does so at least two thousand times per year in the United States.[48] Iron overdose is a leading cause of hospitalization of young children. It most often results from the ingestion of iron supplements found in the home. The lethal dose of iron for a two-year-old is around 3 grams, the amount present in twenty-five pills that contain 120 mg of iron each.[47] Iron supplements containing 120 mg of iron are commonly prescribed during pregnancy and, because of the side effects of this high dose, they are often not taken. The unused pills frequently end up in medicine cabinets and therefore are available to the curious preschooler.

### *Zinc*

Zinc was not recognized as an essential nutrient until 1958. Before that, zinc was considered not essential, but toxic. The primary knowledge scientists had about zinc and health was based on zinc toxicity that occurred in workers who smelted zinc ores. We now know that zinc is, well, an "essential poison." Zinc deficiency is recognized as being an important cause of poor growth in children in many parts of the world, including some U.S. locations.[49]

Zinc is a component of over two hundred enzymes, most of which are involved in the manufacture of body proteins. It is incorporated into the structure of the enzymes, and enzyme levels decrease if zinc is not available when the enzymes are produced. Reduced levels of the zinc-containing enzymes cause a slowdown in the production of protein by the body. Consequently, normal growth and the repair and maintenance of tissues depend on an adequate supply of zinc.

#### ZINC: WHERE TO GET IT

As shown in table 29, meats are the best food sources of zinc, just as they are for iron. Many other types of food contain small amounts of zinc, and their contribution to our total zinc intake largely depends on how frequently they are consumed. Milk and milk products are the second leading sources of dietary zinc, not so much because they are rich sources, but because we tend to consume them often.

Whether zinc is principally obtained from meats or plants is an important issue. Not all zinc is equally well absorbed. Much of the

TABLE 29. FOOD SOURCES OF ZINC
*(RDA for women = 12 mg)*

| FOOD | AMOUNT | ZINC MG |
|---|---|---|
| *Meat*[a] | | |
| Liver | 3 oz. | 4.6 |
| Beef | 3 oz. | 4.0 |
| Crab | ½ cup | 3.5 |
| Lamb | 3 oz. | 3.5 |
| Turkey ham | 3 oz. | 2.5 |
| Pork | 3 oz. | 2.4 |
| Chicken | 3 oz. | 2.0 |
| *Legumes* | | |
| Dried beans (cooked) | ½ cup | 1.0 |
| Split peas (cooked) | ½ cup | 0.9 |
| *Grains* | | |
| Fortified breakfast cereals | 1 cup | 1.5–4.0 |
| Wheat germ | 2 T. | 2.4 |
| Brown rice | 1 cup | 1.2 |
| Oatmeal | 1 cup | 1.2 |
| Bran flakes | 1 cup | 1.0 |
| White rice | 1 cup | 0.8 |
| *Nuts and seeds* | | |
| Pecans | ¼ cup | 2.0 |
| Cashews | ¼ cup | 1.8 |
| Sunflower seeds | ¼ cup | 1.7 |
| Peanut butter | 2 T. | 0.9 |
| *Milk and milk products* | | |
| Cheddar cheese | 1 oz. | 1.1 |
| Milk (whole) | 1 cup | 0.9 |
| American cheese | 1 oz. | 0.8 |

[a]*Octopus anyone? Did you know that octopus is a very rich source of zinc? Three ounces of it contains about 38 mg of zinc. Octopus was not listed in the table because it is rarely eaten in the United States.*

zinc consumed in meats is present in zinc-containing enzymes. Zinc contained in enzymes is easily detached during digestion, making it available for absorption. The zinc contained in grains, beans, and other plants is firmly bound to substances that don't readily release it. Consequently, only a small amount of zinc from plants becomes available for absorption. Iron supplements decrease zinc absorption, so iron supplements should be taken between meals and not at the same time as supplemental zinc.[50]

It is estimated that only 8 percent of people in the United States consume the RDA of zinc.[51] On average, we consume around 10 mg of zinc per day—enough to meet day-to-day needs but not enough to maintain zinc stores.[52] Vegetarians need to consume considerably more than the recommended 15 mg of zinc per day because of the poor absorbability of zinc in plants.

#### ZINC DEFICIENCY

Zinc deficiency is fairly prevalent throughout the world, and mild forms of zinc deficiency have been identified in 2 to 3 percent of U.S. infants and children.[31] The mild forms of zinc deficiency occurring in the United States produce slow growth and poor appetite. Zinc deficiency associated with high dosages of iron supplements, which interfere with zinc absorption, has been observed among pregnant women in the United States.[50] Severe cases of zinc deficiency produce profound effects on growth and sexual maturation.

#### ZINC OVERDOSE

*Zinc may be only a poor relation of gold in the mineral world, but in the health food market it has financial clout.*

*"Nutrition Therapy,"* Consumer Reports, *v. 45, no. 1, 1980, p. 23.*

Zinc has been widely promoted as an antistress and provirility mineral. Although false, these claims have made the use of zinc supplements very attractive, while the negative effects of zinc supplements have not been heard of. Self-medication with zinc at levels greater than 15 mg per day is unwise because of the effects of high levels of zinc on blood lipids.[53] Supplemental zinc at doses of about 15 mg per day appears to block the positive effects of exercise on increasing HDL-cholesterol level (the lipoprotein you want to have in high amounts in your blood). Zinc doses of 150 mg or more per day raise LDL-cholesterol[54] (the wrong one to go up) as well as produce a drop in HDL-cholesterol.[53]

### *Iodine*

The story behind iodine is rich and intriguing. Shortly after it was discovered in 1811, iodine became a very popular disease remedy and was used in vapors and pills to cure a wide assortment of illnesses. In French hospitals, strips of gauze saturated with iodine would be hung like flypaper from the ceilings to rid the air of germs. Iodine was thought to be so powerful against disease that people would hang a bottle of it around their necks.[55] Iodine is still widely used as a disinfectant in medicinal lotions and cleaning solutions.

In addition to its germ-destroying property, iodine is known for its deficiency disease, goiter. (*Goiter* means an enlargement of the thyroid gland.) Iodine deficiency goiter has been a public health problem since at least 3000 BC.[56] The cure, iodine-rich foods or extracts, has been known for hundreds of years and yet the disease still affects millions of people throughout the developing world.[57]

Iodine is distributed throughout the body, but is concentrated in the thyroid gland. (The thyroid gland is a pink pad of tissue at the base of the neck that is wrapped around the esophagus and windpipe.) The thyroid is the only tissue known to require iodine, and the only known role of iodine is in the formation of two very potent thyroid hormones.

Iodine-containing thyroid hormones regulate the rate at which energy and protein formation take place within cells. (Adding iodine to a diet doesn't increase the level of the activity of these hormones, however.) During growth, the thyroid hormones increase the pace at which energy and protein are formed by cells. They decrease the rates when growth is not occurring. Without sufficient iodine, too little of the thyroid hormones are produced and growth and development become slow and proceed abnormally. In adults, low levels of thyroid hormones produce sluggishness, sleepiness, and often weight gain.

#### IODINE: WHERE TO GET IT?

The sea is the source of most of the iodine that enters the food chain and eventually our diet. Plants from the sea rarely eaten in the United States are the only naturally rich sources of dietary iodine. Other than many types of ocean fish and shell fish, which contain moderate amounts of iodine, most foods are naturally low in iodine.

Iodine is added to foods in several ways. It is purposefully added to salt, and it incidentally ends up in milk, bread, and some artificially colored foods. Iodized salt has been available in the United States since 1924. It was introduced to halt the spread of cases of goiter in sections of the country referred to as the "goiter belt." The widespread use of iodized salt by people in the goiter belt led to a decline in goiter, and today it is a rare problem. About 50 percent of all salt manufactured in the United States is iodized, and on average, people receive around 150 mcg (or the adult RDA level) of iodine from iodized salt each day.[58] The addition of iodine to salt is voluntary, and the word *iodized* is clearly printed on the labels of those salts that are.

Iodine incidentally ends up in foods by three major routes. The dairy industry uses it to disinfect vats for pasteurizing milk. Some of the iodine in the disinfectant adheres to the vats and enters the milk. Many commercial bakeries use iodine to improve the texture of bread dough, and iodine is a component of food dyes such as Red Number 3. Iodized salt and incidental sources of iodine are the major contributors to the iodine intake of people in the United States.[58]

Much more iodine is available in the food supply than was the case just twenty years ago. Rather than being concerned about iodine deficiency, the current issue is whether we're getting too much of it. Although no solid evidence exists to show that current levels of iodine intake are hazardous to health, a note of caution has been sounded about further increases in iodine intake in the United States.[9]

Habitual intakes of over 2,000 mcg (2 mg) of iodine per day may be toxic. Daily intakes of iodine in the United States run between 500 and 1,900 mcg.[59] (The RDA for adults is 150 mcg.) It doesn't appear necessary to go out of your way to find more iodine for your diet.

#### IODINE OVERDOSE

People with iodine toxicity look like their eyes are bulging from their sockets, are thin, high strung, and anxious. Large outbreaks of iodine overdose have occurred in countries where iodine fortification of foods has been overdone and, in Japan, among people eating too much seaweed.[60]

### *Fluoride*

Fluoride is best known for its use in the prevention of tooth decay. About 50 percent of the supply of drinking water in the United States is fluoridated, and sodium fluoride compounds are widely used in toothpastes and mouth rinses. These uses have contributed to an impressive reduction in the incidence of tooth decay in the United States, Europe, and many other countries. Fluoride has the overall effect of strengthening bones and making teeth resistant to decay caused by bacteria in the mouth.

Teeth get fluoride both from the mouth and through the fluoride content of blood, which nourishes teeth. Children who regularly drink fluoridated water or use fluoridated toothpaste or mouth rinse have more fluoride in their teeth and 40 to 70 percent fewer cavities than people without access to fluoride.[61] Adults benefit from fluoridated water, too, but fluoride is incorporated into adult teeth at a slower pace than in children.

Although fluoridation has greatly reduced the incidence of tooth decay, it is still an important public health problem among that half of the U.S. population that lacks access to fluoridated water. Some communities are reluctant to add fluoride because of fears that it may promote cancer and other diseases. Such fears are unfounded. Fluoridated water has not been shown to be even weakly related to the development of cancer, heart disease, birth defects, or other health problems.[62] Furthermore, only trace amounts of fluoride are used to fluoridate water: Municipal water supplies contain one part fluoride per million parts of water, the equivalent of about four grains of salt per quart of water.

Water fluoridation is the least expensive (it costs about thirty cents per person per year) and most effective way of preventing tooth decay, but other approaches are needed in areas where water is not fluoridated. Fluoride supplements and fluoridated toothpaste and mouth rinses have been successfully used to fill the "fluoride gap." The regular use of fluoridated toothpaste or mouth rinses can decrease dental decay in children by 40 percent.[63]

#### FLUORIDE: WHERE TO GET IT

Fluoridated water is our largest source of fluoride; commercial products made with fluoridated water are the second. There are no excellent food sources of this mineral, but milk, spinach, eggs, and some teas contain small quantities of fluoride.

#### FLUORIDE DEFICIENCY/OVERDOSE

The only known effect of fluoride deficiency is an increased susceptibility to tooth decay. As much as half of the U.S. population may fail to consume the recommended level of fluoride. *Fluorosis*, the development of "mottled" teeth with rusty-colored stains, occurs among children raised in communities where the water is naturally high in fluoride. Mild fluorosis, the kind that produces a light staining of teeth, occurs when children regularly consume water containing over 2 parts per million (ppm) of fluoride, instead of the 1 ppm used to fluoridate water supplies. Because the stains are part of the tooth structure, they are permanent. Adults don't develop mottled teeth as a result of fluorosis; it occurs only during tooth formation. Mottled teeth may be unattractive, but they are highly resistant to decay. Aside from cosmetic concerns, fluorosis appears to have no other undesirable effect.

### *Selenium*

Selenium was not identified as an essential nutrient until the early 1970s, and many pages in its book of functions are still blank. Only one function of selenium in human nutrition is known with certainty: it is part of an enzyme that functions as an antioxidant. This selenium-containing enzyme acts as an antioxidant in much the same way as vitamin E. Both selenium and vitamin E repair damage to molecules in cell membranes caused by oxygen. Roles of selenium in the development of muscular dystrophy, in sperm production, and in the body's response to infection have been proposed, but these functions are yet to be confirmed. Lack of detailed knowledge about the many possible roles of selenium in human health, however, has not interfered with the work of the pervasive peddlers of nutrition nonsense. Selenium has been touted as a cure for cancer, heart disease, sexual problems, and poor eyesight, and as effective in preventing aging. The book on selenium, once written, is likely to be an interesting one indeed.

#### SELENIUM: WHERE TO GET IT

A food's selenium content varies a lot depending on soil and water. Animals reared on plants grown in selenium-rich soil contain more selenium than animals that eat plants grown in selenium-poor soil. As shown in table 30, meats are the best food sources of selenium. How much selenium ends up in meats varies substantially, however, depending on growing conditions. For example, the selenium content of 3 ounces of beef ranges from 0.05 to 0.42 mg; in 3 ounces of tuna, it ranges from 0.04 to 0.1 mg.

Most people in the United States who eat meat regularly are likely getting an adequate supply of selenium.[64] Although there are selenium-rich and selenium-poor growing conditions in the United States, frank selenium deficiency is rarely diagnosed in this country.

#### SELENIUM OVERDOSE

Prior to 1970, selenium was thought of as a toxic substance, and one especially dangerous to livestock. We now know that selenium is an essential nutrient that can have toxic effects. The line between health and toxicity disease is drawn by the amount of selenium consumed.

Selenium toxicity is called *selenosis*. The signs of selenosis in cattle have been known for decades, but those occurring in humans were not well defined until a recent accident. Due to a manufacturing error, a supplement containing 25 to 35 mg of selenium per tab-

TABLE 30. FOOD SOURCES OF SELENIUM
*(RDA for women = 55 mcg)*

| FOOD | AMOUNT | SELENIUM MCG |
|---|---|---|
| *Seafood* | | |
| Lobster | 3 oz. | 66 |
| Tuna | 3 oz. | 60 |
| Shrimp | 3 oz. | 54 |
| Oysters | 3 oz. | 48 |
| Fish | 3 oz. | 40 |
| *Meats* | | |
| Liver | 3 oz. | 56 |
| Ham | 3 oz. | 29 |
| Beef | 3 oz. | 22 |
| Bacon | 3 oz. | 21 |
| Chicken | 3 oz. | 18 |
| Lamb | 3 oz. | 14 |
| Veal | 3 oz. | 10 |
| *Egg* | 1 medium | 37 |

let (rather than the dose of less than 0.2 mg) reached the market. The dose was sufficient to cause signs of selenium overdose. The first sign observed was breath that smelled like garlic. Other signs of selenium overdose included hair and fingernail loss, discolored skin, weakness, and liver damage.

Early signs of selenosis have been observed with daily intake of 900 mcg (0.9 mg) selenium over a two-year period.[65] Selenium supplements should be used with caution; intake should not exceed 200 mcg (0.2) mg per day.

### *Sodium*

Sodium: On the one hand, it can be considered a gift from the sea, on the other, a hazard to health brought to us by the salt shaker. The life- and health-sustaining functions of this mineral are frequently overshadowed by the effects of excessive sodium on blood pressure.

Much of the sodium present on this planet is in the form of sodium chloride, or table salt. The oceans are far and away the leading source of sodium; they contain enough salt to cover the surface of the earth to a depth of over four hundred feet. Although found in abundance in the oceans, humans have not always had access to enough salt to satisfy their taste for it. In earlier times, wars were fought over salt shortages. During such times of scarcity, a pocketful of salt was as good as a pocketful of cash. *Salt* originally came from the word for *salary.*

#### THE POWER OF SALT

*There are six flavours, and of them all, salt is the greatest.*

*Sanskrit proverb, circa 800* BC

Ah, for the taste of salt. Throughout the ages, humans have gone to great lengths to get and maintain a supply of it. Now that salt is cheaply and readily available, the challenge is to reduce intakes to levels closer to those consumed when salt was scarce.

Due to the naturally low sodium content of foods and the important roles of sodium in the body, humans appear to have evolved powerful mechanisms that enhance sodium intake and conserve it once absorbed. Humans are born with a preference for the taste of salt, and it is the only substance for which humans will develop an appetite in response to need. You could be seriously ill from scurvy, severely iron deficient, or suffer from pellagra, but you would not seek out or spontaneously prefer foods that would cure your deficiency. Only sodium has built-in safeguards that encourage consumption. Unfortunately, the body lacks mechanisms that decrease our appetite for salt when we consume more of it than we need or is good for us.[66]

The safeguards that encourage salt consumption likely developed in response to a shortage of sodium in the diets of early humans. Our ancestors' total dietary supply of sodium came from meats and plants, and probably amounted to less than 2 grams of sodium per day. In contrast to the sodium intake of hunter-gatherers, people in industrialized western societies consume an average of 8 or more grams of sodium a day.[66] Obviously, the biological mechanisms put in place forty thousand years ago did not prepare humans for the day when they could eat all the salt they wanted.

#### WHAT THE BODY DOES WITH SODIUM

It's hard to discuss the functions of sodium in the body without also discussing potassium's functions. The two work closely together on one major role: the maintenance of the right amount of water in different compartments of the body. Nearly all of the body's sodium supply is located in blood and the fluid that surrounds cells, whereas potassium is located inside cells. Cells need a balance of water between their outside and inside to function normally, and sodium and potassium help achieve that balance. Both minerals chemically attract water to the outside or inside of cells to maintain a healthy balance. Water balance and cell functions can be upset when there's an imbalance in the body's supply of sodium and potassium. When there is more sodium on the outside of cells than potassium inside, the sodium on the outside draws water away from the inside of the cell. The buildup in water on the outside of cells increases the pressure on the cells. This situation affects the pressure of blood inside of blood vessels. Blood pressure goes up in the presence of an oversupply of sodium compared to potassium. The effect of high sodium levels on increasing the pressure of fluid between cells and on the blood and chemical changes induced by the presence of high levels of sodium are thought to be directly related to the development of high blood pressure or, as it is otherwise known, *hypertension*.

#### SOURCES OF SODIUM

Very few foods naturally contain much sodium. In fact, only 5 to 10 percent of the sodium in the U.S. diet consists of sodium that is originally present in food. The rest is added to foods during processing or preparation or at the table.[67] Diets in the United States would contain levels of sodium equivalent to a highly restricted sodium diet (one similar to that consumed by our hunter-gatherer ancestors) if we did not add salt to our foods.

Food sources of sodium are listed in table 31. Most of the high sources of sodium are miscellaneous foods, those that cannot be neatly assigned to a particular food category. Among the richest sources of sodium are table and sea salt, smoked and canned foods, sauces, and salty snacks.

Most people in the United States consume at least 8,690 mg, or 8.69 grams, of sodium from food each day (that includes about 2,000 mg—2.0 grams—added at the table).[67] The range of recommended intake level for adults is 1,100 to 3,300 mg per day. Humans actually need only 500 mg per day to maintain the normal functions of sodium in the body. Intakes of sodium up to 3,300 mg per day do not appear to increase the risk of developing hypertension.[9]

#### SODIUM DEFICIENCY/OVERDOSE

Most cases of sodium deficiency are caused by problems that increase sodium loss, such as diarrhea, vomiting, and some types of kidney disorders. Heavy sweating can also cause sodium deficiency if the sodium lost is not replaced by foods or fluids. People with sodium deficiency feel weak and shaky. These symptoms disappear seconds after consuming salt or another source of sodium.

The primary consequence of excessive sodium intake appears to be hypertension. Consuming high amounts in a short period of time (such as taking too many salt tablets) can cause dehydration.

### *Potassium*

Potassium is found in all cells, but most of our body's 4½-ounce supply is located inside muscle cells.

Potassium's primary role in the body is to assist in the maintenance of an appropriate level of fluid inside of cells. The attraction

TABLE 31. FOOD SOURCES OF SODIUM
*(Recommended intake for adults = 1,100–3,300 mg)*

| FOOD | AMOUNT | SODIUM MG |
|---|---|---|
| *Miscellaneous* | | |
| Salt | 1 tsp. | 2,132 |
| Dill pickle | 1 (4½ oz.) | 1,930 |
| Sea salt | 1 tsp. | 1,716 |
| Chicken broth | 1 cup | 1,571 |
| Ravioli, canned | 1 cup | 1,065 |
| Spaghetti w/sauce, canned | 1 cup | 955 |
| Baking soda | 1 tsp. | 821 |
| Beef broth | 1 cup | 782 |
| Gravy | ¼ cup | 720 |
| Italian dressing | 2 T. | 720 |
| Pretzels | 5 (1 oz.) | 500 |
| Green olives | 5 | 465 |
| Pizza w/cheese | 1 wedge | 455 |
| Soy sauce | 1 tsp. | 444 |
| Cheese twists | 1 cup | 329 |
| Bacon | 3 slices | 303 |
| French dressing | 2 T. | 220 |
| Potato chips | 10 pieces | 200 |
| Catsup | 1 T. | 155 |
| *Meats* | | |
| Corned beef | 3 oz. | 808 |
| Ham | 3 oz. | 800 |
| Canned fish | 3 oz. | 735 |
| Meat loaf | 3 oz. | 555 |
| Sausage | 3 oz. | 483 |
| Hot dog | 1 | 477 |
| Smoked fish | 3 oz. | 444 |
| Bologna | 1 oz. | 370 |
| *Milk and milk products* | | |
| Cream soup | 1 cup | 1,070 |
| Cottage cheese | ½ cup | 455 |
| American cheese | 1 oz. | 405 |
| Cheese spread | 1 oz. | 274 |
| Parmesan cheese | 1 oz. | 247 |
| Gouda cheese | 1 oz. | 232 |
| Cheddar cheese | 1 oz. | 175 |
| Skim milk | 1 cup | 125 |
| Milk, whole | 1 cup | 120 |

TABLE 31. CONTINUED

| FOOD | AMOUNT | SODIUM MG |
|---|---|---|
| *Grain products* | | |
| Bran flakes | 1 cup | 363 |
| Cornflakes | 1 cup | 325 |
| Croissant | 1 medium | 270 |
| Bagel | 1 | 260 |
| English muffin | 1 | 203 |
| White bread | 1 slice | 130 |
| Whole wheat bread | 1 slice | 130 |
| Saltine crackers | 4 squares | 125 |

of potassium for water inside cells is balanced by the water-attracting property of sodium on the outside of cells. The fluid content inside and outside of cells is maintained in a healthy balance through the shifting of potassium and sodium across cell membranes. Due to this important function, the major role of potassium in the body is referred to as maintaining the body's "fluid balance." Like calcium, potassium plays a role in the conduction of nerve impulses and muscle contractions.

#### POTASSIUM: WHERE TO GET IT

The best food sources of potassium are shown in table 32. Bananas are the single best source of potassium in the U.S. diet. Most vegetables and fruits are particularly good sources of potassium, but this mineral is widely distributed in many types of foods. A relatively new source of dietary potassium is gaining popularity in the United States—salt substitutes. Many types of salt substitutes provide around 200 mg of potassium with every shake. Low-sodium salts are often produced by replacing the *sodium* in sodium chloride with potassium.

The average intake of potassium in the United States falls at the low end of the RDA range of 1,875–5,625 mg per day.[68] Humans can biologically adjust to a wide range of potassium intakes, and deficiency or overdose has never been related to foods eaten by healthy people. They have, however, been related to disease states and the overzealous use of potassium supplements.

#### POTASSIUM DEFICIENCY

Potassium deficiency related to excessive loss of body potassium does occur. Many cases of potassium deficiency are related to the

TABLE 32. FOOD SOURCES OF POTASSIUM
*(Recommended Intake for adults = 1,875–5,625 mg)*

| FOOD | AMOUNT | POTASSIUM MG |
|---|---|---|
| *Vegetables* | | |
| Potato | 1 medium | 780 |
| Winter squash | ½ cup | 327 |
| Tomato | 1 medium | 300 |
| Celery | 1 stalk | 270 |
| Carrots | 1 medium | 245 |
| Broccoli | ½ cup | 205 |
| *Fruits* | | |
| Avocado | ½ medium | 680 |
| Banana | 1 medium | 440 |
| Orange juice | 6 oz. | 375 |
| Raisins | ¼ cup | 370 |
| Watermelon | 2 cups | 315 |
| Prunes | 4 large | 300 |
| *Meats* | | |
| Fish | 3 oz. | 500 |
| Hamburger | 3 oz. | 480 |
| Lamb | 3 oz. | 382 |
| Pork | 3 oz. | 335 |
| Chicken | 3 oz. | 208 |
| *Grains* | | |
| Bran buds | 1 cup | 1,080 |
| Bran flakes | 1 cup | 248 |
| Raisin bran | 1 cup | 242 |
| Wheat flakes | 1 cup | 96 |
| *Milk and milk products* | | |
| Yogurt | 1 cup | 531 |
| Skim milk | 1 cup | 400 |
| Whole milk | 1 cup | 370 |
| *Other* | | |
| Salt substitutes | 1 tsp. | 1,300–2,378 |

use of certain types of diuretics (water pills) used to control high blood pressure. Over 100 million prescriptions for diuretics are written each year. Potassium supplements or instructions for a high-potassium diet are generally provided along with diuretic pills that can cause an excessive loss of body potassium. Prolonged bouts of vomiting and diarrhea can also lead to potassium loss and deficiency. The most noticeable effects of low blood-potassium levels are weakness and irregular heart beats.

#### POTASSIUM OVERDOSE

Excessive amounts of supplemental potassium are highly toxic and can cause death due to heart failure. Oral doses of 18 grams (a whopping dose compared to the 0.5 to 2 grams needed to replace potassium loss due to diuretic pills) can make the heart stop beating.

## PILLS AS A SOURCE OF VITAMINS AND MINERALS

Adults tend to be rather heavy users of vitamin and mineral supplements. About 58 percent of women and 45 percent of men in the United States take one or more vitamin or mineral supplement at least occasionally.[69] Sales of vitamin and mineral supplements are expected to increase by 15 percent each year until 2000.[70]

For the most part, supplemental vitamins and minerals are used as a nutritional insurance policy, as protection against accidents caused by inadequate diets. Some people take supplements to prevent colds and other diseases, to improve the complexion, to get a dose of zip and energy, or because it's better than having to eat vegetables! Most supplement users choose a single vitamin or mineral, and of the individual nutrients, vitamin C supplements are the most popular for men, and calcium and iron for women.

### *Can We Supplement Our Way into Balanced Diets?*

The path to balanced diets is generally not paved by vitamin and mineral supplements. No supplement provides 100 percent of all the nutrients needed daily. Most multivitamin and mineral supplements contain seven to seventeen of the forty essential nutrients, and even that level of nutrient variety is missed by the majority of users because individual nutrient supplements are most commonly used. Some supplements include biotin, molybdenum, and pantothenic acid—elements that are very rarely in short supply in diets. Other supplements contain ingredients that are not essential and have never been shown to be related to deficiency diseases or improvements in health. A fifty-pill bottle of *rutin*, for example, can be purchased in some health food stores. But what's rutin? A nonessential nutrient that costs $4.95 a bottle.

The availability of vitamins and minerals contained in supplements has been questioned. It is known that the availability of minerals decreases as the number included in a supplement increases.[71] Taking vitamin C with iron causes a destruction of vitamin

C, iron plus zinc reduces the absorption of zinc, and the presence of calcium carbonate decreases the amount of iron absorbed from a supplement by over half.[72] Most vitamins and minerals appear to be more completely absorbed if taken with food than on an empty stomach. The absorption of calcium from a supplement is increased if taken with milk. You can substantially increase iron absorption if you take the supplement with orange or grapefruit juice, or if you take the iron with a meal containing meat but not tea. (If you take more iron than you need, your body will let you know. You'll get black and tarry stools, gas, and cramps.) Smaller doses of vitamins and minerals (those providing 100 percent of the U.S. RDA or less) are more completely absorbed than are higher doses.

Several studies have shown a mismatch between the vitamin and mineral supplements taken and those that are in short supply in diets.[73,74] Supplements are often taken by people who have adequate dietary intakes of the vitamins and minerals contained in them. Deficient intake levels are often not "supplemented" by the supplements chosen.

SITUATIONS IN WHICH VITAMIN AND MINERAL SUPPLEMENTS MAY BE BENEFICIAL[75]

| *Situation* | *Supplement Type* |
|---|---|
| Oral contraceptive use | Folic acid, vitamin $B_6$ |
| Pregnancy | Iron, folic acid |
| High menstrual blood loss | Iron, folic acid |
| Diagnosed deficiency disease (e.g. anemias) | As indicated |
| Vegan diets | Vitamin $B_{12}$, vitamin D, zinc, iron |
| Osteoporosis | Calcium, vitamin D |
| Chronic dieting, caloric intakes below 1,600 calories per day | Multivitamin and mineral |
| Use of drugs that interfere with the body's use of vitamins and minerals (some blood pressure drugs, antidepressants, and antibiotics) | As indicated by type of drug |
| Diseases that produce malabsorption (e.g. cystic fibrosis, celiac disease) | Multivitamin and mineral |
| Inadequate diets due to food allergies, alcoholism, or a narrow selection of food types | Multivitamin and mineral, or as indicated |

### WHO BENEFITS FROM SUPPLEMENTS?

Some situations call for either the selective use of vitamins or minerals or the use of a multivitamin and mineral supplement. Follow the accompanying guide for selecting over-the-counter vitamin and mineral supplements. Dietary improvements should go hand-in-hand with supplement use in cases where faulty diets produced the need for supplements.

### SUPPLEMENT CHOICES

Hundreds of different supplements and supplement combinations are available for over-the-counter sale. Depending on the type and amount of vitamins and minerals included, a supplement can represent money ill spent, a benefit if the nutrients are needed, or a hazard in the form of overdosing. The primary health concerns related to supplements are the dangers of overdosing and their use for self-treatment of diseases for which they are ineffective.

High doses (those that are two to ten times the RDA) of certain vitamins and minerals may cause toxic reactions if taken habitually. Vitamins A and D, selenium, iodine, and zinc are of particular concern because they have narrow margins of safety around the RDA levels.

### GUIDE FOR SELECTING OVER-THE-COUNTER VITAMIN AND MINERAL SUPPLEMENTS

1. Avoid supplements labeled "megadose," "therapeutic," or "high potency." They are likely to contain levels of vitamins and minerals that exceed the body's ability to use them, and may precipitate toxic overdosing. Pass them by for lower dose levels.
2. Select supplements that contain vitamins and minerals recognized as essential. Para-aminobenzoic acid (PABA), inositol, and enzymes included on labels should serve as a strong clue as to whether unessential nutrients are being purchased.
3. Examine the label for the percentage of the RDA for each micronutrient. The supplement to choose is the one that has a balance of vitamins and minerals that do not exceed 100 percent of the U.S. RDA.
4. Buy the least expensive supplement that meets the criteria in number 3. *Natural* and *organic* are sales terms. The average markup on vitamins is 43 percent, but can go as high as 500 percent in health food stores. Don't pay extra for a meaningless label.
5. Note the expiration date given on the label. Buy "fresh" supplements.

### MEGADOSES

Levels of vitamins and minerals in supplements that exceed ten times the RDA are considered *megadoses*. Such supplements are most likely to lead to overdoses because they exceed levels the body can use to maintain health. Instead of promoting the normal functions of vitamins and minerals, megadose supplements may negate them, and produce adverse effects totally unrelated to the normal functions of vitamins and minerals. It has been suggested that because of the druglike effects of very high levels of vitamins and minerals, megadoses should be sold on a prescription basis. The reality is that, with the exception of folic acid, manufacturers are free to formulate and sell vitamin and mineral supplements at any dose level.

The labels on vitamin and mineral supplement bottles are generally informative. Some of the information on labels is required by law, and some is listed voluntarily. All supplement labels must indicate how many pills are in the container, which vitamins and minerals are included and their doses, the expiration date, and the name and address of the manufacturer. Supplement labels or packaging cannot state unproven health claims about the vitamins and minerals contained, but manufacturers are free to present such information elsewhere.

### WATER: THE FORGOTTEN NUTRIENT

Water: It's not to be taken for granted. Water qualifies in all respects as an essential nutrient. It is required for growth and health; it performs specific, required functions in the body; and deficiency and toxicity signs develop when we consume too little or too much of it. Without water, our days are numbered to about six.

The physical and chemical properties of water have made it the basic required substance for all forms of life as we know it. Water is needed as a medium for most chemical reactions that take place within the body, and it functions as the body's cooling system. Water in our blood collects heat generated by the body and releases it on the surface of the skin.

On average, we consume around 6 cups per day from water and beverages, 4 cups from foods, and our bodies produce a cup as a result of energy formation. Most beverages contain over 85 percent water, and fruits and vegetables are 75 to 90 percent water. Meats, depending upon their type and how well done they are, contain from 50 to 70 percent water. Although it is nearly impossible to meet your need for water from solid foods, the water composition of foods does make an important contribution to our daily intake.

A new source of water has hit the U.S. market with a wallop. A wide assortment of gourmet, bottled waters are now available in most supermarkets, and Americans are downing them by the ton.

About twenty-five years ago, the French made drinking "fine waters" very stylish. In Paris, boulevardiers crowded sidewalk cafés for hours while they nursed along bottles of Perrier, chilled and served with thinly sliced lemon. The popularity of bottled waters skyrocketed in many western countries, and in the United States *mineral*, *spring*, and *seltzer* waters have become bestsellers.

Ever wonder what the differences are among mineral, spring, and seltzer water? True mineral water is taken from underground reservoirs that are lodged between layers of rocks. The water dissolves some of the minerals found in the rocks and as a result contains a higher amount of minerals than most sources of surface water. Spring water is that taken from fresh water springs that form pools or streams on the surface of the earth. It may be mineralized or not, depending on the conditions present in the spring. True seltzers (and not the kind you often find for sale that may be sweetened) are naturally carbonated sparkling waters. Most seltzers, however, become bubbly through the addition of pressurized carbon dioxide.

A type of bottled water not sold in supermarkets is "pure" water. All types of naturally occurring water contain gases and minerals. Even distilled water is not 100 percent pure water. In order for water to become pure, it must be distilled around forty-two times. Water is considered pure when it no longer conducts electricity. It is quite likely that none of us has ever drunk pure $H_2O$, or ever will.

The trend toward consuming bottled waters is a healthy one. Bottled waters contain no sugar, are generally low in sodium, and quench a thirst better than their major competitor, soft drinks.

### *Hard and Soft Water*

Water is often classified by whether it is *hard* or *soft*. Hard water generally comes from underground wells and characteristically contains calcium, magnesium, and iron. The mineral content of hard water interacts with the minerals in soap and detergents, inhibiting the chemical reactions that cause a lather to form and cleaning to occur. You know your water supply is hard if you need a lot of soap to get a good lather, if you have mineral deposits forming in your teakettle or bath tub, or if your clothes start turning grayish after repeated washings. Hard water can be made soft by water conditioners that replace calcium, magnesium, and iron with sodium. Sodium does not interfere with the chemical actions of soap, and does not precipitate out of water and leave deposits. Unfortunately, the sodium content of very hard water that has been softened may contribute to an excessively high dietary sodium intake and the risk of developing hypertension.[76] Because of the sodium content of softened water, it is customary to condition hot water, and not cold water used for cooking and drinking.

### *The Earth's Supply of Water*

Water covers about three-fourths of the earth's surface, yet very little of it is drinkable. Nearly 97 percent of the total supply is salt water, and only 3 percent is fresh. Of the fresh water supply, only one-fourth is available for use; the rest is located in polar and glacier ice. Although fresh water is abundant in most locations in the United States, this is not the case in a number of other countries.

Water is sufficiently scarce in parts of the Soviet Union that drinking-water dispensers are coin operated. Fresh water is so highly prized in sections of the arid Middle East that fountains decorating homesites are considered a sign of affluence. Drinking water is sampled, judged, and celebrated in Middle East countries as ceremoniously as are fine wines in France.

Although water is still abundant in the United States, there are concerns about the quality and safety of our water supply. The detection of hydrocarbons, chloroform, radioisotopes, and asbestos fibers in drinking water in parts of Canada and the United States has focused attention on the potential health effects of contaminated water. The list of chemicals identified in samples of drinking water in the United States includes sixty-four that are suspected of promoting cancer.[77] Whether environmentally contaminated water causes cancer in humans is not yet clear. However, it is clear that action needs to be taken to clean up the water supply in certain parts of the country before complete information on health effects becomes available.

### *How Much Water Is Best?*

Physically inactive adults living in moderate climates need about 10 cups of water each day to replace that lost in urine, perspiration, stools, and exhaled air. For individuals in other circumstances, the requirement for water is met when the amount ingested equals the amount lost. People who are physically active, who live in hot climates, or who have illnesses that produce vomiting, diarrhea, or fever need more water to replace the losses than other people.

*Water Deficiency*

Built-in mechanisms that trigger thirst generally protect people from consuming too little water and becoming dehydrated. However, some people lose more water through physical activity and sweating than can be compensated for by thirst mechanisms. In hot weather heavy work, athletic or otherwise, means you have to drink beyond your thirst to make up for water lost in sweat. One runner competing in the grueling Death Valley race—a fifty-five-mile, seventeen-hour event, had to drink 30 pounds of water (the equivalent of almost 4 gallons) to keep up with his water losses. If fluid losses are not replaced, you get *heat cramps*, which cause muscle spasms that put you out of the running.

Prolonged bouts of vomiting, diarrhea, and fever can also produce dehydration, as can high-protein diets and alcohol binges. Both protein and alcohol consumption increase urine production. That is why people on high-protein diets are encouraged to drink a lot of water, and people get very thirsty after overindulging in the spirits. Dehydrated people feel very sick—weak, dizzy, and nauseated. But they feel better quickly after replenishing their water supply.

*Water Overdose*

It may sound fantastic, but people can overdose on water. Water intoxication occurs when people consume more water than can be readily excreted. Deaths from overdoses of water have been reported, but they resulted from rapid intakes of water measured by the bucket, not the cup.

# Chapter 7

## *Nutrition and the Prevention and Management of Disease throughout Life*

*I had the good fortune of being seated next to Joyce on a flight from Minneapolis to Dallas. Joyce was returning from a vacation in the Midwest and I was on my way to give a talk about nutrition and women. Noticing the words* Nutrition and Women *on my papers, Joyce asked what I did. Her interest peaked when she heard I was writing a book on nutrition for women. She was very interested in the topic and shared her story with me.*

*Joyce, at the age of 57, was overweight and had high cholesterol. She was on a weight-loss diet (she had pretty much stuck to the diet while on vacation) and was cutting down on fat and cholesterol. Joyce belonged to a weight-loss group and was on a 1,000-calorie diet. She also had a staple placed in her ear to help her lose weight, but admitted she wasn't sure if it was the diet or the staple that was causing the weight loss. Joyce wanted to know more about oat bran. She had recently switched to oat bran from cholesterol-lowering drugs because they "tore her up inside" and cost $72 per month. In addition to two tablespoons of oat bran every morning, Joyce regularly took L-tryptophan to help her sleep at night, 2 grams of calcium to prevent osteoporosis, 500 IU of vitamin E to ward off cancer, 2 grams of vitamin C to prevent infections, and a multivitamin and mineral supplement for overall health. As far as* *vitamins and minerals are concerned, Joyce believed the more, the better.*

*Our discussion was interrupted by the in-flight lunch service. After lunch was served, we continued to chat. The two of us started lunch by dissecting the fried batter from the chicken and by tilting our plates to allow the fat to drain off the overcooked green beans and rice. We had more in common than an interest in nutrition and health. We were pros at eating airline food.*

▼ Perhaps in no other area representing such importance to health have decision makers like Joyce been provided with so little reliable and helpful information. The role of nutrition in the development, prevention, and management of eight conditions of primary concern to women are presented in this chapter. The conditions are osteoporosis, heart disease, hypertension, cancer, diabetes, hypoglycemia, obesity, and lactose intolerance. (Relationships between nutrition and other conditions are discussed in the book; refer to the index.) You can read more about food sources and other information regarding the nutrients discussed here by referring back to chapters 4 through 6.

## OSTEOPOROSIS

*Osteoporosis* means porous bones. It develops over years due to losses in the mineral content of bone, and appears to have a number of causes.

Approximately twenty million adults in the United States have osteoporosis, and one million have suffered a fracture of the wrist, hip, or other bone because of the disease. One out of four women and one in every eight men in the United States will develop osteoporosis. The risk of developing osteoporosis greatly increases among women after menopause, a period in life when estrogen levels fall. By the time women reach ninety, most will have experienced a fracture due to osteoporosis.[1]

The consequences of osteoporosis are much more serious than bone fractures, however. Nearly 20 percent of elderly people experiencing a hip fracture die from complications within six months. Osteoporosis is a serious condition and one that can be prevented in most people.

### *Calcium and Bone Formation*

Bone is not as solid and dead as it looks. Bone is living tissue infiltrated by blood vessels, nerves, and specialized cells. About half of the content of bone is water, and half solids.

The solid part of bones is made from a network of strong protein fibers, the *protein matrix*, that are embedded with mineral crystals. Calcium is by far the most abundant type of mineral found in bones. The combination of the tough protein matrix and the mineral crystals makes bone very strong, yet shock absorbing and slightly flexible. Bones lose these characteristics when osteoporosis develops.

Bones slowly but continually go through a repair-and-replacement process known as remodeling. During remodeling, the old protein matrix is replaced with newly produced protein and the minerals in bones are renewed. A continual supply of calcium and other nutrients is needed to support the activities of bone cells in forming and maintaining bone tissue. Bones stay dense and strong as long as mineral replacement takes place.

Certain hormones and physical activity affect bone remodeling. For example, estrogen and growth hormone increase bone formation, and physical inactivity decreases it. For reasons yet unknown, bone formation is stimulated by putting bones under pressure. The greater the physical strain on bones, the greater the formation of bone. As a result, bones of physically active or heavy people are usually thicker and stronger than bones of inactive or light people. Bones not used at all, such as the bones of a leg in a plaster cast or those in people who are bedridden, lose calcium and slowly decrease in size and strength.

### *Preventing Osteoporosis*

Bone formation begins early in life, during the fourth to sixth week of pregnancy, and does not stop until well into adulthood. Bones grow in length and width up to about age twenty, and then, although they stabilize in size, continue to mineralize until about age thirty. Peak bone mineral density is achieved at about the age of thirty, and the density of bones around this age is an important predictor of who will develop osteoporosis. In general, the higher the peak bone density, the less likely it is that osteoporosis will develop.

Bone size and density normally remain fairly stable from age thirty to the mid-forties. After that, bones tend to demineralize and weaken with increasing age. An inch or two of height is generally lost during old age due to the compacting of weakened bones in the spine. By the age of ninety, the bone density of women in the United States is, on average, half of what it was when peak bone density was achieved.[1]

Some thinning of bone with aging occurs in almost everyone. But the extent of the loss in bone density can be lessened in both women and men by lifelong dietary adequacy of calcium.[2] Adequate calcium intake is especially important during the first thirty years of life, when bones are increasing in mineral content and peak bone density is achieved. It appears to be much easier for the body to use calcium to mineralize bone that is forming and developing than it is to remineralize bones that have undergone extensive calcium losses. Recent evidence indicates, however, that hip fractures between the ages of fifty and seventy-nine are 60 percent more common among people who regularly consume less than about 800 mg of calcium per day.[3]

### *Treating Osteoporosis*

Scientists have yet to find a treatment to reverse bone demineralization totally once it is established. Current recommendations call for treating postmenopausal osteoporosis with 1,200 to 1,500 mg of calcium daily. Vitamin D (400 IU) is recommended in addition to calcium if a person does not drink vitamin-D-fortified milk or if she doesn't get enough exposure to sunshine.[4] (Read more about the sun as a source of vitamin D on pages 115–16.) Small doses of estrogen and progesterone (not estrogen alone) are recommended, along with calcium, in advanced cases of osteoporosis.[5] The effectiveness of calcium in reducing bone loss is enhanced by regular, weight-bearing exercise, such as walking or tennis.[1]

### *Supplemental Calcium*

Calcium is needed in large amounts each day—amounts that are difficult to fit into one pill. The required size of the pill is made larger by the fact that calcium supplements are not 100 percent calcium. To increase its chemical stability, calcium in supplements comes combined with other substances. The most common type of calcium supplement is calcium carbonate.

Oyster shells and the bones of animals are also used to make supplements. Because these "natural" sources of calcium contain many minerals, only about 250 mg worth of calcium can fit into a pill of the size that can be more-or-less easily swallowed. The other mineral ingredients of shells and bones is of concern. Some calcium supplements made from shells and bones contain excessive amounts of arsenic, mercury, and lead. Much of the calcium found in shells and bones is in the form of calcium phosphate, the main type of mineral crystals found in bones. It is one of the least easily absorbed forms of calcium, making the availability of calcium in shells and bones an additional problem area.

Antacids have become a popular, although expensive, route to calcium supplementation. Pharmacists and others have expressed concern about the habitual use of antacids among people who have no need for them. Antacids lower the acidity of fluids in the stomach, and habitual use may lower acidity to levels that interfere with normal digestion. Calcium is among the nutrients whose absorption is decreased by lower-than-normal levels of acidity in the stomach. The routine use of antacids as calcium supplements may pose a particular problem in old people. The acidity of the stomach generally declines during old age, and antacids may aggravate existing digestive problems due to an inadequate level of acidity.

Vitamin D, needed for the absorption of calcium, is only occasionally included in calcium supplements. When it is, it can be found in reasonable to irrational amounts. One calcium supplement on the market contains 112 mg of calcium and 400 IU of vitamin D in each tablet. To get 1,000 mg (or 1 gram) of calcium from this supplement, a person would have to take nine tablets, and they would be getting too much vitamin D—3,600 IU. Examples of the calcium and vitamin D content of supplements are shown in table 33.

If calcium supplements are required, calcium carbonate, and not supplements made from shells or bones, is generally recommended. The amount of calcium absorbed from supplements declines after 1,200 mg, and little additional calcium is absorbed if intake exceeds about 1500 mg. Taking calcium supplements with

TABLE 33. CALCIUM AND VITAMIN D CONTENT OF SUPPLEMENTS

| SUPPLEMENT | CALCIUM PER TABLET (MG) | VITAMIN D PER TABLET (IU) |
|---|---|---|
| Centrum® | 162 | 400 |
| One-A-Day® Plus Iron | 300 | 400 |
| Lilly® Multiple Vitamin-Mineral Supplement | 29 | 33 |
| Calcium (generic) | 600 | 0 |
| Caltrate™ 600 + D | 600 | 125 |
| Tums® (chewable) | 200 | 0 |

milk assures that vitamin D and other substances in milk that promote calcium absorption are available.

The shift from food sources of calcium to supplements should not be made without considerable thought. Food sources of calcium are generally rich in a variety of nutrients that can contribute to a well-balanced diet. In addition, the calcium found in milk (and that includes chocolate milk), yogurt, cheese, and calcium-fortified juices and dairy products is more completely absorbed than the calcium in supplements.[6] A list of the best food sources of calcium is given in table 25 in chapter 6. The caloric values of foods providing about 300 mg of calcium in a serving are presented in table 34. Of the food sources of calcium, milk is the only one that is routinely fortified with vitamin D. Milk provides 100 IU of vitamin D per cup.

## HEART DISEASE

Heart disease is often thought of as primarily a male condition. That is by no means the truth. Heart disease is a leading cause of death in women; it's just that it strikes women about ten years later than men.[7]

Atherosclerosis is the leading form of heart disease in the United States and is a leading contributor to strokes. It results from a buildup of a solid material called *plaque* in and around the walls of blood vessels. The largest single ingredient of plaque is cholesterol. The accumulation of cholesterol plaque within the walls of blood vessels causes them to become narrow and may eventually plug them up. At least a 50 percent narrowing of arteries is required before symptoms of atherosclerosis appear. Two of the first symptoms that occur are frequent chest pains and shortness of breath. These symptoms are due to the reduced blood flow to the heart caused by the narrowed arteries. People who experience these symptoms are said to have *angina*. When one or more arteries in the heart becomes plugged, a heart attack may occur. The stoppage in blood flow may cause the affected part of the heart to die and the whole heart may stop beating. The reduced diameter of the arteries leading to the brain also increases the chances that either a blood clot will get stuck in a vessel or a blood clot will form and clog the vessel. When this happens, a person experiences a *stroke*. The severity of a stroke depends on which part of the brain has its blood supply cut off.

TABLE 34. CALORIC CONTENT OF 300 MG CALCIUM FROM MILK AND MILK PRODUCTS

| FOOD | AMOUNT TO PROVIDE APPROXIMATELY 300 MG CALCIUM | CALORIES |
|---|---|---|
| Skim milk | 1 cup | 90 |
| 1% milk | 1 cup | 102 |
| Low-fat yogurt | ¾ cup | 110 |
| Swiss cheese | 1¼ oz. | 138 |
| 2% milk | 1 cup | 140 |
| 3.25% milk (whole) | 1 cup | 160 |
| Cheddar cheese | 1½ oz. | 175 |
| American cheese | 2 oz. | 220 |
| Low-fat yogurt with fruit | 1 cup | 225 |
| Pudding | 1½ cups | 240 |
| Cream soup | 1 cup | 248 |
| Cottage cheese, low-fat | 1 cup | 324 |
| Frozen yogurt | 1½ cups | 324 |
| Milk shake | 1¼ cups | 336 |
| Ice cream | 1½ cups | 403 |
| Cottage cheese | 2 cups | 480 |

### *Risk Factors for the Development of Heart Disease*

The major risk factors for the development of heart disease in adults are:

Elevated blood cholesterol (over 200 mg/dl)
Low HDL-cholesterol level (under 35 mg/dl)
Hypertension
Family history of early heart disease
Smoking
Diabetes (particularly in women)
Type "A" personality
Obesity (particularly in women)

Diabetes and obesity have a stronger impact on women than on men. Women with the highest risk of developing heart disease work for, or live with, men with the highest heart disease rates. In one sense, heart disease is contagious.

Women tend to have higher levels of the good lipoprotein, HDL, than men. High levels of HDL, over 50 mg/dl, strongly reduce the risk of heart disease.[7] However, if HDL is low (less than 35 mg/dl), women are at greater risk of developing heart disease than men with the same HDL level.[8] Elevated cholesterol levels (over 200 mg/dl) are also related to heart disease, but more strongly for men than women and for premenopausal than postmenopausal women. The strength of cholesterol level as a risk factor for heart disease decreases somewhat as women pass the age of fifty.[9]

High triglyceride levels (those over 300 mg/dl) appear to be a risk factor for heart disease in women and not men.[7] Blood levels of triglycerides of over 150 mg/dl pose a strong risk if combined with low HDL levels. Elevated triglyceride levels in women are also closely related to the development of diabetes and hypertension.[8] They may also be related to having a blood-triglyceride test done after eating. Blood for a triglyceride measurement should be taken after a fourteen-hour fast.

Obesity is clearly a risk factor for the development of heart disease in women.[8] If combined with diabetes, high LDL, and low HDL levels, a woman would be at very high risk of having a heart attack.

### *Cholesterol and Heart Disease*

The likelihood of developing atherosclerosis and of dying from heart disease increases as blood-cholesterol levels increase. Approximately 40 percent of adults aged twenty-five to twenty-nine in the United States have some degree of atherosclerosis, and most adults have blood-cholesterol levels over 200 mg/dl that put them at risk for developing heart disease.[10,11] Total cholesterol levels of about 160 mg/dl in adults, and 110 in youth aged five to eighteen correspond to a substantially below-average risk of developing heart disease.[11]

Our bodies get cholesterol from two sources: our diets and our livers. In people who don't have a family history of very high blood-cholesterol levels, the amount of cholesterol produced by the liver will decrease if dietary intake of cholesterol is high. So, although the liver produces cholesterol, the amount produced varies depending on the amount and type of fat and how much cholesterol we eat.

Because cholesterol is fat soluble, it has to be transported in blood and other body fluids attached to a water-soluble particle. To do this, cholesterol and many other types of fatty substances become attached to *protein carriers* that mix with water. When a fat or fatlike substance is combined with a protein carrier, the result is *lipoprotein*. It turns out that lipoprotein levels are actually the important measures as far as dietary fat/heart disease relationships are concerned.

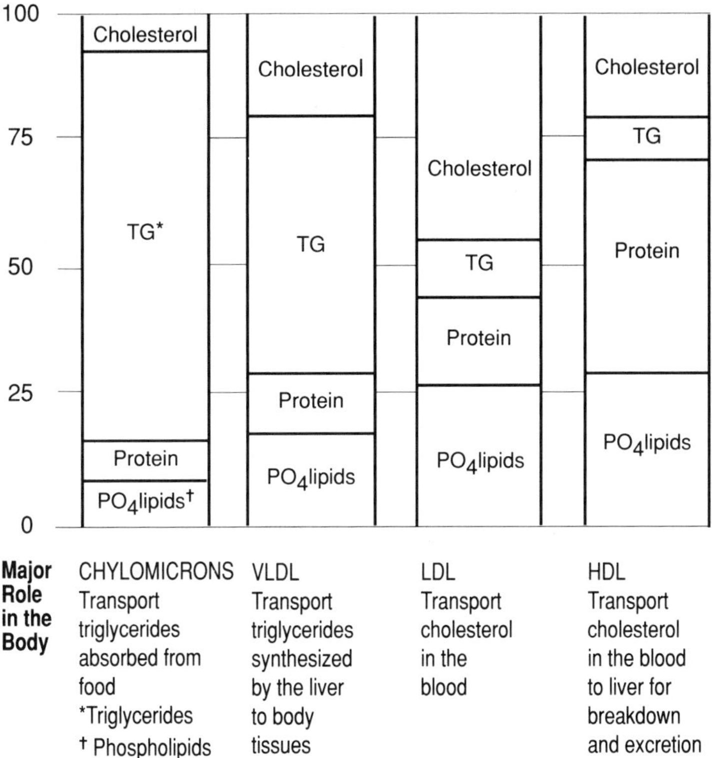


**FIGURE 6. COMPOSITION AND FUNCTIONS OF THE FOUR MAJOR CLASSES OF LIPOPROTEINS**

LIPOPROTEINS

There are four major types of lipoproteins that transport fats and fatlike substances in the blood. They are classified by their density, or their weight relative to other substances of equal volume. Lipoproteins containing a large proportion of fat have low densities, while those containing relatively large amounts of protein have higher densities. Figure 6 presents the four types of lipoproteins and shows the proportion of cholesterol, triglycerides, protein, and phosopholipids in each.

Chylomicrons are the least dense lipoprotein—they come close to floating in blood. They are packed with triglycerides and contain very little cholesterol or protein. Chylomicrons are responsible for transporting many of the end products of fat digestion through the blood. Very low-density lipoproteins (VLDL) also consist primarily of triglycerides, but they contain less of them than the chylomicrons. VLDL is formed by the liver and transports triglycerides made in the body to fat and other cells. Low-density lipoproteins (LDL) contain the highest proportion of cholesterol of all the lipoproteins. They are the major transporters of cholesterol in the blood and high blood-cholesterol levels are generally due to high levels of LDL (above 150 mg/dl).[7] High-density lipoproteins (HDL) contain the largest amount of protein. They are considered the "good lipoproteins" because they protect against heart disease. HDL removes cholesterol from the blood by transporting it to the liver, where it is broken down and eventually excreted.

BLOOD-CHOLESTEROL TESTS

*Madalyn came into the office with a very concerned look on her face. She had just finished talking with her doctor about her blood test results. "Oh no," Madalyn groaned to her friend. "It finally happened. I got a positive result on my blood test—my cholesterol is high. The results of those tests have* always *been negative. It must be because I'm fifty!"*

*You could see Madalyn was devastated. It hadn't occurred to her that the positive result might not last forever. It also hadn't occurred to her that the high cholesterol level could be due to some of her lifestyles, and not to aging. When she realized that it might be, Madalyn went on the offensive. She cut down on the amount of fat in her diet, started to walk the two miles to work and back every day, and lost twenty unneeded pounds. Within six months, her cholesterol level was back to normal. She felt better too.*

Abnormal blood test results come as quite a shock. For many of us, the first shock is delivered by news of a high cholesterol level. Fortunately, high blood levels of cholesterol are not an inevitable consequence of aging; they can often be reduced if improvements in diet and other habits are made.

Blood-cholesterol level is most commonly assessed by determining the total amount of cholesterol in the blood. Total cholesterol level measures the amount of cholesterol in chylomicrons, LDL, VLDL, and HDL. Fasting before the test is not required. At least two separate measurements of total cholesterol are

MODIFYING BLOOD LIPID LEVELS IN ADULTS

| *Blood lipid* | *Factors tending to increase levels* | *Factors tending to decrease levels* |
|---|---|---|
| Total cholesterol | • High-saturated-fat intake<br>• Low P/S ratio (i.e., more saturated fats are consumed than polyunsaturated fats) | • Low-saturated-fat diet<br>• High P/S ratio |
| | • High-cholesterol intake | • Low-cholesterol diet |
| | • Family history of elevated cholesterol levels | • Soluble fibers such as oat bran |
| | • Excess body fat* | • Sequestrants (cholesterol-lowering drugs) |
| | • Physical inactivity<br>• Oral contraceptives* | • Estrogen*<br>• Loss of excess body fat* |
| | • Progestins*<br>• Testosterone<br>• Stress<br>• Menopause*<br>• Some antihypertension drugs | • Physical fitness |
| HDL-cholesterol (Remember, you want this lipid to be high or increase) | • Loss of excess body fat | • Excess body fat |
| | • Physical fitness<br>• Estrogen*<br>• Moderate alcohol intake† | • Progestins*<br>• Testosterone<br>• Diabetes*<br>• Physical inactivity<br>• Zinc supplements (over 50 mg per day)<br>• Oral contraceptives* |
| Triglycerides | • Excess intake of simple sugars and calories<br>• Hypertension<br>• Diabetes* | • Fish oil (omega-3-fatty acids, particularly EPA)<br>• Physical fitness<br>• Normal body-fat content |

- Fasting, low-calorie diets
- High-fat meals
- Excess body fat
- Oral contraceptives*
- Low simple-sugar intake

**Factors apply particularly to women or have a stronger impact on blood lipids in women than in men.*
*†Moderate alcohol intake is defined as the consumption of two standard-sized drinks per day. It is not meant to be a dietary recommendation. The results of research indicate, however, that moderate alcohol consumption tends to increase the level of a particular type of HDL. That type is the HDL-cholesterol that contains a protein called* apolipoprotein I. *Increased levels of this form of HDL are associated with a reduced risk of heart disease. Alcohol appears to change the type of HDL formed, rather than HDL-cholesterol levels.*[12]

needed to confirm a result. If total cholesterol is above 200 mg/dl, a follow-up test is generally done. This blood test measures LDL- and HDL-cholesterol. These are meaningful tests because a high total cholesterol level that is accompanied by a high HDL level may not increase the risk of developing heart disease. A total cholesterol/HDL ratio (or total cholesterol ÷ HDL) of less than 4.5 is not associated with an increased risk of heart disease.[7]

#### CONDITIONS THAT AFFECT CHOLESTEROL LEVELS

The levels of total cholesterol, HDL-cholesterol, and triglycerides in blood are affected by a number of conditions. For people without a family history of high levels, the primary factor that affects total cholesterol is the amount of saturated fat in the diet.

#### SATURATED FAT INTAKE AND CHOLESTEROL LEVEL

*Not long ago I was interviewed by a health reporter who was preparing a two-minute TV spot on diet and blood cholesterol. After we had discussed the relationships between saturated fat intake and blood cholesterol, the reporter concluded: "So, the bottom line is that saturated fats have a stronger impact on blood cholesterol than does dietary cholesterol." "Right!" I said. "Too bad," the reporter replied. "I only have two minutes and the public just wants the bottom line. They would never understand that and I don't have time to explain it."*

*The report that aired on the local news gave a bottom line: "Reduce your saturated fat intake." After the report was over, I imagined hearing thousands of viewers saying to themselves, "Huh? What's a saturated fat?"*

TABLE 35. FAT PROFILES OF SELECTED FOODS

| *Food* | *Amount* | *Fatty Acids* | | |
|---|---|---|---|---|
| | | □ SATURATED | □ MONOUNSATURATED | □ POLYUNSATURATED |
| DAIRY PRODUCTS | | | | |
| Brick cheese | 1 oz. | 67 | 30 | 3 |
| Cheddar cheese | 1 oz. | 67 | 30 | 3 |
| Cottage cheese | 1 cup | 67 | 30 | 3 |
| American cheese | 1 oz. | 67 | 30 | 3 |
| Milk, whole | 1 cup | 65 | 31 | 4 |
| Butter | 1 T. | 65 | 31 | 4 |
| HUMAN MILK | 1 cup | 48 | 40 | 12 |
| EGG | 1 med. | 37 | 48 | 15 |
| OILS AND MARGARINES | | | | |
| Coconut oil | 1 T. | 92 | 6 | 2 |
| Corn oil | 1 T. | 13 | 25 | 62 |
| Corn oil margarine | 1 T. | 17 | 61 | 22 |
| Olive oil | 1 T. | 14 | 77 | 9 |
| Palm oil | 1 T. | 52 | 38 | 10 |
| Peanut oil | 1 T. | 18 | 48 | 34 |
| Soybean oil | 1 T. | 15 | 25 | 60 |
| Soybean oil margarine | 1 T. | 22 | 50 | 28 |
| Sunflower oil | 1 T. | 11 | 21 | 68 |
| MEATS | | | | |
| Hamburger, regular (21% fat) | 3 oz. | 53 | 43 | 4 |
| Chicken, roasted (no skin) | 3 oz. | 26 | 46 | 28 |
| Pork chop | 3 oz. | 39 | 49 | 12 |
| Turkey, roasted | 3 oz. | 40 | 25 | 35 |
| NUTS AND SEEDS | | | | |
| Cashews | 1 oz. | 21 | 62 | 17 |
| Macadamia nuts | 1 oz. | 16 | 82 | 2 |
| Peanuts, dry roasted | 1 oz. | 15 | 52 | 33 |
| Peanut butter | 1 T. | 18 | 51 | 32 |
| Sunflower seeds, dried | 1 oz. | 11 | 20 | 69 |

*Source: USDA ©8, vols. 1, 4, 5, Washington, D.D., 1980–85.*

[a]*P/S = the ratio between polyunsaturated and saturated fatty acid content. A ratio of 1 or greater is recommended.*

Dietary fats come in two basic types: *saturated* and *unsaturated*. Unsaturated fats are subdivided into those that are *monounsaturated* and *polyunsaturated*. Saturated fats tend to be solid at room temperature, whereas unsaturated fats are liquid.

Saturated fats are present in the highest amounts in foods of animal origin, such as dairy products and meat. With the exception of palm and coconut oils, they make up only a small proportion of the fat content of plants (see table 35). Saturated fat can be converted to cholesterol by the body, whereas unsaturated fats cannot be. Consequently, high saturated fat intakes tend to raise cholesterol levels in almost all individuals.[13]

Blood-cholesterol levels can generally be decreased if more unsaturated than saturated fat is consumed. Although monounsaturated fat has a cholesterol-lowering effect, this type of fat reduces blood cholesterol to a lesser extent than do polyunsaturated fats. People who consume more polyunsaturated fat than saturated fat in their diet (or who achieve, therefore, a P-to-S ratio of 1 or higher) tend to have lower total cholesterol levels than people who consume more saturated than polyunsaturated fat. The relatively high intakes of saturated fat by Americans is considered to be an important reason for the prevalence of heart disease in the United States. Heart disease rates tend to be substantially lower in countries where people consume less saturated fat and more unsaturated fat.[14]

Most people who reduce their saturated fat intake also lower their total intake of calories, fat, and cholesterol. You can observe the effects of a low-fat diet on caloric, fat, and cholesterol intake by reviewing the menus on page 165. You will notice that the P-to-S ratio of the lower-fat diet is 0.9, which is very close to the recommended figure of 1. Substituting low-fat cheese for regular cheese and sherbet for the ice milk in the lower-fat menu would bring the P-to-S ratio to over 1 and would further reduce the fat and caloric content of the menu.

Five effective ways to reduce your intake of saturated fat are to:

> Use low-fat dairy products such as skim milk and low-fat cheese and yogurt.
>
> Limit beef consumption to two meals per week. (Choose lean cuts of beef such as flank and round steak.) Use fish, poultry, and dried beans in place of beef.

COMPARISON OF THE FAT CONTENT OF TWO MENUS

| *Meal* | *High fat* | *Lower fat* |
|---|---|---|
| Breakfast: | Orange juice, 6 oz. | Orange juice, 6 oz. |
| | Cornflakes, 1 cup | Cornflakes, 1 cup |
| | Whole wheat toast, 2 slices | Whole wheat toast, 2 slices |
| | Margarine, 2 tsp. | Margarine, 2 tsp. |
| | Milk, 1 cup | Skim milk, 1 cup |
| Lunch: | Cream of tomato soup, 1 cup | Vegetable soup, 1 cup |
| | Grilled cheese sandwich | Cheese sandwich |
| | Potato chips, 1 oz. | Tomatoes, ½ cup |
| | Milk, 1 cup | Skim milk, 1 cup |
| Snack: | Peanut butter, 2 T. | Orange, 1 |
| | Ritz crackers, 4 | Whole wheat crackers, 4 |
| Dinner: | Tossed salad, 1½ cups | Tossed salad, 1½ cups |
| | Salad dressing, 2 T. | Salad dressing, 2 tsp. |
| | Fried chicken, 4 oz. | Baked chicken, 4 oz. |
| | French fries, 1 cup | Boiled potatoes, 1 cup |
| | Green beans, ½ cup | Green beans, ½ cup |
| | Margarine, ½ tsp. | Margarine, ½ tsp. |
| | Ice cream, 1 cup | Ice milk, 1 cup |
| | Milk, 1 cup | Skim milk, 1 cup |

*NUTRIENT ANALYSIS*

| | *High-Fat Menu* | *Lower-Fat Menu* |
|---|---|---|
| Calories | 2,800 | 1,800 |
| Carbohydrate | 38% of calories | 53% of calories |
| Protein | 14% of calories | 21% of calories |
| Fat | 48% of calories | 29% of calories |
| P/S[a] | 0.7 | 0.9 |
| Cholesterol | 390 mg | 210 mg |

[a]*P/S = ratio of grams polyunsaturated to saturated fats. A P/S ratio of at least 1 is recommended.*

Trim the fat off meats. Choose lean cuts of pork (tenderloin, chops) and lamb (leg). Remove visible fat and skin from chicken and other poultry products.

Limit your intake of meats such as cold cuts (bologna, salami), sausage, bacon, hot dogs, and hamburger.

Use low-fat sauces and gravies or limit their use to small portions.

A by-product of these changes is a reduction in cholesterol intake. You can get more information about dietary fat by reading pages 86 to 92.

### DIETARY CHOLESTEROL INTAKE AND CHOLESTEROL LEVEL

Total cholesterol level in some people (but not in everyone) is influenced by cholesterol intake.[13] For people who are *cholesterol sensitive*, diets that provide more than 300 mg of cholesterol per day tend to raise blood-cholesterol level, and lower intakes to lower blood cholesterol.

Cholesterol is a clear, oily substance found only in animal products. (Have you seen "no cholesterol" labels on bananas and breakfast cereals? Cholesterol would have to be *added* to these nonanimal products to be present in them.) Cholesterol is found in animal cell membranes and in the coating that surrounds nerves. Consequently, it is found in both the flesh and fat components of animal products. The best way to identify high-cholesterol foods is to look them up in a table of the leading food sources of cholesterol. Such a table appears on page 92. If you have a total cholesterol level of over 200 mg/dl, the wisest action would be to reduce saturated fat and cholesterol intake.

### OTHER FACTORS THAT AFFECT TOTAL CHOLESTEROL LEVEL

In addition to low saturated fat and cholesterol intakes, blood-cholesterol levels can be lowered in most people by a loss of body fat, if overweight, and the regular ingestion of oat bran or a similar type of fiber (flaxseed bran, pectin, and guar gum, for example). Oat and similar brans bind with cholesterol in the intestine and carry it out of the body in the stools rather than allowing the cholesterol to be absorbed. About 2 tablespoons of oat bran per day are effective in reducing cholesterol level in many people.

Blood-cholesterol reductions can be achieved by drugs. Except for people with very high blood-cholesterol levels, however, dietary changes are the recommended route to lowering cholesterol. Many of the drugs used to lower cholesterol have side effects that make them worth the risks they present only for people who can't lower their cholesterol levels by diet. They are also expensive.

Estrogen, either as normally produced by the body or in pill form, reduces cholesterol level. It decreases LDL-cholesterol while increasing HDL-cholesterol. One study showed that the maximum reduction in LDL-cholesterol combined with the maximal increase in HDL-cholesterol occurred with estrogen doses of 1.25 mg per day.[15] The use of estrogen is not risk free, however. For every one thousand estrogen users, the number of cases of endometrial cancer in women increases by one.[15] Estrogen therapy is not currently recommended for the reduction of cholesterol levels.[15]

Certain types of blood-pressure-lowering drugs, oral contraceptives, progestins, testosterone, and psychological stress increase blood-cholesterol levels. A large study showed that the risk of heart disease in women aged thirty-five to sixty-four years is doubled among those with *Type A* personalities.[16] People with Type A personalities tend to be aggressive, competitive, and ambitious, and are driven by the urgency of time. People who have a feeling of control over their environment appear to be at lower risk of high cholesterol levels and heart disease than people who feel they have little control.[16]

#### FACTORS THAT AFFECT HDL

Excess body fat appears to exert a major influence on HDL level.[17] The well-publicized, positive effect of physical activity on HDL levels may actually be due to the effect of exercise on reducing body fat levels. In addition, the decrease in HDL level that occurs with age in most people and the increase in HDL levels noted with weight loss are both likely due to changes in body fat content.[18]

The moderate consumption of alcohol-containing beverages (one to two drinks per day) appears to protect against the development of heart disease. Alcohol appears to enhance the effect of HDL in lowering blood cholesterol.[12]

Zinc supplements in doses of 50 mg per day given for twelve weeks to men, and doses of 100 mg zinc in women, have been found to lower HDL-cholesterol levels by 10 percent.[19]

#### FACTORS THAT AFFECT TRIGLYCERIDES

Elevated triglyceride levels (over 300 mg/dl) are often present in adults who are obese or who have diabetes or hypertension. (As mentioned in chapter 5, triglycerides are the most prevalent type of fat in our bodies.) Blood-triglyceride levels are elevated by an excessive calorie or simple sugar intake, fasting, high-fat meals, cigarette smoking, and oral contraceptives.[20] They can usually be reduced by physical activity, weight loss (if overweight), and a reduction in simple sugar intake.[21] Fish oils and an increased consumption of fish have also been found to reduce triglyceride levels.

It has been recognized for many years that Eskimos consuming a traditional diet are at low risk of developing heart disease, hypertension, and a number of other diseases common in the United States. It appears that part of the protection Eskimos receive against these diseases is related to their high-fish diet. Eskimos in Greenland, for example, eat about a pound of fish a day. Their high fish intake supplies a constant source of the omega-3-fatty acids. Fish oils are particularly rich in eicosapentaenoic acid (EPA), a specific type of the omega-3-fatty acids thought to be responsible for the beneficial effects of fish oils on health. People consuming a western-type diet don't get nearly as much of the omega-3-fatty acids as the Eskimos. This type of unsaturated fat is primarily found in fish and seafood; only trace amounts of them are contained in some other foods. In general, fatty fish like mackerel and lake trout are better sources of the omega-3-fatty acids than drier fish such as perch or haddock.

Omega-3-fatty acids influence health by altering the types of prostaglandins that are produced by the body, much like aspirin does. Prostaglandins are hormonelike substances that affect everything from blood pressure to our response to pain. Over sixty prostaglandins have been identified, and each has a different effect on body processes. The types of prostaglandin affected by omega-3-fatty acids are those that influence blood pressure, blood clotting, and the deposition of cholesterol into the walls of arteries.[22] A number of studies have shown that omega-3-fatty acids can decrease blood pressure and lower triglyceride levels.[23] When consumed at a level of 2 to 5 grams per day by both women and men, omega-3-fatty acids inhibit the production of the prostaglandins that increase blood pressure and promote the formation of cholesterol plaques.[23] One study undertaken in the Netherlands reported that the habitual consumption of as little as two fish meals a week was protective against heart disease.[24]

The increased consumption of fish by Americans is being encouraged, but the use of concentrated sources of fish oils is not. The effects of excessive intake of fish oils may include slowed blood clotting, an induced deficiency of vitamin E, toxicities of vitamins A and D (two vitamins that are stored in fish oils), high intake levels of environmental contaminants that accumulate in the fat stores of fish, and fragile cell membranes.[25] (The omega-3-fatty acids become part of cell membranes and may make cells less resistant to certain disease processes, as well as more resistant to others.) As for all nutrients, there is an optimal range of intake of the omega-3-fatty acids and more is not necessarily better.

OMEGA-3-FATTY ACID CONTENT OF FISH AND SEAFOODS

| *Seafood (3½-oz. serving)* | *Omega-3-fatty acids (grams)* |
|---|---|
| Mackerel, Atlantic | 2.6 |
| Scad | 2.1 |
| Spiny dog fish | 2.0 |
| Lake trout | 2.0 |
| Herring | 1.8 |
| Tuna | 1.5 (0.4-1.6) |
| Salmon | 1.5 (1.0-1.5) |
| Whitefish, lake | 1.5 |
| Sturgeon | 1.5 |
| Anchovy | 1.4 |
| Bluefish | 1.2 |
| Mullet | 1.1 |
| Conch | 1.0 |
| Oyster | 0.6 |
| Brook trout | 0.6 |
| Squid | 0.6 |
| Catfish | 0.5 |
| Shrimp | 0.5 (0.2-0.5) |
| Perch | 0.4 |
| Crab | 0.3 |
| Pike, walleye | 0.3 |
| Cod | 0.3 |
| Flounder | 0.2 |
| Haddock | 0.2 |
| Lobster | 0.2 |
| Scallops | 0.2 |
| Swordfish | 0.2 |

## HYPERTENSION

*Excess of salty flavor hardens the pulse.*

*The Yellow Emperor's Classic of Internal Medicine, circa 1000 BC*

High salt intake has been thought to cause high blood pressure for over two thousand years. However, only in the past fifty years has the relationship between blood pressure and the sodium component of salt been clarified.

Hypertension is considered a major public health problem in the United States and other countries where salt intake tends to be high.[26] Although not considered a disease by itself, the presence of hypertension substantially increases the risk of developing heart disease or kidney failure, or experiencing a heart attack or stroke. Hypertension occurs in about 24 percent of U.S. adults and is more likely to develop as people age. About one in fourteen eighteen-year-olds are hypertensive, whereas one in three people over the age of seventy-four have the disorder. Hypertension becomes an especially important problem for women as they age. Hypertension is more common among men up to the age of fifty, but then the situation reverses.[27]

Although a common health-threatening disorder, little is known about what causes hypertension. Only 5 percent of hypertension cases can be linked directly to a cause. It's not yet clear what causes the other 95 percent of cases, referred to as *essential* hypertension. Because this is the most prevalent type of hypertension, it is essential hypertension that we shall consider here. Potential causes for hypertension in adults are:

Family history of hypertension
High sodium intake
Excess body fat
Low potassium intake
Physical inactivity
Excess alcohol intake
Smoking

Dietary factors appear to be among the most important. Of the dietary factors, the link between sodium intake and hypertension is the strongest.[28]

Several lines of evidence strongly indicate that high-sodium diets are a leading factor in the development of hypertension. Foremost among the evidence is the finding that the incidence of hypertension increases within populations as the average daily intake of salt goes up. People living in societies where salt intake is low, such as the Greenland Eskimos, African Pygmies, and Australian aborigines, experience very little hypertension. They tend to develop hypertension, however, when they switch to a high-salt diet.[29]

### *The Effects of Salt Restriction on Hypertension*

Low-sodium diets tend to reduce blood pressure among people with hypertension, and they may also help to maintain normal blood pressure levels among people with a family history of hypertension.[30] Mild hypertension, the diagnosis in over 75 percent of hypertension cases, can often be lowered to normal by a diet that contains around 2 mg of sodium per day in normal-weight adults.[28] That amount of sodium equals roughly 1 teaspoon a day. A 2-gram sodium diet can be achieved by avoiding processed foods and foods with added salt such as salty snacks, smoked meats, pickled foods, and convenience dinners, and by not adding salt during food preparation or at the table. To achieve a 2-gram sodium diet:

> Eat fresh or frozen unprocessed or lightly processed foods.
>
> Limit intake of salty snacks, canned soups, and cured and smoked meats.
>
> Take the salt shaker off the table.
>
> Read food labels. (You may be surprised to discover how many foods have added salt.)

Moderate-salt diets that exclude processed foods also offer an important fringe benefit: they tend to be high in potassium. High potassium intake appears to protect against the blood-pressure-raising effects of high-sodium diets.[30,31] Diets that are most likely to be low in potassium and high in sodium are those that rely heavily on processed convenience foods. Processing generally reduces the potassium content of foods significantly while increasing the sodium content by the addition of salt. For example, the 135 mg of potassium in ½ cup of fresh corn is decreased to 24 mg in ½ cup of cornflakes. At the same time, the sodium content increases from less than a few milligrams in fresh corn to 325 mg in cornflakes.

People on moderate-salt diets often replace processed foods with fresh and unprocessed vegetables, fruits, and meats that have more potassium than sodium. To get a notion of how the inclusion or exclusion of processed and salty foods affects dietary intake of sodium and potassium, review the two menus shown below.

The amount of sodium in the high-salt menu about equals the average U.S. intake, determined before salt is added to foods at the table. The high-sodium menu contains three and one-half times the sodium, and one-fourth less potassium, than the moderate-salt menu. As shown in figure 7, the moderate-salt menu contains more potassium than sodium—a combination that helps to lower blood pressure in many people with hypertension.

It is just as important to know about foods containing low amounts of sodium as to know about high-sodium foods. Table 36

EXAMPLES OF HIGH- AND MODERATE-SALT MENUS
*(Menus do not include salt added at the table.)*

| *High-salt menu* | *Moderate-salt menu* |
| --- | --- |
| Orange juice, 6 oz.<br>Egg sandwich, 1<br>(egg, Canadian bacon,[a] American cheese, and butter on English muffin)<br>Coffee, 1 cup | Orange juice, 6 oz.<br>Egg, 1<br>Whole wheat toast, 2 slices<br>Margarine, 2 tsp.<br>Coffee, 1 cup |
| Hot dog,[a] 1, on bun<br>Catsup,[a] 1 T.<br>Dill pickle,[a] ¼ whole<br>Potato chips,[a] 1 oz.<br>Milk, 1 cup | Hamburger, 3 oz., on bun<br>Sliced tomatoes, ½ cup<br>Coleslaw, ½ cup<br>Milk, 1 cup |
| Tomato soup,[a] 1 cup<br>Meat loaf,[a] 3 oz.<br>Scalloped potatoes, ½ cup<br>Gravy,[a] ¼ cup<br>Peas (canned), ½ cup<br>Milk, 1 cup | Tossed salad, 1½ cup with Italian dressing,* 2 T.<br>Pork chop, 3 oz.<br>Baked potato, 1 medium<br>Green beans, frozen, ½ cup<br>Milk, 1 cup |
| American cheese, 1 oz.<br>Saltine crackers,[a] 4 squares<br>Tea, 1 cup | Peanuts (unsalted), ¼ cup<br>Apple, 1 medium<br>Tea, 1 cup |

[a]*Main contributors to sodium level of diet.*

lists a number of low-sodium fruits and vegetables, all of which are also good sources of potassium. These foods are excellent examples of good food choices and may be particularly appropriate for people with hypertension and for those at risk of developing hypertension because of their family history. A recent study found that adults aged fifty to seventy-nine years who consume one more serving of fruits and vegetables than the average intake (about four servings per day) experienced 40 percent fewer strokes than adults who consume the average amount. The protective effect of the additional fruit or vegetable was stronger for women than men in this southern California study.[32]

*Calcium and Blood Pressure*

Is calcium related to high blood pressure? The answer is a resounding, scientifically determined *maybe.*

Research results suggesting that habitually low intake of dietary calcium may be related to the development of hypertension came as quite a shock to many scientists. All previous research had firmly pointed accusing fingers at sodium. Why would low calcium intake, and not high-sodium diet, be related to hypertension in these studies?

Those initial studies were conducted with male participants. Later research studying female subjects failed to show any effect of dietary or supplemental calcium on blood pressure in women.[33,34] It is generally concluded that it is premature to recommend using calcium supplements to prevent or treat hypertension. It is not premature, however, to recommend that people with hypertension limit their salt intake and that all women and men consume enough calcium in their everyday diet.

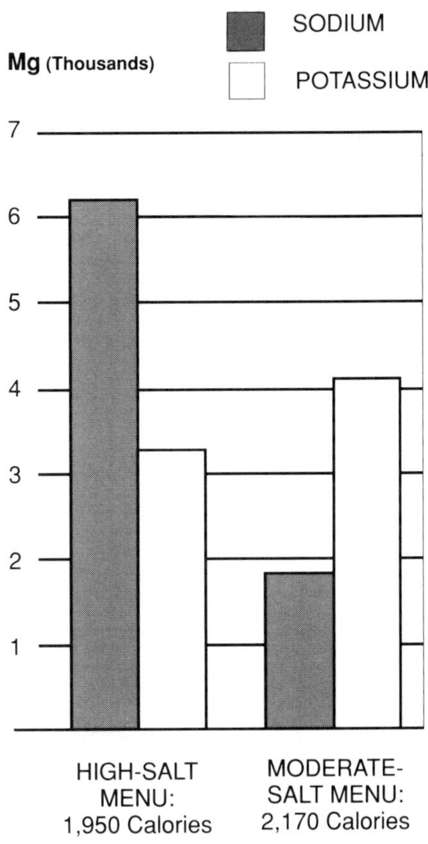


**FIGURE 7. CALORIC, SODIUM, AND POTASSIUM CONTENTS OF THE TWO MENUS SHOWN ON PAGE 172.**

*Other Factors Related to the Development of Hypertension*

Hypertension appears to have many causes. In addition to the effects of sodium and potassium, factors such as smoking, stress, physical activity, being overweight, and alcohol intake may contribute to its development.

People who quit smoking, lower their day-to-day level of stress, and increase their physical activity level are less likely to develop hypertension than if they had not changed their lifestyles.[34]

Overweight and obesity are clearly related to hypertension, and the risk of becoming hypertensive increases with body weight.[34] In

TABLE 36. SOME LOW-SODIUM FRUITS AND VEGETABLES THAT ARE ALSO GOOD SOURCES OF POTASSIUM

| FOOD | AMOUNT | SODIUM MG | POTASSIUM MG |
|---|---|---|---|
| *Fruits* | | | |
| Banana | 1 medium | 1 | 440 |
| Blueberries | ½ cup | 1 | 60 |
| Cherries | ½ cup | 1 | 130 |
| Grapefruit | ½ whole | 1 | 130 |
| Peach | 1 medium | 1 | 200 |
| Strawberries | ⅔ cup | 1 | 165 |
| Pear | 1 medium | 3 | 215 |
| *Vegetables* | | | |
| Corn | ½ cup | 1 | 135 |
| Green beans | ½ cup | 2 | 95 |
| Tomato | 1 medium | 4 | 300 |
| Cucumber | ½ medium | 4 | 125 |
| Potato | 1 medium | 5 | 780 |
| Cauliflower | ½ cup | 5 | 150 |
| Broccoli | ½ cup | 8 | 205 |
| Green pepper | ½ cup | 10 | 155 |
| Lettuce | 1½ cups | 10 | 160 |

contrast to underweight and normal-weight individuals, people who are overweight benefit little from reductions in dietary sodium intake. For them, weight loss is the best antihypertension medicine. Even small amounts of weight loss generally reduce blood pressure in overweight and obese people with hypertension.[30] Weight loss in the range of sixteen pounds has been shown to produce a greater fall in blood pressure than antihypertensive drugs.[35] And the effect of weight loss on reducing hypertension is stronger for women than men.[36]

Excessive alcohol consumption has also been related to hypertension. Habitual alcohol use exceeding two drinks per day is associated with above-average blood pressure levels. Blood pressure of heavy drinkers generally returns to normal when intake is reduced to two or fewer drinks per day.[28]

### *Why Not Just Use Drugs to Lower Blood Pressure?*

Dietary changes may be difficult for some people to achieve. So why put them through the trouble? Why not just use antihypertensive drugs? These are good questions, and they have good answers. Antihypertensive drugs have effects on the body other than reducing blood pressure. These side effects include raising blood cholesterol and decreasing potassium levels.[37] The elevated cholesterol levels increase the risk of heart disease among people already at risk because of hypertension. Potassium losses caused by some of the antihypertensive drugs increase the risk of potassium deficiency, a potentially fatal disorder. One type of drug, *beta blockers*, reduces libido in men, making the trade-off between blood pressure and sex drive potentially unacceptable. In contrast to the antihypertension drugs, moderate-salt diets effectively reduce blood pressure in people with mild hypertension and do not appear to pose any health risk. The combination of weight loss, dietary changes, and increased physical activity is as effective as drugs in treating most cases of high blood pressure in women, without the undesirable side effects of drugs.[38] Antihypertensive drugs plus dietary sodium reduction or weight loss are the accepted treatments for severe forms of hypertension.[28]

Many people initially find moderate-sodium diets difficult to stick to because they miss the taste of salt. People who can hang in with the diet for two months, however, find the going gets easier. After getting used to a moderate-salt diet, low amounts of salt taste "saltier" than before and less salty foods tend to be preferred.[39]

## CANCER

Cancer of the breast and reproductive system is the number-one cause of death in women under forty years of age. Only heart disease kills more women (it is the leading cause of death after age forty).[40] Rates of cancer among women vary substantially within population groups and from country to country, indicating that environmental factors play important roles in its development. The relationships among cancer and dietary fat intake, obesity, low fiber and vegetable intake, and diets that provide low amounts of vitamins A, C, and E and the mineral selenium are presented here.

### *Dietary Fat and Cancer*

The single most common type of cancer in women is cancer of the breast. Of the factors related to a woman's risk of developing breast cancer, fat intake is among the strongest. The relationship between a high-fat diet and the risk of breast cancer is especially strong for premenopausal women.[41] Reducing fat intake after breast cancer diagnosis appears to decrease the risk of death from the cancer.[41,42] The association between fat intake and cancer in women may be due to fat's tendency to cause elevated estrogen levels, which may enhance tumor growth.[43]

A number of years ago, caffeine intake was suspected of being related to the development of cancer by way of fibrocystic breast disease, a disease that is relatively common among U.S. women. It is characterized by small, hard, and painful knots of tissues in the breast. The disease commonly occurs among women who are heavy coffee drinkers, or who habitually use medicines that contain caffeine. Recent evidence indicates that fibrocystic breast disease is probably not a precursor of breast cancer.[44] A sharp reduction in caffeine intake, such as switching to decaffeinated coffee, is the treatment of choice for many cases of fibrocystic breast disease. It is important, however, that all knots or lumps in the breast are examined and identified.

### *Other Nutrition Facts about Cancer in Women*

Obesity, dietary fiber, and vegetable intake have been related to the development of cancer of the breast, endometrium, cervix, and colon. Obesity has been associated with cancer of the female reproductive system.[45] Dietary fiber intake of over 25 grams per day in women appears to confer some protection against colon cancer.[46] Women who favor vegetables—and eat them frequently—may be less susceptible to breast cancer than women who avoid them.[46,47] Women in the United States who are vegetarians have 60 to 80 percent less breast cancer than U.S. women in general.[48] High vegetable intake may reduce cancer risk by increasing the content of vitamin A or beta-carotene in diets, or by reducing blood levels of estrogen. Diets rich in vegetables tend to be low in fat and calories, and these attributes may also contribute to the reduced rates of breast cancer in women who love their vegetables.[46]

### *Vitamin A, Beta-Carotene, and Cancer*

The role of vitamin A in the formation and maintenance of cells that line the respiratory, reproductive, and digestive tracts, and the protective effects of beta-carotene on body cells have made them prime targets for cancer research. About half of all fatal cancers start in cells of the skin and in those that line the respiratory, reproductive, and digestive tracts. Vitamin A and beta-carotene appear to slow down the development of cancers that originate within these cells. They may, however, have little effect on halting the spread of established cancer.[49]

Above-average intakes of vitamin A and beta-carotene have been specifically shown to provide protection against the development of lung cancer in women.[50] Vitamin A and beta-carotene intakes are above average if two servings of dark-colored vegetables, such as carrots, broccoli, squash, and spinach, are consumed each day. (See table 23 for a list of rich food sources.)

### *Is Vitamin E Related to Cancer?*

Many studies have examined vitamin E and cancer development, and none have shown a strong relationship between them. It is generally concluded that if there is a link between vitamin E and cancer in humans, it is a very weak one.[51]

### *Vitamin C and Cancer*

There is no strong evidence in favor of or against a role of vitamin C in the prevention of cancer. The results of a few studies have indicated that vitamin C protects against the development of some types of cancer, whereas other studies have shown either no relationship or harmful effects.[52,53] Whereas this vitamin appears to be of no benefit in the treatment of advanced cancer,[54] because of its antioxidant functions few scientists are willing to rule out the possibility that it may protect against the development of certain types of cancer.

### *Selenium and Cancer*

Because selenium functions as an antioxidant, scientists suspect that it may play a role in cancer development. Research results clearly indicate a role of selenium in the development of cancer in laboratory animals, but the few studies involving humans have not produced such clear-cut results. It appears, however, that people who habitually consume around the RDA level of selenium from foods (0.05 to 0.2 mg) experience less cancer than those who consume less.[55] (Food sources of selenium are given in table 30.)

## DIABETES

Diabetes is the seventh leading cause of death in the United States and is an important contributor to hypertension and heart disease among women in particular.[56] Women under the age of fifty who do not have diabetes or hypertension are, on the other hand, strikingly resistant to heart disease.[7] The relative protection women have against heart disease compared to men is erased by the presence of diabetes.[7] Diabetes is a complex, chronic disease for which there is care but currently no cure. It affects an estimated eleven million people in the United States.[57]

In people with diabetes, either the pancreas does not produce enough insulin, or the body does not properly use the insulin that is produced. As a result, excess glucose accumulates around cells and in the blood, and overflows into the urine. (Many years ago, diabetes would be diagnosed by tasting urine. If it was sweet, the diagnosis was made. Whether ants gathered in mass around the outhouse was also used in the diagnosis.) Diabetes due to an inadequate supply of insulin appears to result from a viral infection or other disease that causes damage to the pancreatic cells that produce insulin.[58] The other type of diabetes, due to poor use of existing insulin, is thought to be related to a decreased sensitivity of cells to insulin. Consequently, although insulin is present, it does not perform its usual function of transporting glucose across cell membranes and into cells. Without the action of insulin, glucose piles up in the fluid surrounding cells and in the blood, and leaves the inside of cells starved for glucose.

Diabetes due to insulin deficiency—*insulin-dependent diabetes mellitus*—accounts for around 10 percent of all cases. Diabetes occurring in the presence of insulin production—called *non-insulin-dependent diabetes mellitus*—accounts for the other 90 percent of cases. The majority of people with non-insulin-dependent diabetes mellitus are obese and have measurable or even excessive amounts of insulin.[58] The problem appears to be that their cells are not sensitive to the action of insulin. Overeating, excessive body fat, and low activity levels contribute to the cause of this common type of diabetes. Cells become more sensitive to the action of insulin with body fat loss and exercise.[58]

### *Dietary Management of Diabetes*

The diets of people with diabetes used to be rigorously controlled. A high-fat, high-protein, low-carbohydrate diet was the standard fare. The use of simple sugars was strongly discouraged. Emerging evidence on the effects of a high-fat diet on heart disease, the high prevalence of heart disease among people with diabetes, and research results on the influence of different types of carbohydrates on blood-glucose levels have produced a radical change in diet therapy for diabetes. The focus is now on achieving a match between caloric intake and insulin doses that maintains the blood-glucose level within the normal range. The new guidelines and procedures for managing diabetes give people a lot more control over their condition. A low-fat, moderate-protein, and high-carbohydrate diet (that may include some simple sugars with meals if desired) is the currently recommended diabetic diet. Diets should be limited in alcohol because it directly affects blood-glucose levels.

Dietary intake built around the "healthy eating" pattern presented in chapter 4 is well suited to meeting the needs of people with diabetes. Guidance on weight-loss strategies is also covered later in this book. Of the possibilities, diabetes prevention and weight control would probably do more to benefit women's health than anything else.

AMERICAN DIABETES ASSOCIATION DIETARY RECOMMENDATIONS FOR PERSONS WITH DIABETES

| *Dietary factor* | *Recommendation* |
|---|---|
| Calories | Should be prescribed to achieve and maintain a desirable body weight. |
| Carbohydrate | Should comprise 55 to 60 percent of the calories with the form and amount to be determined by individual eating patterns and blood glucose and lipid responses. Unrefined carbohydrates should be substituted for refined carbohydrates to the extent possible. Modest amounts of sugars may be acceptable as long as metabolic control and desirable body weight are maintained. |
| Protein | Should follow the Recommended Dietary Allowance (NRC 1980) of 0.8 g/kg body weight for adults, although more may be needed for older persons. Some reduction in protein intake may prevent or delay the onset of the kidney complications of diabetes. |
| Fat | Should comprise 30 percent or less of total calories, and all components should be reduced proportionately. Replacement of saturated with polyunsaturated fat is desirable to reduce cardiovascular risk. |
| Cholesterol | Should be restricted to 300 mg/day or less to reduce cardiovascular risk. |
| Alternative sweeteners | Both nutritive and nonnutritive sweeteners are acceptable in diabetes management. |

| | |
|---|---|
| Sodium | Should be restricted to 1,000 mg/1,000 kcal, not to exceed 3,000 mg/day, to minimize symptoms of hypertension. Severe sodium restriction, however, may be harmful for persons whose diabetes is poorly controlled and for those with postural hypotension (low blood pressure and consequent dizziness when first standing up) or fluid imbalance. |
| Alcohol | Should be moderate and may need to be restricted entirely by persons with diabetes and insulin-induced hypoglycemia, neuropathy, or poor control of blood sugar, blood lipids, or obesity. |
| Vitamins and minerals | Should meet recommended levels for good health. Supplements are unnecessary for persons with diabetes except when caloric intake is exceptionally low or the variety of food intake is limited. Calcium supplements may be necessary under special circumstances. |

*Source: American Diabetes Association Task Force on Nutrition and Exchange Lists, 1987. Nutritional recommendations and principles for individuals with diabetes mellitus; 1986.* Diabetes Care *10:126–32. Reproduced with permission from the American Diabetes Association, Inc.*

## HYPOGLYCEMIA

Hypoglycemia is a rare condition most often caused by an excess availability of insulin. It is accompanied by abnormally low blood-glucose levels, weakness, and behavioral signs such as nervousness and irritability. These signs disappear rapidly after eating.[59] It has been speculated that a high simple sugar intake stimulates the excessive secretion of insulin and may cause hypoglycemia. This notion has not been verified among healthy people in research settings, however. The diagnosis of diet-related hypoglycemia requires that blood samples used to test for hypoglycemia should be taken when the symptoms are present.[59]

Standard diet therapy for hypoglycemia is five well-balanced, small meals per day and avoidance of sweet snacks.[60] People who feel very hungry, tense, and weak shortly after consuming a highly sugared snack may benefit from this type of diet. Consuming snacks that are low in simple sugars, such as peanuts, cheese and crackers, milk, and yogurt, and not skipping meals may solve the problem. The cause of the symptoms should, of course, be medically investigated.

## OBESITY

Perhaps no other area within the field of nutrition is more intensively researched and written about than the subject of obesity. But, for all the research and writing that goes on, it remains a disorder for which there is no clear cause or reliable treatment. It is a major health problem and one of the most complex and misunderstood disorders of our time. Approximately 22 percent of men and 24 percent of women in the United States are obese, or weigh 20 percent more than their desirable weight.[61]

Interest in solving the mysteries surrounding the cause and cure of obesity is intense because this common disorder poses serious threats to health. Although it is rarely the direct cause of death, obesity is associated with a wide range of problems, including:

- Shortened life span
- Heart disease
- Diabetes
- Certain types of cancer
- Hypertension
- Depression
- High blood-cholesterol levels
- Gallbladder disease
- Infertility
- Complications during pregnancy
- Injury to weight-bearing joints
- Varicose veins
- Accidents
- Complications from surgery
- Gout
- Skin disorders

The increased risk of developing heart disease, diabetes, certain types of cancer, hypertension, and other disorders may contribute to a shortened life span and decreased quality of life for people who are obese.

A consequence of obesity that perhaps has the greatest impact on quality of life stems from people's attitudes about it. Obesity is a visible disorder and one against which many Americans hold strong biases. These biases may subtly or overtly translate into job discrimination, social isolation, ridicule, and rejection.

The consequences of obesity are much better understood than its causes. However, the scientific literature does offer several theories about the causes of obesity.

Two main theories have been presented about the causes of obesity; each has contributed to filling in part of the gap in our knowledge. One theory centers around causes related to *nature* and the other to *nurture*. The nature theory attempts to explain obesity by genetic, or inborn traits. The nurture theory examines the roles of environmental factors, such as early childhood food experiences and exercise, in obesity development. Neither theory fully explains why people become obese. It appears that both play a role.

*The Nature Theory of Obesity Development*

Are people born with a tendency to become obese? Evidence that supports a ''perhaps—for some people'' answer to this question has been found by studies of obesity in families.

Obesity tends to run in families. One well-known study published some twenty-five years ago found that children raised in families where both parents were obese had an 80 percent chance of being obese. If one parent was obese, then 40 percent of the children were also obese. If, however, neither parent was obese, only 14 percent of the children were.[62] These results do not provide conclusive evidence that obesity is inherited. It is frequently argued that the children may have adopted the overeating and underactivity patterns of their parents. Families have a lot more in common than their genes.

Inborn differences in *dietary thermogenesis*, the calories expended for digestion and absorption after a meal, may also be related to obesity. People whose thermogenesis thermostats are set on low use up fewer than average calories for the digestion of foods and the absorption and processing of nutrients. The difference in caloric expenditure may be great enough to lower the total caloric requirement and make it easier for some people to gain weight than others with a higher rate of dietary thermogenesis.[63]

The possible genetic links to obesity uncovered in studies of families and research that shows individual differences in thermogenesis strongly argue in favor of a genetic component to obesity. They do not, however, explain all cases of obesity. Only four out of ten obese children become obese adults; most people who are obese as adults were normal weight as children and infants.[64] The incidence of obesity is on the rise in children and men in the United States and genetics is clearly not the sole cause.[65]

*The Nurture Theory of Obesity Development*

Two important factors, apparently unrelated to genetic traits, have been associated with the development of obesity. They are dietary and physical activity behaviors.

Children learn to eat to satisfy hunger as well as for other reasons. Instead of eating to cure hunger pangs, they may learn to eat to relieve boredom, to escape a stressful situation, or to please their parents. Consider parents who insist that children clean their plates or who reward good behavior with cookies, candy, or other high-calorie treats. The child's natural eating cue, hunger, may come in second place to emotional signals to eat. The same sort of inappropriate eating cues may be related to obesity in adults. Food may be used to cope with stress, depression, and boredom. Women are much more likely than men to cope with stress by eating.[66]

The types of food available may influence whether a person eats too much and becomes obese.[67] Most children and adults in the United States live in environments where much more tempting food is available than they need. The opportunity to overeat is generally no further away than the refrigerator, a vending machine, the corner grocery, or the dining table. Continuous access to highly preferred foods may lead to overeating and obesity. Research has shown that when normal-weight and obese human volunteers are given a monotonous but nutritionally adequate liquid diet, normal-weight subjects will consume enough to maintain their weight. Obese volunteers, on the other hand, will consume less and lose weight rapidly.[68] In other experiments, both normal-weight and obese humans were found to gain weight if offered unlimited amounts of highly preferred foods.[69] These results may help explain why some people with no family history become obese while others with a genetic tendency towards obesity may remain obese. They have led Theodore Van Itallie, a leading obesity researcher, to conclude:

> There may not be anything basically wrong with most obese people. The problem simply may lie in the fact that human beings have had to learn how to store fat in order to survive. When it becomes easy rather than difficult to obtain extra calories from the environment, obesity is the natural outcome. Perhaps *thin* people are the ones who are abnormal.[65]

### *Physical Activity Patterns and Obesity*

Physical inactivity has been directly related to the development of obesity in children and adults. For some people, a very low level of physical activity may be a primary reason for obesity, while for others, a high level of physical activity may be the reason they aren't obese.

A number of surveys have shown that groups of people with relatively high caloric intakes are less likely to be obese than people with lower caloric intakes. The people with high caloric intakes tend to be the same ones who are physically active. So you can't predict obesity based on caloric intake alone. Some obese people don't eat more than normal-weight people—they simply are much less physically active.

### *Do Obese People Have More Fat Cells?*

Observations that obese people tend to have more fat cells than normal-weight people led many to believe that how many fat cells a person forms during growth is responsible for obesity. It was assumed that fat cells, like nerve or muscle cells, increase in number only during growth. If a person overate while a child, it was reasoned, they would form an excess number of fat cells, which would tend to make and keep them obese.

It now appears that humans can add fat cells throughout life if they continue to overeat.[70] Once a person's existing fat cells reach the maximum size—or become filled with storage fat—the body will produce new cells to handle the overflow. The presence of many fat cells may make it difficult to lose weight. It has been suggested that the body may trigger eating signals when the amount of fat stored in the fat cells begins to decrease.[65] Rather than responding to reduced caloric intake by decreasing the body's supply of fat cells, the body may act to protect the cells present by keeping them well stocked with fat.

### *Set-Point Theory*

The *set-point* theory of obesity holds that each of us is programmed to weigh a certain amount. If you weigh less or more than this predetermined amount, your body will automatically make adjustments in food intake so that you get back to your set-point weight. According to this theory, people end up obese because they have high set-points.

Very little scientific evidence exists to support the set-point theory, but it offers an attractive explanation for why most people gain back weight they lose. People who manage to reduce their body weight and keep it at a new, lower level commonly report they have to diet constantly. If they ate at a level that satisfied their desire for food, they would gain weight rapidly.

Why people tend to defend a particular body weight is not at all clear. It is clear, however, that people have a strong tendency to maintain a particular weight and that this tendency is not easily modified.

Examinations of the possible causes of obesity, such as the ones just covered, generally end with the same major conclusion: It is better to prevent obesity from developing than to try to undo its causes once it is established.

### *Trends in Body Weight*

A very positive trend is developing in the body weights of women. The trend suggests that women are becoming more physically active with age than in the past. Women over the age of twenty-five years weigh less on average now than they did in 1959. As shown in table 37, the average weight-for-height of women between twenty-five and sixty-nine years of age is declining. The same trend does not appear for men; as a group they have gained in weight-for-height since 1959. It should be pointed out that the weights given in the table represent average weights, not the desired weights listed in chapter 2; desired weights are generally at least several pounds lower than average weights.

## FOOD ALLERGIES AND INTOLERANCES

Adverse reactions to specific components of food come in two major forms: allergic reactions and nonallergic reactions, or *food intolerances*. The difference between an allergy and a food intolerance is that the body's immune—or disease defense—system becomes involved in allergic reactions only. The immune system becomes involved in allergic reactions because it produces antibodies to neutralize the invading antigen, or the offending component of food that has entered the body proper. While present in the body, antigens cause disruptions in normal cell functions that can result in diarrhea, hives, rashes, a runny nose, sneezing, wheezing, and irritated eyes. Adverse reactions to cow's milk protein, soy protein, the gluten component of wheat, and egg white protein are appropriately termed allergic reactions. The vast majority of allergic reactions that occur are due to the ingestion of one or more of these four substances. Peanut butter and nuts and other substances in food may also cause allergic reactions.

Food intolerances are caused by the lack of specific digestive enzymes or the direct effects of absorbed substances on body processes. The "Chinese restaurant syndrome" that develops in people sensitive to MSG (monosodium glutamate); headaches that occur in tandem with the consumption of chocolate, red wine, and aged cheese; and the flatulence that some individuals develop after eating dried beans are examples of food intolerances. The most common type of food intolerance, however, is lactose intolerance. Lactose is the main type of carbohydrate found in milk and milk

TABLE 37. CHANGES IN AVERAGE WEIGHTS FOR MEN BETWEEN 1959 AND 1979
*(Weight in pounds, without clothing, according to height and age)*

| HEIGHT (WITHOUT SHOES) | | AGES 20–24 | | AGES 25–29 | | AGES 30–39 | | AGES 40–49 | | AGES 50–59 | | AGES 60–69 | |
|---|---|---|---|---|---|---|---|---|---|---|---|---|---|
| FEET | INCHES | AVERAGE WEIGHT 1979 | CHANGE SINCE 1959 | AVERAGE WEIGHT 1979 | CHANGE SINCE 1959 | AVERAGE WEIGHT 1979 | CHANGE SINCE 1959 | AVERAGE WEIGHT 1979 | CHANGE SINCE 1959 | AVERAGE WEIGHT 1979 | CHANGE SINCE 1959 | AVERAGE WEIGHT 1979 | CHANGE SINCE 1959 |
| 5 | 1 | 125 | 4 | 129 | 2 | 133 | 3 | 135 | 2 | 136 | 1 | 135 | 3 |
| 5 | 2 | 131 | 6 | 135 | 4 | 138 | 4 | 139 | 2 | 140 | 2 | 139 | 4 |
| 5 | 3 | 134 | 5 | 138 | 4 | 142 | 4 | 144 | 3 | 145 | 3 | 144 | 5 |
| 5 | 4 | 138 | 6 | 142 | 5 | 146 | 4 | 149 | 4 | 150 | 4 | 148 | 5 |
| 5 | 5 | 143 | 8 | 147 | 6 | 151 | 5 | 153 | 4 | 154 | 4 | 153 | 6 |
| 5 | 6 | 148 | 10 | 151 | 7 | 155 | 5 | 158 | 4 | 159 | 4 | 158 | 6 |
| 5 | 7 | 152 | 10 | 156 | 8 | 160 | 6 | 162 | 4 | 163 | 4 | 162 | 6 |
| 5 | 8 | 158 | 12 | 161 | 9 | 165 | 7 | 167 | 5 | 168 | 5 | 167 | 6 |
| 5 | 9 | 162 | 12 | 166 | 10 | 169 | 6 | 171 | 4 | 172 | 4 | 171 | 5 |
| 5 | 10 | 166 | 12 | 170 | 10 | 174 | 7 | 176 | 5 | 177 | 4 | 176 | 5 |
| 5 | 11 | 171 | 12 | 176 | 11 | 179 | 7 | 181 | 5 | 182 | 4 | 181 | 5 |
| 6 | 0 | 177 | 14 | 181 | 11 | 185 | 9 | 187 | 7 | 188 | 6 | 186 | 5 |
| 6 | 1 | 182 | 15 | 186 | 11 | 190 | 9 | 192 | 7 | 193 | 6 | 191 | 5 |
| 6 | 2 | 188 | 17 | 192 | 13 | 196 | 10 | 198 | 8 | 199 | 7 | 195 | 4 |
| 6 | 3 | 193 | 19 | 197 | 14 | 201 | 9 | 203 | 7 | 204 | 6 | 202 | 5 |

*Source of basic data:* Build Study, 1979 *and* Build and Blood Pressure Study, 1959. *Society of Actuaries and Association of Life Insurance Medical Directors of America.*
*Note: Prepared by Metropolitan Life Insurance Company.*

TABLE 37. (CONTINUED). CHANGES IN AVERAGE WEIGHTS FOR WOMEN BETWEEN 1959 AND 1979
*(Weight in pounds, without clothing, according to height and age)*

| HEIGHT (WITHOUT SHOES) | | AGES 20–24 | | AGES 25–29 | | AGES 30–39 | | AGES 40–49 | | AGES 50–59 | | AGES 60–69 | |
|---|---|---|---|---|---|---|---|---|---|---|---|---|---|
| FEET | INCHES | AVERAGE WEIGHT 1979 | CHANGE SINCE 1959 | AVERAGE WEIGHT 1979 | CHANGE SINCE 1959 | AVERAGE WEIGHT 1979 | CHANGE SINCE 1959 | AVERAGE WEIGHT 1979 | CHANGE SINCE 1959 | AVERAGE WEIGHT 1979 | CHANGE SINCE 1959 | AVERAGE WEIGHT 1979 | CHANGE SINCE 1959 |
| 4 | 8 | 98 | 0 | 103 | 0 | 107 | −4 | 111 | −7 | 115 | −6 | 117 | −6 |
| 4 | 9 | 102 | 1 | 107 | 1 | 110 | −3 | 115 | −5 | 118 | −5 | 120 | −5 |
| 4 | 10 | 107 | 3 | 109 | 0 | 112 | −4 | 118 | −5 | 122 | −4 | 124 | −3 |
| 4 | 11 | 109 | 1 | 111 | −1 | 115 | −4 | 120 | −6 | 124 | −5 | 127 | −3 |
| 5 | 0 | 113 | 2 | 116 | 1 | 118 | −4 | 124 | −5 | 128 | −4 | 130 | −3 |
| 5 | 1 | 117 | 3 | 118 | 0 | 121 | −4 | 126 | −6 | 130 | −6 | 133 | −4 |
| 5 | 2 | 121 | 4 | 122 | 1 | 125 | −3 | 130 | −6 | 134 | −6 | 137 | −4 |
| 5 | 3 | 124 | 3 | 125 | 0 | 128 | −3 | 133 | −6 | 138 | −6 | 140 | −5 |
| 5 | 4 | 127 | 2 | 129 | 0 | 131 | −4 | 136 | −7 | 141 | −7 | 144 | −5 |
| 5 | 5 | 130 | 2 | 131 | −1 | 134 | −4 | 140 | −7 | 144 | −8 | 147 | −6 |
| 5 | 6 | 134 | 2 | 135 | −1 | 138 | −4 | 144 | −7 | 149 | −7 | 152 | −5 |
| 5 | 7 | 138 | 2 | 139 | −1 | 142 | −4 | 147 | −8 | 153 | −7 | 155 | −5 |
| 5 | 8 | 143 | 3 | 145 | 1 | 147 | −3 | 152 | −8 | 156 | −9 | 158 | * |
| 5 | 9 | 146 | 1 | 147 | −2 | 150 | −5 | 155 | −10 | 159 | −11 | 160 | * |
| 5 | 10 | 152 | 2 | 153 | −1 | 156 | −4 | 159 | −11 | 163 | −13 | 164 | * |

*Source of basic data:* Build Study, 1979 *and* Build and Blood Pressure Study, 1959. *Society of Actuaries and Association of Life Insurance Medical Directors of America.*
*Note: Prepared by Metropolitan Life Insurance Company.*
**Not calculated because of insufficient data in 1959.*

products. It requires the enzyme lactase for its digestion. People with lactose intolerance produce too little lactase for the complete digestion of lactose.

LACTOSE INTOLERANCE

Symptoms of lactose intolerance occur within fifteen minutes to several hours after an individual consumes more lactose than their lactase supply can handle. The reaction produced can be very painful, and some people with very low levels of lactase report that drinking milk makes them feel like a total intestinal revolt is taking place. Symptoms of lactose intolerance include bloating, diarrhea, gas, and cramps. These symptoms are all related to the effects of undigested lactose. Free lactose in the large intestine is a favorite food of bacteria that reside there. Unfortunately, bacteria don't completely break down lactose, either. When bacteria in our large intestine consume lactose, they excrete fat particles and gases. The gas accumulates and causes cramps and diarrhea.

Not all of the side effects associated with lactose intolerance are considered undesirable—at least they aren't by one researcher:

> Although we think of lactose intolerance as a cause of distressing symptoms, some degree of incomplete absorption of carbohydrates is not only common, but also desirable. In our constipated society, it may be ingestion of milk and other sources of poorly absorbed carbohydrates that keeps us regular.[71]

Most lactose-intolerant individuals can consume small amounts of milk and milk products because they produce some lactase. Many can tolerate aged cheese and fermented or cultured milk products, such as yogurt and buttermilk, because the lactose has been partially broken down during processing. Lactase-treated milk and the enzyme lactase are commercially available and are becoming popular products in the United States among people with lactose intolerance. Lactase-treated milk tastes a little differently than regular milk—it's sweeter. The lactose in treated milk has been converted to glucose and galacatose, which are sweeter tasting than lactose.

It's important that people with lactose intolerance consume foods with adequate amounts of calcium, such as lactase-treated milk. Studies have shown that they are at risk of consuming too little calcium and are more likely to develop osteoporosis than people without this intolerance.[72]

# Chapter 8

## *What Works for Weight Control*

*"Linda, did you just say you wanted to lose some weight? It happens I know about a terrific diet. A couple of months ago, I went on Dr. Smith's Amino Acid Diet and lost twenty pounds! You eat nothing but fish, papaya, and broccoli and the pounds just drip off!"*

*Linda was shocked. Kathy didn't look any lighter than when she last saw her. "But Kathy," Linda inquired, "what happened to the weight you lost?" Kathy's reply: "Oh, I gained it back."*

*Both Kathy and Linda were silent for a few seconds while the same thought ran through their heads. "Fish, papaya, and broccoli for a couple of months and then you get to gain the weight back. Why do we let ourselves in for that kind of dietary torture?"*

*"There's got to be a better way," said Linda. "You've got that right," Kathy replied. "I want the next diet I go on to be the last."*

▼ Does this conversation have the ring of reality? Women are surrounded by popular weight-loss books, articles, and advice. But the vast majority of the revolutionary-breakthrough-really-works diets are missing the one crucial element: they don't help you keep the weight off.

Any approach to weight loss (and some get pretty spectacular) that calls for a reduction in caloric intake can produce weight loss. It's not the gimmicks, the special fat-burning or appetite-suppressing foods that are allowed, or the herbal tablets that cause weight to be lost. It's the low-calorie diet that's hidden behind the gimmicks. The approaches crumble under the burden of scientific proof required to show that they work in the long run. Many don't even pass the safety test. Diets are sometimes so bizarre that health can be compromised on the way to weight loss.

There is a "diet" that helps people more than it hurts. You won't see it in paperback at your local bookstore, however. It's the weight-control plan favored by those who know that weight loss is 1 percent of the issue and weight maintenance the remaining 99 percent.

## THE SENSIBLE DIET

Although the title is not very catchy, the sensible diet is still the preferred approach to weight loss and control. Sensible diets are like sensible shoes. They aren't very flashy but they're better for you in the long run.

The basic components of the sensible diet are:

- Eating to satisfy hunger, not other needs
- Maintaining a regular eating schedule (no fasts or skipped meals)
- Paying more attention to food portion sizes than to calories
- Increasing physical activity
- Not torturing yourself—being able to live with the diet chosen.

The people who choose to follow this type of recipe for weight control are often the most successful at losing weight and keeping it off.[1]

### *Separating Hunger and Appetite*

Separating hunger from appetite is a key ingredient of the sensible approach to weight control. When you are hungry, you feel physical pain, or "hunger pangs," in your stomach. The feeling goes away within several minutes after you start eating. Appetite is in your head and not your stomach. It's a desire for food and the pleasure it brings. Appetite may stay with you even after you've eaten. Many events can trigger appetite: stress, the thought or sight of food, or even reading about it. Separating appetite from hunger and limiting food intake to times when you are hungry can make a substantial dent in caloric intake.

*Keep to the Meal Plan*

It appears that many people start diets in the morning—and then go off them by early afternoon. Although experience tells a different story, it seems to be widely thought that skipped meals won't be missed. This sort of impulsive dieting usually backfires. People get so hungry that they eat more following the skipped meals than they would had they eaten three portion-controlled, square meals and a snack. A regular eating pattern prevents ravenous hunger and the rebound eating that may follow it.

*The Smaller, the Better*

As a general rule, the smaller the changes in personal behavior required by a weight-control program, the greater the chance that the program will succeed. It is generally much easier to adjust to modest changes, such as reducing portion sizes of foods usually consumed or cutting down on fat, than it is to drastically change habits. Weight-loss programs that require major changes overnight are almost certain to fail. The closer the changes are to behaviors a person finds acceptable and can live with, the greater her sticking power. The sensible approach to weight control calls for small and acceptable changes in eating and physical activity habits.

Unlike the quick results promised by many weight-loss programs, the sensible diet is planned around a gradual weight loss of a pound or two a week. Diets that produce a higher rate of weight

IMPROVING EATING AND BEHAVIOR PATTERNS FOR WEIGHT CONTROL: SMALL CHANGES FOR LASTING EFFECTS

Separate hunger from the desire to eat. Eat when hungry.
Keep to a regular eating pattern. Don't skip meals.
Serve yourself smaller portion sizes and don't take second helpings.
Stop eating before you feel too full.
Increase your intake of vegetables and fruits you like.
Limit the availability of high-calorie snacks and desserts.
Roast, broil, or steam foods rather than fry them.
Select lean cuts of meat and low-fat dairy products.
Go easy on butter, margarine, sauces, and gravy.
Eat slowly. Give your stomach a chance to notify your brain about how much you've eaten.
Walk more.
Make a habit of using stairs whenever possible.
Make time to participate in your favorite sport more often.
If you watch TV, do floor exercises while you watch.

loss are generally so different from a person's usual diet that they are totally abandoned after weight loss is achieved. The reintroduction of old habits leads to a regain in weight.

Some people can successfully lose weight and maintain the loss by following the guides just given. However, other people do better if they start with a more structured plan. The next section gives a nuts-and-bolts approach to planning for weight loss and control.

### *The Calculating Sensible Diet*

You lose weight by consuming fewer calories than needed to maintain your current weight. You can estimate how many calories you need each day to maintain your current weight by identifying your activity status category.

- ☐ Inactive: Sitting most of the day, with less than two hours of moving about slowly or standing.
- ☐ Average activity: Sitting most of the day, walking or standing two to four hours each day, but not involved in strenuous activity.
- ☐ Active: Physically active four or more hours each day, little sitting or standing, involved in some physically strenuous activities.

If you classify as physically *inactive*, multiply your weight in pounds by 13. The result is approximately the number of calories you need to maintain your weight. For example, if you weigh 160 pounds, the number of calories roughly needed to maintain your weight is: 160 × 13 = *2,080*. If you are moderately active, then you should multiple your weight by 15.5, and if very active by 18.2, to calculate calories needed to maintain weight. Since a deficit of about 3,500 calories is needed to produce a pound of weight loss, if you consume 500 fewer calories than needed for 7 days, you would achieve a loss of about a pound a week. If you were to cut back by 750 calories per day, you'd lose about a 1½ pounds per week. It should be pointed out that calories expended by increasing physical activity count toward the calorie deficit. So, instead of consuming 750 fewer calories per day, you could, for example, increase energy expenditure by 200 calories per day and only reduce intake by 550 calories. See the accompanying list of the caloric value of a wide variety of activities.

Once you have reached your weight-loss goal, you can maintain that weight by consuming the level of calories needed for someone

AVERAGE ENERGY OUTPUT PER POUND OF BODY WEIGHT FOR VARIOUS TYPES OF EXERCISES

| *Exercise* | *Calories/lb/hr* |
|---|---|
| Walking | |
| 3 mph (20 min/mi.) | 1.6 |
| 3½ mph (17 min/mi.) | 1.8 |
| 4 mph (15 min/mi.) | 2.7 |
| 4½ mph (13 min/mi.) | 2.9 |
| Jogging | |
| 5 mph (12 min/mi.) | 4.1 |
| 5½ mph (11 min/mi.) | 4.5 |
| 6 mph (10 min/mi.) | 4.9 |
| 7 mph (8½ min/mi.) | 5.2 |
| Running | |
| 8 mph (7½ min/mi.) | |
| 8½ mph (7 min/mi.) | 6.7 |
| 9 mph (6⅔ min.mi.) | 7.1 |
| 9½ mph (6⅓ min/mi.) | 7.4 |
| 10 mph (6 min/mi.) | 7.8 |
| 11 mph (5½ min/mi.) | 8.5 |
| 12 mph (5 min/mi.) | 9.5 |
| Rebound trampoline | |
| 50–60 steps/min. | 4.1 |
| Cycling (stationary) | |
| mild effort | 2.9 |
| moderate effort | 3.4 |
| vigorous effort | 4.3 |
| Cycling (level) | |
| 6 mph (10 min/mi.) | 1.5 |
| 8 mph (7½ min/mi.) | 1.8 |
| 10 mph (6 min/mi.) | 2.0 |
| 12 mph (5 min/mi.) | 2.8 |
| 15 mph (4 min/mi.) | 3.9 |
| 20 mph (3 min/mi.) | 5.7 |
| Skating | 2.9 |
| Wrestling | 6.2 |
| Handball | |
| moderate | 4.8 |
| vigorous | 6.2 |
| Swimming | |
| resting strokes | 1.4 |
| 20 yd/min. (mod.) | 2.9 |
| 40 yd/min. (vig.) | 4.8 |
| Rowing | |
| sculling or machine | 4.8 |
| Downhill skiing | 3.8 |
| Cross-country skiing (level) | |
| 4 mph (15 min/mi.) | 4.3 |
| 6 mph (10 min/mi.) | 5.7 |
| 8 mph (7½ min/mi.) | 6.7 |
| 10 mph (6 min/mi.) | 7.6 |
| Aerobic Dancing | |
| moderate | 3.4 |
| vigorous | 4.8 |
| Raquetball/Squash | |
| moderate | 3.4 |
| vigorous | 4.3 |
| Tennis | |
| moderat | 3.4 |
| vigorous | 4.3 |
| Volleyball | |
| moderate | 3.4 |
| vigorous | 3.8 |

| Activity | |
|---|---|
| **Calisthenics** | |
| moderate | 2.4 |
| vigorous | 2.9 |
| **Rope skipping** | |
| moderate | 4.8 |
| **Bench stepping** | |
| 12'' high, 24 steps/min. | 3.2 |
| **Other** | |
| weight lifting | 2.9 |
| soccer/hill climbing | 5.3 |
| baseball/golf/woodcutting/ horseback riding/badminton/ canoeing | 2.4 |
| **Other (continued)** | |
| fencing/judo/snowshoeing/ bowling/archery/pool | 1.2 |
| **Basketball** | |
| moderate | 3.8 |
| vigorous | 4.3 |
| **Football** | |
| moderate | 3.8 |
| vigorous | 4.3 |

*Values calculated from:* Guidelines for Graded Exercise Testing and Exercise Prescription, *2d ed. American College of Sports Medicine, Philadelphia: Lea & Febiger, 1984.*

of your weight and activity level. For example, if you reach a goal of 130 pounds and are physically inactive, you should be able to maintain your weight by consuming 1,690 calories per day on average. By the time you reach your weight, you probably won't have to count calories. You'll know from experience when your diet is on track.

An example of a calculated, sensible weight-loss plan is shown below. The menus shown average 1,379 calories per day if the snacks listed are included and 1,262 calories if they are not. You'll notice that the menus provide a wide assortment of common foods that contribute to a balanced diet. For a person who maintains her weight with an intake of around 1,900 calories a day, adherence to the menus would lead to about a pound of weight loss per week. For some people who are tall or physically active, the menus shown would be too low in calories. Portion sizes would have to be increased to ensure a healthy and gradual weight loss.

*Don't Go Too Low on Calories*

Reducing caloric intake to below 1,200 calories per day is not advised for at least three reasons. First, it's nearly impossible to get the nutrients you need from food at such low levels of calories. Second, limiting food intake to very small amounts may represent too radical a departure from usual eating patterns to have much staying power.

EXAMPLE OF A SEVEN-DAY LOW-CALORIE MENU

*Average calorie level: Including snacks: 1,379*

*Excluding snacks: 1,262*

*(Caloric value of food is given in parentheses.)*

| | DAY 1 | DAY 2 |
|---|---|---|
| Meal 1 | Orange juice, 6 ounces (85)<br>Cheerios, 1 ounce (97)<br>Whole wheat bread, 1 slice (65)<br>Margarine, 1 teaspoon (35)<br>Skim milk, 1 cup (90) | Cantaloupe, ¼ whole (50)<br>Bran flakes, 1 cup (127)<br>English muffin, 1 (138)<br>Margarine, 1 teaspoon (35)<br>Skim milk, 1 cup (90) |
| Meal 2 | Hamburger (lean), 3 ounces (190)<br>Bun, 1 (112)<br>Tomato, ½ (13)<br>Skim milk, 1 cup (90) | Bean soup, 1 cup (170)<br>Crackers, 4 pieces (50)<br>Ham, 1 ½ ounces (96)<br>Rye bread, 1 slice (65)<br>Mustard, 1 teaspoon (4)<br>Skim milk, 1 cup (90) |
| Meal 3 | Baked chicken (no skin), 3 ounces (164)<br>Peas, ½ cup (60)<br>Macaroni, ½ cup (98)<br>Skim milk, 1 cup (90)<br>Margarine, 1 teaspoon (35) | Chow mein, 1 cup (95)<br>Rice, ½ cup (113)<br>Fortune cookie, 1 (43)<br>Tea, 1 cup (0) |
| | Calories before snack: 1,224 | 1,166 |
| Snack | Banana (100) | Peanuts, 1 ounce (165) |
| | Calories including snack: 1,324 | 1,331 |

| | DAY 3 | DAY 4 |
|---|---|---|
| Meal 1 | Peanut butter, 1 tablespoon (190)<br>Whole wheat bread, 1 slice (130)<br>Orange, 1 (80)<br>Skim milk, 1 cup (90) | Orange juice, 6 ounces (85)<br>Bran muffin, 1 (100)<br>Margarine, 1 teaspoon (35)<br>Skim milk, 1 cup (90) |

| | | |
|---|---|---|
| Meal 2 | Chef's salad, 2 cups (285) (includes 1 ounce of ham, turkey, and cheese, 1½ cups of lettuce, ½ egg)<br>Salad dressing, 1 tablespoon (130)<br>Skim milk, 1 cup (90) | Vegetable-beef soup, 1 cup (80)<br>Turkey, 3 ounces (150)<br>Mayonnaise, 1 teaspoon (30)<br>White bread, 2 slices (140)<br>Skim milk, 1 cup (90) |
| Meal 3 | Baked chicken (no skin), 3 ounces (163)<br>Sweet potatoes, ½ cup (117)<br>Green beans, ½ cup (15)<br>Skim milk, 1 cup (90) | Spaghetti, ½ cup (95)<br>Tomato sauce, ½ cup (43)<br>Meatballs, 1 (159)<br>Corn, ½ cup (70)<br>Roll, 1 (112)<br>Margarine, 1 teaspoon (35)<br>Tea, 1 cup (0) |
| | Calories before snack: 1,380 | 1,314 |
| Snack | Fudgesicle, 1 (91) | Low-fat yogurt, 1 cup (145) |
| | Calories including snack: 1,471 | 1,459 |

| | DAY 5 | DAY 6 |
|---|---|---|
| Meal 1 | Orange juice, 6 ounces (85)<br>Cornflakes, 1 cup (95)<br>Whole wheat toast, 1 slice (65)<br>Margarine, 1 teaspoon (35)<br>Skim milk, 1 cup (90) | Pineapple juice, 6 ounces (105)<br>Low-fat yogurt, 1 cup (145)<br>Graham cracker, 1 (55) |
| Meal 2 | Low-fat cottage cheese, ½ cup (81)<br>Peaches, ½ cup (75)<br>Grapes, 10 pieces (35)<br>Roll, 1 (112)<br>Margarine, 1 teaspoon (35)<br>Iced tea, 1 cup (0) | Hamburger (lean), 3 ounces (190)<br>Bun, 1 (112)<br>Catsup, 1 Tablespoon (15)<br>Coleslaw, ½ cup (59)<br>Skim milk, 1 cup (90) |

| | | |
|---|---|---|
| Meal 3 | Lettuce, 1 cup (6)<br>French dressing, 1 tablespoon (65)<br>Beef (lean), 3 ounces (220)<br>Peas, ½ cup (55)<br>Roll, 1 (112)<br>Margarine, 1 teaspoon (35)<br>Skim milk, 1 cup (90) | Tomato soup, 1 cup (90)<br>Macaroni and cheese, ½ cup (215)<br>Spinach (cooked), ½ cup (20)<br>Beets, ½ cup (30)<br>Margarine, 1 teaspoon (35)<br>Skim milk, 1 cup (90) |
| | Calories before snack: 1,291 | 1,251 |
| Snack | Apple, 1 (80) | Sherbet, ½ cup (134) |
| | Calories including snack: 1,371 | 1,385 |

DAY 7

Meal 1
Orange juice, 6 ounces (85)
Poached egg, 1 (80)
Whole wheat toast, 1 slice (65)
Margarine, 1 teaspoon (35)
Skim milk, 1 cup (90)

Meal 2
Chicken salad, 1 cup (254)
Whole wheat crackers, 4 (64)
Pineapple, ½ cup (95)
Skim milk, 1 cup (90)

Meal 3
Pork (lean), 3 ounces (201)
Noodles, ½ cup (95)
Broccoli, ½ cup (20)
Margarine, 1 teaspoon (35)
Tea, 1 cup (0)

Calories before snack: 1,209

Snack
Pear, 1 (100)

Calories including snack: 1,309

The third reason has to do with why some people have to "eat like a bird" to lose weight. The practice of going on and off very low-calorie diets may lower your basal metabolic rate by 10 to 30 percent and cause your body to burn fewer calories. That makes it easier to gain weight on relatively low caloric intakes.[2]

### *A Plug for Physical Activity*

Weight-control efforts that include a physical activity program offer several bonuses. Exercise can help burn off calories and contribute to weight loss and to weight control in the long run. Muscular bodies require more calories for metabolism than fatter bodies. Regular exercise improves circulation, stamina, and often a person's alertness and feeling of well-being. It may also decrease appetite. Obese women who get involved in exercise tend to have less appetite and a lower food intake than those who don't exercise.

### *Dieting for Dollars: An Examination of Popular Approaches to Weight Loss*

There are a lot of people in the United States who want to lose weight, and most of them are women. On any given day, about 46 percent of all U.S. women are dieting.[3] We want to lose weight quickly, painlessly, and permanently. It hasn't seemed to strike most U.S. dieters yet that popular approaches to weight loss don't work very long. Many people are so anxious about their weight that they appear to be much more interested in getting it off than keeping it off. Admittedly, most of the popular diets that hit the market do help people lose weight. As a nation, people lose millions of

FOODS THAT REALLY DO HAVE CALORIES: A TONGUE-IN-CHEEK REPORT

Cookie pieces
Food "sampled" when you're preparing a meal
Food that doesn't taste very good
Candy, popcorn, soft drinks consumed in a movie theater
Foods eaten while discussing weight-control diets
Foods you grab and eat on-the-run
Alcohol-containing drinks
Foods eaten along with grapefruit or a diet soda
Foods eaten directly from their storage container
Foods you eat when you're not thinking about eating

pounds every year while following popular diets. The problem is that the weight is not really lost. It's found again. If popular diets worked, new ones wouldn't keep popping up on the market.

A number of popular schemes and last-ditch approaches to weight loss are presented here. As you read through them, ask yourself two questions: Are extreme changes in eating behavior required? Is exercise omitted from the plan? If the answer to either of these questions is yes, then the approach lacks a key ingredient for weight-loss maintenance.

*Approach #1: Weight-Loss "Diets"*

Examples include:

Beverly Hills Diet
Dr. Stillman's Diet
Grapefruit Diet
Protein-Sparing Modified Fast
High-Fiber Diet
Last-Chance Diet
Hogwash

Popular weight-loss diets generally have several features in common that give them away.

A GIMMICK

The gimmick separates a new book from those that preceded it. It is often advertised as the "unique" ingredient of the approach offered and provides the reason why the diet works whereas the others have failed. Gimmicks used in the past have included:

The Grapefruit Gimmick—grapefruit "burns up fat."

The High-Carbohydrate Gimmick—it improves your mood so you're happier and won't eat so much.

The High-Protein Gimmick—it spares your muscles while using up your fat.

The Doctor Gimmick—the book was written by a doctor, so it must be good.

There are many others.

QUICK RESULTS

Can you imagine a weight-loss book selling if it promised "slow" results? It has to be quick or it may not seem worth it.

EASY TO DO

Popular diets frequently offer black-and-white advice that is highly structured. It's generally simple to follow but impossible to live with.

CALORIE CUT-BACK

All of the popular diets include the feature of being low in calories. Although this component of the approach may be overshadowed by the gimmick presented, it is the reason people lose weight if they follow the book's advice.

### *Approach #2: Fasting*

The most extreme type of weight-loss diet is fasting. It can either be a total fast, in which only water is allowed, or a partial fast that includes several hundred calories a day. Either type should be undertaken only in a hospital with medical supervision.

Obese people can, and have, lost a tremendous amount of weight by fasting. It appears to be worth the effort and expense when used to get a person's weight down so that required surgery can be performed. People who have lost large amounts of weight by fasting have reported that it is easier to get a job and to increase their earnings than before they fasted.[4]

Although there may be benefits, there is one major problem that plagues this and other approaches. It is the problem of regaining weight. Fasting does not correct the underlying causes of a person's obesity and it is not effective in preventing a rebound in body weight. Most people who lose weight by fasting regain all or most of the weight back within two to three years.[4]

THE LIQUID-PROTEIN DIET

*Haste makes waist.*

In the mid-seventies, a "liquid-protein" diet made from the incomplete protein collagen (also known as gelatin) was sold over-the-counter for weight loss. Despite promotional claims for this product, body protein was not spared from use as an energy source among people on the diet and muscle protein was used to supply the essential amino acids that people needed. The protein quality of gelatin is too low to support protein tissue construction in the body. Women who used the liquid-protein diet lost muscle mass, including that from the heart. Although the diet was often undertaken under the supervision of a doctor, by early 1978 at least fifty-eight deaths occurred among women who had been on the diet for three months. The exact causes of death aren't known, but excessive use of the heart muscle as a source of protein may have played a role.[5] Liquid-protein diets are no longer recommended for use, even while being monitored by a physician.

#### PROTEIN-SPARING MODIFIED FAST (PSMF)

The PSMF approach to weight loss is relatively new. This approach utilizes very low-calorie formulas that include approximately 400 calories as high-quality protein and 200 to 400 calories worth of carbohydrates and fat. By including high-quality protein and some carbohydrates and fat, the PSMF diet was supposed to avoid the loss of muscle mass that occurred with the liquid-protein diet. Because it now appears that it does not, it is only recommended for use for short periods of time (three to four weeks) by severely overweight people, under medical supervision.[6,7]

Protein-sparing modified fast formulas and similar products can be purchased over-the-counter (Slim Fast™), through distributors (the Cambridge Diet™ and Genesis™), and through medically supervised sources (Optifast™, for example). This type of diet should not be used by the vast majority of overweight Americans; it has been recommended that they should not be made directly available to the public.[6,7]

### *Approach #3: Organized Weight-Loss Programs*

Group approaches to weight loss are widely available in the United States and Europe. Programs such as Overeaters Anonymous®, TOPS® (Take Off Pounds Sensibly), and WeightWatchers® tend to offer reasonably balanced low-calorie diets as well as group support and encouragement for weight loss. Some group programs are beginning to emphasize exercise and positive behavioral changes as core components of their approach. Their primary negative is the lack of scientific data that shows their approaches help people keep the weight off.

### *Approach #4: Drugs for Weight Loss*

Pills are easier to swallow than most weight-loss diets. We have pills that can cure an infection, rid us of headaches, and take the worry out of sex. Why isn't there one that can fix obesity? There isn't because the "cure" for obesity is a long-term change in eating and activity patterns. People, not pills, have to do that.

Several types of pills that suppress appetite are available for sale over-the-counter. Most contain the chemical *phenylpropanolamine* (PPA). (Amphetamines were used in the past, but because of the high potential for addiction, they are no longer allowed for use in weight loss.) They may be effective in helping people lose weight for a few months, but then they lose their effectiveness. People who take diet pills may experience a rapid heartbeat, nervousness, irritability, insomnia, and other side effects. Diet pills have not been shown to be effective in preventing weight regain. They are one of the rhythm methods of girth control.

### *Approach #5: Surgery and Other Drastic Measures*

Included in this category of weight-loss approaches of last resort are jaw wiring, stomach balloons, and surgery.

Jaw wiring entails the partial closing of a person's jaw with wire so the mouth can't open very wide. Only enough of an opening is left so a person can drink with a straw. People who have their jaws wired have trouble speaking, sneezing, coughing, yawning, and keeping up good oral hygiene. Because they are at risk of choking, people with wired jaws are generally given pliers and taught how to undo them if they start to choke. So much for eliminating the chance to overeat. The opportunity to go off their liquid diets is only as far away as the pliers or liquids in the form of milk shakes.

Stomach balloons are actually rubber tubes that are inserted into a person's stomach. They reduce the amount of food the stomach can hold. Although effective in reducing food intake, stomach balloons are no longer used because they can be stretched and popped and because they may leave the stomach and form an obstruction in the intestines.

*Lipectomy* is a type of surgery that is intended to help normal-weight people "spot reduce" for cosmetic reasons. Also called liposuction, this method involves vacuuming out fat cells that cause undesirable bulges around the thighs, stomach, buttocks, or arms. It appears to keep people shapely only if they don't gain the fat back. If they overeat, fat will again accumulate in the fat cells that remain after liposuction and new fat cells may eventually form. Liposuction is a form of cosmetic surgery and is not recommended for weight control. It is a very expensive procedure.

In the past, surgery that reduced the length of the small intestine would be performed for weight loss. This type of surgery led to so many complications that it has been abandoned. The current, most common surgical approach for weight loss is a procedure called *stomach stapling* or *gastric bypass*.

Stomach stapling is usually reserved for the highest-risk, most stubborn cases of obesity. The procedure is generally restricted to people who weigh twice their normal weight or more and who, because of poorly controlled diabetes, joint problems, or other medical indication, would likely benefit from the procedure. Based on body weight, only 0.5 percent of U.S. women qualify for the surgery.[8]

The purpose of stomach stapling is to reduce the size of the stomach. By stapling closed around 90 percent of the stomach, people are only able to eat 1 or 2 tablespoons of food at a time. If people exceed this amount, especially in the first few months following surgery, they get sick to their stomachs. People who have had their stomachs stapled often find they are no longer able to tolerate certain foods such as meats, milks, breads, sweets, and fried foods. Their diets tend to be highly inadequate.

Food intake is drastically reduced by stomach stapling, and weight loss tends to be rapid during the first few months. By stretching the stomach with more food as time goes on, however, people can eat larger amounts of food and gain weight. One study reported food intake to increase from an average of 745 calories per day three months after surgery to 1,089 calories after a year.[9] Weight loss tends to plateau after a year and most people regain some of the weight that was lost.[10] Two years after surgery, however, people still tend to weigh less than their presurgery weight.[11]

Surgery and other drastic measures of weight loss may be particularly attractive to obese people who have repeatedly had little success losing weight by dieting. Stomach stapling, jaw wiring, or stomach balloons may be viewed as their only chance to lose weight. According to Dr. Philip White, formerly a nutrition expert with the American Medical Association, this situation makes for a good deal of abuse. White has noted that these radical approaches keep obesity specialists busy treating over 10 million patients and billing at a level of 1 to 2 billion dollars annually.

# Chapter 9

## *Women Sweat: Nutrition, Physical Fitness, and Performance*

*per•spi•ra•tion (pûr' spərā'shən), n. 1. the act or process of perspiring. Syn.* SWEAT. *Refers primarily to moisture extruded from the pores of the skin.* PERSPIRATION *is the more refined and elegant word, and is often used overfastidiously by those who consider* SWEAT *coarse; but* SWEAT *is a strong word and in some cases obviously more appropriate.*

Random House Dictionary, Unabridged, *1979, p. 1075*

▼ Women sweat. Thank goodness, it's in fashion. Exercise and sweating are good for women at all ages and stages. It's one of the most important things we can do to take care of ourselves, yet it is as likely to take the form of a good intention as reality. This chapter aims to charge the batteries of women who are sitting on the fence. For the seasoned athlete, the chapter attempts to provide facts and figures that will broaden current understanding of nutrition, fitness, and performance. It looks at the benefits of nutrition and physical fitness, aerobic conditioning, glycogen loading, protein and performance, "magic bullets," what to eat before and during strenuous events, and sports drinks. Perhaps the best place to be while you read this chapter is on an exercise bicycle, sweating.

### THE BENEFITS OF PHYSICAL FITNESS: A PRELUDE TO THE FACTS

Remember hearing the parental order: "Go outside and play." That has been shown to be excellent advice for both children and adults. Our parents were on to something. For most children *playing* means physical activity, and our parents knew that was good for us. Unfortunately, the play we thoroughly enjoyed as children often turns out to be a chore later on. Maybe it's because we're too rushed and run low on energy. Or, maybe we run low on energy because we're too rushed and physically inactive. We forget how to play.

The benefits of physical fitness that have been studied concern health. But there's another, important benefit that hasn't been the subject of research. It's getting to play again—to skate, run, ski, sled, swim, or jump rope—and remembering how much fun that is.

## THE BENEFITS OF PHYSICAL FITNESS: THE FACTS

Regular physical activity, like a balanced diet, reduces a person's chances of developing heart disease, hypertension, diabetes, osteoporosis, and obesity. It can reduce the symptoms of depression and anxiety, and help people cope with stress. Exercise improves circulation, helps to increase HDL-cholesterol, and increases caloric need, which means you can eat more and wear it less. You get all of this for the price of sweating while you play.

### *Getting Fit, Staying Fit*

There are two basic types of exercise that affect energy formation and fitness level: *aerobic* and *anaerobic*. Exercise fueled by energy-forming processes in the body that require oxygen are called aerobic. The body's source of stored fuel used to form energy in the presence of oxygen is fat. The body will use fat as the main source of energy for exercise as long as we can breathe in and deliver to our muscles enough oxygen to make energy from fat. Since most of our physical activity is light, fats serve as the primary source of energy for physical movement. When we exercise beyond our body's ability to deliver oxygen for energy formation from fat, the body switches to using glucose. Glucose, mainly obtained from the approximately 1,000-calorie store of glycogen in muscles, doesn't require the presence of oxygen to be converted into energy. It is used to fuel anaerobic (without oxygen) exercise. Intense activities of short duration, such as slamming on the brakes, sprinting, and tennis serving, cannot be supplied with energy from fats quickly enough. Glucose is used to fuel these bursts of muscular activity.

You know when you've relied too much on glucose for energy formation—or overdone vigorous exercise—when you wake up with stiff muscles. A by-product of overusing glucose for fuel is lactic acid. It accumulates in muscles that have used glucose extensively for energy formation and makes them feel stiff. The lactic acid buildup can take a day or two to disappear, depending on how much has accumulated.

THE TYPES OF ACTIVITIES FUELED PRIMARILY BY AEROBIC OR ANAEROBIC ENERGY FORMATION

| *Aerobic* *(With oxygen; energy source is fat)* | *Anaerobic* *(Without oxygen; energy source is glucose)* |
|---|---|
| Long-distance running | Sprinting |
| Long-distance swimming | High jumping |
| Jogging | Golf swinging |
| Walking | Weight lifting |
| Hiking/backpacking | Push-ups |
| Bicycling (level) | Pull-ups |
| Ice skating | Kicks |
| Basketball | Full court press |
| Tennis volleying | Tennis serving |
| Reading | Wrestling |
| Waiting | Diving |

### ANAEROBIC CONDITIONING

Since glycogen is the primary source of glucose used to fuel strenuous bursts of exercise, you can increase your endurance by increasing your stores of glycogen. You can approximately double your glycogen stores and substantially increase endurance with a moderately high-carbohydrate diet and physical training.[2]

During training, a diet that provides around 60 to 70 percent of total calories as carbohydrate leads to much higher levels of glycogen stores than does an average or low-carbohydrate diet.[4] It should be emphasized that dietary carbohydrates increase glycogen stores above normal levels when combined with a training program. During training, glycogen stores accumulate only in muscles that are exercised. This fact was demonstrated forcefully in a study where a subject was given a high-carbohydrate diet and then allowed to exercise only one leg on a stationary bicycle. The muscles in the leg that had done the work had increased glycogen stores, while the other didn't.[3] So glycogen stores will increase on a carbohydrate-rich diet only in the muscles that are used during the training program. That's a big part of the reason why coaches don't emphasize weight lifting for long-distance runners. Athletes are generally coached to exercise and develop the same muscles they use the most in their particular events.

It used to be thought that the best way to increase glycogen stores was to first deplete them with exercise and a low-carbohydrate diet, and then to eat a very high-carbohydrate diet for several days before an event. This method of glycogen loading works, but it produces too many undesirable side effects. So much glycogen may be stored by this approach that muscles become stiff from the excess glycogen. People who are superloading with glycogen feel heavy and tired. Muscle tissue may be lost by overloading them with glycogen, and chest pains and depression may also occur.[4] For these reasons and others, this traditional approach to glycogen loading is no longer recommended. It has been replaced with a safer method that effectively increases glycogen stores and endurance. This method calls for consuming an above-average amount of carbohydrates during training along with a well-balanced diet. The diet should provide between 60 and 70 percent of total calories as carbohydrates, rather than the usual level of around 50 percent. The food sources of the carbohydrates should be mainly breads, pastas, rice, cereal, and starchy vegetables like potatoes and squash, rather than sweets or sweetened beverages. This type of diet should be maintained up to the time of the event, but the intensity of training should be tapered off a few days before a competition.[5]

Glycogen loading can be a safe way to increase glycogen stores while allowing for the selection of a balanced variety of foods. Because diets that supply 60 to 70 percent of total calories as carbohydrate tend to be low in animal products (which, with the exception of skim milk, are poor sources of carbohydrates), the diet may be low in iron, zinc, and vitamin $B_{12}$. These nutrients are primarily supplied by meats. The menu shown on the facing page, for example, is a bit low in zinc (it provides 88 percent of the RDA for women). It contains adequate amounts of the other nutrients with RDAs, however. Care should be taken to eat a variety of foods while following a moderately high-carbohydrate diet.

### AEROBIC CONDITIONING

The primary goals of aerobic conditioning, or aerobic fitness, are to increase your body's ability to deliver oxygen to muscle cells and to use fats as a fuel source. The extent to which this happens is measured by ***maximal oxygen consumption***. (You may see this term abbreviated as "$VO_2$ max.") Maximal oxygen consumption is the highest amount of oxygen a person can deliver to her muscles for use in energy formation. When we reach that level, we are no longer able to fuel increases in activity with fat, and have to switch to glucose. Aerobic conditioning increases maximal oxygen consumption by expanding the network of blood vessels that infiltrate muscle tissues. It also conditions the heart to deliver a larger

A HIGH CARBOHYDRATE DIET
(Carbohydrates make up 68% of the 2,420 calories provided in the foods listed; protein accounts for 11% and fat 21% of total calories.)

*Breakfast*

Orange juice, 1 cup
Oatmeal, 1 cup
Brown sugar, 1 T.
Skim milk, 1 cup
Banana, 1

*Snack*

Granola, ½ cup
Apple juice, 1 cup

*Lunch*

Tossed salad, 1 cup
Salad dressing, 1 T.
Macaroni and cheese, 1 cup
Crackers, 4 squares
Sliced tomato, ½
Skim milk, 1 cup

*Dinner*

Spanish rice, 1 cup
Baked potato, 1
Corn, ½ cup
Apple crisp, ½ cup
Iced tea, 2 cups

*Snack*

Cornflakes, 1 cup
Peaches, ½ cup
Skim milk, 1 cup

amount of blood with every beat. Consequently, with aerobic conditioning, more oxygen is delivered to muscles and more fat is used for energy formation than before. The net effect is that you can exercise longer and harder because you can get additional energy from fat. This type of training program is commonly recommended for athletes who undertake endurance events, as well as for dieters and people who have had heart attacks. You should get your health care provider's okay before beginning an aerobic training program. The activity program described below may be overstrenuous for some people with heart or kidney disease or other health problems.

COMPONENTS OF AN AEROBIC FITNESS PROGRAM

Most programs oriented toward improving aerobic fitness emphasize exercises that maintain a person's heart rate for about thirty minutes at a particular level. The desired heart rate is usually calculated as 60 percent of *maximum heart rate* for beginners, and as 70 to 85 percent of maximum for people who are physically fit. Maximum heart rate is the highest number of beats per minute that doesn't overly strain the heart. It is frequently estimated at 220 minus a person's age in years. Estimates of 60 percent and 80 percent of maximum heart rates for people of various ages is given in Table 38. People involved in aerobic exercise are advised to monitor their heart rate occasionally to see if it is close to the target rate. You can calculate your heart rate by counting the number of heart beats, or pulses you feel with a finger *gently* pressed on the front side of your neck or the inside of your wrist for ten seconds. By multiplying that number by 6, you get your heart rate per minute. You can often tell how aerobically fit a person is by how fast their heart beats at rest and during exercise. Many seasoned long-distance runners have resting heart rates that are at least twenty beats per minute less than the average of seventy to eighty beats per minute. Aerobic fitness is usually achieved by a regular program of moderate exercise that maintains heart rate at the target level for thirty minutes, three to five times per week.[4]

### PROTEIN AND PERFORMANCE: IS THERE A MATCH?

Muscles contain a lot of protein, right? So, if you eat a high-protein diet, you'll make more muscles, right? These two *rights* add up to a *wrong*. And here's why.

The body needs a certain amount of protein when muscle cells are forming and when the cells are increasing in size. How much protein we eat in excess of the required level in no way affects how many muscle cells we have or how big they are. The protein content of diets of most people in the United States far exceeds the level required to develop muscle cells. The only way muscle size can be increased (short of the very dangerous use of steroid hormones) is to exercise them on a regular basis. Exercise programs that emphasize muscle development increase the size and strength of muscle cells, but not their numbers. Body-building exercises work because they make muscle cells larger and therefore muscles become stronger.

High-protein diets and protein supplements may have a negative effect on performance. High-protein foods such as meat and dairy products tend to be high in fat and low in glycogen-forming carbohydrates. High protein intake prior to an event increases the body's requirement for water, making dehydration a more likely possibility during exercise than if less protein is consumed. It is clear that high-protein diets and supplements should not be given a second thought by athletes. An adequate diet that provides ample amounts of carbohydrates for glycogen stores and a weight-training program are the actions that give the biggest payoff for endurance during strenuous exercise and muscle strengthening.

TABLE 38. AGE-PREDICTED MAXIMUM HEART RATE ADJUSTED FOR PEOPLE GETTING AEROBICALLY FIT AND THOSE WHO ARE

| AGE IN YEARS | MAXIMUM HEART RATE | BEGINNER 60% OF MAXIMUM | EXPERIENCED 80% OF MAXIMUM |
|---|---|---|---|
| 15 | 205 | 123 | 164 |
| 18 | 202 | 121 | 162 |
| 20 | 200 | 120 | 160 |
| 22 | 198 | 119 | 158 |
| 24 | 196 | 118 | 157 |
| 30 | 190 | 114 | 152 |
| 40 | 180 | 108 | 144 |
| 50 | 170 | 102 | 136 |
| 60 | 160 | 90 | 128 |

*Magic Bullets or a Bunch of Hooey?*

| | |
|---|---|
| Wheat germ oil | Vitamin E |
| Bee pollen | Royal jelly |
| Enzyme supplements | B-complex vitamins |
| Honey | Vitamin C |

Can women look to any of these to improve physical performance? The promoters of these and similar types of products would like you to think so, and many athletes believe in them. But none of these products has been shown to improve physical performance. There is no hard evidence to suggest that vitamin or mineral supplements improve athletic performance in people without nutrient deficiencies. However, if a woman is deficient in vitamin C or iron, for example, improving intake or taking supplements does remove the problem that was hindering performance in the first place.

*Pre-Event Meals*

What the body needs before an event are foods that are low in fat and high in carbohydrates. Carbohydrates spend the least amount of time in the stomach and are the most readily digested of the energy nutrients. High-fat foods such as steak, hot dogs, pizza, and hamburgers take longer to digest and may still be in the stomach when the event begins.

Pre-event meals should be eaten about two hours before the activity and highlight foods such as cereal, muffins, breads, potatoes, fruit, and juices. These light foods are much less likely to cause stomach upsets and cramping during and after an event than a steak-type of meal. Athletes feel and perform better on high-carbohydrate pre-event meals.[4]

### *Eating between Events*

For events such as swim meets, play-offs, and track and field meets, athletes have to participate in several competitions a day. To keep going, they need to eat between events. Carbohydrates are once again the food of choice. Crackers, fruit, cereals, breads, and juices are good examples of foods that "go down easy" and help keep your energy level up between events.

### *What about Sports Drinks?*

The best sports drink yet discovered is water. For most athletic events, it is all that is needed. Physical performance is improved if athletes remain hydrated, that is, maintain normal levels of body water, during exercise. Once the body starts to run low on water, fatigue and weakness set in and performance suffers. Water should be consumed before, during, and after exercise. Particular care should be taken to drink enough water when exercise is prolonged or takes place in hot weather. Very long events, such as marathon races, may deplete your body's reserves of sodium, potassium, and other minerals. In that case, a fruit juice or a low-sugar sports drink may be needed to replace the losses. Salt tablets, however, are no longer recommended.

## EXERCISE DURING PREGNANCY

Is exercise during pregnancy a good idea? There appears to be a simple answer to this question, but it's qualified. The answer is *yes*. The qualifications are:

Exercise should not be too vigorous. It should not exceed the level of exercise called for in a moderate, aerobic fitness program, and should be initiated gradually. (Or, moderate-intensity exercise three times a week for thirty minutes a time. That means a pregnant woman should not exercise to the point of exhaustion.) Exercising too vigorously may divert a woman's blood supply away from the uterus and baby and to the exercising muscles. Physical activity level during pregnancy is too high if it interferes with achieving the recommended amount of weight gain.

The types of exercise should be limited to those that don't jolt the fetus. The baby is cushioned quite securely inside the womb, but it may be harmed if it is physically pressured by activities such as vigorous horseback riding, deep-sea diving, high jumping, and contact sports. Tennis, swimming, walking, jogging, calisthenics, and aerobic dance of low to moderate intensity are good exercise choices for pregnant women.

As pregnancy progresses, the change in a woman's center of gravity calls for caution in exercising. It is easier to lose your balance and fall when you're not used to having more weight in the front of your body than usual. Many formerly pregnant women have stories to tell about how they lost their balance and slipped or tripped during the later part of pregnancy. Changes in balance can take you by surprise. Using handrails and nonslip shoes and boots may help to avoid accidents caused by the shifts in your center of gravity.

Some evidence suggests that maintaining or improving one's level of aerobic fitness during pregnancy may decrease the duration of labor. Women who are physically fit may be better able to withstand this Olympic-caliber event and recover more quickly than women in poor shape.

# Chapter 10

## *When Slimness Is Everything: Eating Disorders*

*Mary was raised by her grandmother and parents on a prosperous ranch on the outskirts of a small town. Her grandmother had a domineering personality and was very influential in guiding and directing Mary's development. Although Mary got along very well with her parents, she felt ignored by her father and unprotected by her mother from the grandmother's demands.*

*Mary showed no signs of an eating disorder until her fourteenth year. That year she had gained some weight and was heavier than many of her classmates. Weighing 120 pounds, she would occasionally be teased by classmates about being "chubby." Mary's response was to withdraw from her friends and to stay away from social events. She made it her full-time job to excel in school work—and to lose weight.*

*As time went on, Mary ate less and less. Within five months, her weight had dropped from 120 to 85 pounds. She would exercise every chance she got. When seen by a doctor ten months after she started to lose weight, Mary weighed 72 pounds and looked nearly starved to death. Although she felt tired all the time and depressed, she continued to maintain her rigorous diet and exercise program. Mary was referred to a psychologist and was diagnosed as having anorexia nervosa.*

*During psychological counseling, it was revealed that Mary deeply resented the lack of attention she got from her parents. She felt she had little control over her life and could not live up to the high expectations of her grandmother. One of the few things Mary had absolute control over was her weight. There was nothing the grandmother could do about that!*

*After counseling and several episodes of gaining and losing weight during adolescence, Mary stabilized her weight at a near-normal level. Spending more time with her parents and gaining independence from her grandmother's demands helped her get past anorexia nervosa.*[1]

▼ Twenty years ago, many nutrition books devoted no more than a paragraph to the subject of eating disorders. Although they have been known to have serious side effects on health for some time, these disorders were considered rare and of passing interest. This is no longer the case. Anorexia nervosa and bulimia, the two major eating disorders, are becoming increasingly common in the United States.[2] It is estimated that one in two hundred teenage girls have anorexia nervosa, and one in twenty teenage and young adult females have bulimia.[2,3] Between 30 and 40 percent of people with anorexia nervosa also show signs of bulimia.

Anorexia nervosa and bulimia are serious conditions that dramatically affect food intake, health, and well-being. Each appears to be the result of deeply rooted psychological disruptions, although physical conditions have not been entirely ruled out as contributing factors. They are conditions that develop during the teen or early adult years, but that may have roots starting as early as age seven.[4] Anorexia nervosa and bulimia are primarily disorders of females from upper-middle and upper-class families.[1] Females are nine times more likely to develop an eating disorder than males,[5] a situation that has been attributed to the greater pressure placed on females to be thin in our society.[6] Among females, professional dancers, dietetics majors, and women in careers that emphasize body size are at especially high risk for developing anorexia nervosa or bulimia.[7,8]

Characteristically, people with anorexia nervosa or bulimia are obsessed with the appearance of their bodies and preoccupied by thoughts of food, eating, and dieting.[5] No matter what their size, they think of themselves as fat. It's hard to believe when you see a person with anorexia that she could possibly think of herself that way. That she does is a good indication of how distorted body image is in people with eating disorders.

## ANOREXIA NERVOSA

People with anorexia nervosa are much more likely to be dangerously thin than are people with bulimia. They act as if they are unaware that the starving bodies they see in mirrors are actually theirs. To them, the mirror shows an overly fat person who must lose weight. In order to lose weight, people with anorexia will follow a strict, very low-calorie diet and exercise at nearly every opportunity. Most are fully informed about the caloric value of foods and will carefully avoid higher-calorie foods and sweets, as well as breads and pastas.[9]

One of the hallmarks of people with anorexia nervosa is their steadfast refusal to eat when offered food. Although preoccupied with eating and intentionally involved with food preparation for others, people with anorexia will deny they are hungry when presented with food. Their persistent refusal to eat is the symptom that causes most concern, frustration, and rage among parents and friends.[1]

Females with anorexia nervosa are generally described as "perfect" children by their parents. In school, they are usually well liked, achieve good grades, are obedient and respectful, athletic, and also stubborn. At home, they tend to be raised by parents who often have unreasonably high expectations for their performance and who are domineering in their control over their children's lives.[1] Rather than fostering self-confidence and independence, the parents of children with anorexia may be unduly critical of the child's performance and decisions. Although she may feel helpless in controlling large parts of her life, the person with anorexia nervosa has definite control over one area—her weight.

### *Consequences of Anorexia Nervosa*

The primary physical effects of anorexia nervosa are the same as those experienced during starvation. Heart rate, basal metabolism, and body temperature decrease; muscle tissue becomes a primary source of body energy; depression settles in; and a preoccupation with food and eating takes over. Growth and sexual maturation come to a halt, as do normal feelings of sexuality.[1] If the weight loss that accompanies anorexia nervosa is not reversed, the most devastating consequences of the disorder occur. Approximately 6 percent of people with anorexia nervosa starve to death.[10]

COMMON ACTIONS AND ATTITUDES OF A PERSON WITH ANOREXIA NERVOSA[7]

Prefers to eat alone
Prepares food for others but doesn't eat what is prepared
Is terrified about being overweight
Is preoccupied with thoughts of food and weight
Binges on occasion
Knows calorie content of foods
Feels "stuffed" after meals
Takes frequent weight measurements
Wakes up early in the morning
Thinks about burning up calories while exercising
Takes a long time to eat meals
Eats "diet" foods
Feels that food controls life
Gets constipated frequently
Regrets eating sweets or "fattening" foods
Feels an impulse to vomit after eating

### *Detecting and Treating It*

Psychotherapy that focuses on the correction of disturbed family interactions and improving a person's self-esteem and confidence level are the cornerstones of the treatment of anorexia nervosa. If these problems are resolved, normal nutrition and weight gain will often follow.[1] About half of people with anorexia recover completely with treatment and half don't. For those who don't recover but survive, the disorder continues well into their adult years.[10] The earlier anorexia nervosa is discovered and treated, the more likely it is that the condition will improve.

A questionnaire has been developed that is widely used to screen possible cases of the eating disorder.[7] It appears in condensed form here. The results, however, do not offer proof-positive that a person has anorexia nervosa; they are only suggestive.

## BULIMIA: THE BINGE-PURGE EATING DISORDER

Unlike people with anorexia nervosa, people with bulimia are often normal weight or slightly overweight, and the signs of bulimia usually don't appear until people are in their twenties or thirties. Instead of dieting constantly, people with bulimia tend to alternate between feasts (*binges*) and famine. During a food binge, a large amount of food is eaten in a short period of time. The foods chosen for binges are usually high-calorie foods such as ice cream, candy,

SNAPSHOT OF THREE DAYS OF FOOD INTAKE BY A PERSON WITH BULIMIA

*Background*: This dietary intake-purge record was submitted by a twenty-six-year-old female who weighs 120 pounds at 5'6".
**Foods in boldface were purged**.

| *Day 1* | *Day 2* | *Day 3* |
|---|---|---|
| | BREAKFAST | |
| Whole wheat toast, 1 piece | **Bread, 1 loaf** | **Bread, 1 loaf** |
| Margarine, 1 teaspoon | **Butter, 1/3 cup** | **Butter, 1/3 cup** |
| Low-cal jam, 1 teaspoon | **Jelly, 2/3 cup** | **Cookies, 1 bag** |
| Strawberries, 3 | **Milk, ? amount** | Apple, 1 |
| Pear, 1 | **Orange juice, ? amount** | Coffee, 1 cup |
| Skim milk, 1 cup | Coffee, 1 cup | |
| Orange juice, 1 cup | | |
| Coffee, 1 cup | | |
| Diet soda, 1 can | | |
| | LUNCH | |
| Minestrone soup, 1 cup | **Chinese food, lots** | **Cookies, 1 bag** |
| Crackers, 2 | **Donut holes, 12** | **M & M's, 1 bag** |
| Turkey and swiss sandwich, 1 with tomatoes, lettuce and mayonnaise | **Soft drinks, ? amount** | **Donut holes, ? amount** |
| Apple, 1 | **Cookies, ? amount** | **Milk, ? amount** |
| | | **Yogurt, ? amount** |
| | DINNER | |
| | **Ice cream, ? amount** | **Girl Scout cookies, ? amount** |
| | **Cookies, ? amount** | **Milk, ? amount** |
| | **Candy bars, ? amount** | **Soft drink, ? amount** |
| | **Soft drinks, ? amount** | **Ice cream, ? amount** |
| | **McDonalds, ? amount** | **Candy bars, ? amount** |
| | **Shakes, ? amount** | |
| | SNACKS | |
| **Butterfinger candy bar, 1** | Apple, 1 | Mixed vegetables, ? amount |
| **10,000 Dollar bar, 1** | Water | Orange juice, ? amount |
| **M & M's, 1 bag** | | |
| **Cookies, 1 bag** | | |
| **Ice cream, 1/2 gallon** | | |
| **Marshmallows, ? amount** | | |
| **Toast, ? amount** | | |
| **Milk, ? amount** | | |
| **Soft drink, ? amount** | | |
| **Orange juice, ? amount** | | |

chips, cookies, and other desserts or sweets. A snapshot of the diet of a woman attending a bulimia clinic appears below. The amounts of some of the foods listed as eaten during the binges were frequently not reported on the dietary record submitted. It is likely that the amounts weren't given a lot of attention during the binges. Although the binges are a source of enjoyment, they are usually followed by overwhelming feelings of guilt. Bulimics appear to have little control over their binges once they start.

Food binges by bulimics are generally followed by self-induced vomiting, laxative or diuretic use, or fasting to prevent weight gain. Of these, only self-induced vomiting successfully spares calories and it is the most common method employed.[11] Laxatives and diuretics may help with weight loss, but the loss is mainly from water. Even the dangerous use of large doses of laxatives only produces a 12 percent loss of food intake.[12] Approximately 78 percent of bulimics vomit daily.[13]

### *Consequences of Bulimia*

Vomiting this often usually leaves a bulimic person's teeth eroded and their salivary glands enlarged. Stomach fluids contain a variety of minerals that are required for the normal functioning of the stomach during digestion. If large amounts of those fluids are lost by repeated vomiting, a deficiency of minerals such as chloride and sodium may develop.

The excessive use of laxatives, diet pills, and diuretics creates a batch of health problems for bulimics. Laxatives, especially in the large doses taken by some bulimics, may lead to a dependence on them for normal bowel function. Diuretics are powerful drugs that can affect blood pressure and mineral balance. Diet pills lose their effect with time, but continue to produce undesired side effects as long as they are taken.

How these general characteristics of people with bulimia may translate into specific behaviors is illustrated in the notes on bulimia cases. The behaviors were reported by four young women with severe bulimia.

Evidence that bulimia may be related to physical conditions is accumulating. It is suggested that bulimia may be related to metabolic changes that produce depression or that trigger a decline in blood-glucose levels and an excessive intake of food.[14] People with bulimia tend to have a strong preference for sweet-tasting foods, and their binge-purge cycles can often be controlled if they maintain a well-balanced, non-junk-food diet.[15]

NOTES ON BULIMIA CASES

The following notes highlight behaviors of several females with bulimia. The notes and the cases are real, but the names are not. They represent mild to extreme examples of behaviors of people with this condition.[16]

Linda and her friend Molly would usually spend their Friday afternoons eating a large bagful of fast foods purchased at the drive-up window. They would vomit the food after their binge.

Sarah, a sixteen-year-old with bulimia for several years, reported eating foods that totaled over 30,000 calories in a day by binging and purging.

Every day after Mary got home from work, she would eat a package of cream-filled cookies and a quart of milk. She was careful to complete her binging and purging before her boyfriend visited her in the evening.

Jane, a seventeen-year-old who had "flunked" treatment in two reputable eating disorders clinics, ended up in a psychiatric institution for treatment. She was very thin and would binge and purge ten to twenty times per day. Jane had to be guarded full time by two attendants to prevent the practice and to allow her extremely irritated throat and stomach to heal. Between bouts of binging and purging, Jane would semistarve herself. She had anorexia nervosa as well as bulimia.

Sandra used laxatives to help rid her body of the food she consumed during binges. Within a year, she needed and used thirty to fifty laxative pills daily to produce diarrhea. Due to her dependence on laxatives, she had lost all normal bowel function.

Joan's bulimia turned out to be a very expensive habit. The fast foods, candy, and ice cream she would routinely binge upon cost her an average of $70 a day. She reported stealing money from the cash register in the restaurant where she worked part time in order to support her food purchases.

The primary approach to treating bulimia is the formation of good eating habits around a nutrient-dense, well-balanced diet.[15] Group and individual therapy sessions that improve a person's sense of self-esteem and confidence, and that modify attitudes about food, eating, and body size, are also important components of treatment.[1]

## PREVENTION OF EATING DISORDERS

Family environment seems to have the greatest influence on the development of eating disorders. Children brought up in families in which "perfection" is life's most important goal, independence and self-confidence are not encouraged, and body weight and dieting are overemphasized are more likely to develop an eating disorder than children reared under different circumstances.[1]

Eating disorders appear to be more common in the United States than in other countries. Part of the cause may be related to social pressures that are antifat and prothin.[17] The prevailing view of a "perfect body" is one that is unhealthfully thin, but it appears that public opinion is changing. Societal norms for body weight during this century have gone from the standard of Mae West and Marilyn Monroe to the very thin profiles of Twiggy, Nancy Reagan, and Victoria Principal. We appear to be headed back toward idealizing slightly fuller figures. Although contestants in the Miss America pageant were, on average, 15 percent underweight in the 1970s, the 1988 winner was only 6 percent underweight for her height. Shifting opinions from "thin is beautiful" to "healthy and fit is better" may help bring society's expectations about desirable body weights into a reasonable and healthful range.

# Chapter 11

## Nutrition and Reproduction

▼ The influence of nutrition on reproduction is broad and starts before pregnancy. Nutrition affects fertility, or the biological ability to conceive and maintain a pregnancy. It influences a woman's health during pregnancy and her ability to breast-feed. There is no other phase in a woman's life during which a larger return is given for nutrition investments than when creating new life.

### THE INFLUENCE OF NUTRITION ON FERTILITY

*To bring on the menses, recover the flesh by giving a woman puddings, roast meats, a good wine, fresh air and sun.*

*Fertility advice from 1847*

That was advice given to restore fertility in the last century. As you will read, "restoring the flesh" remains a basic component of the advice given to some infertile women today.

Infertility is a problem of major proportions. One out of every five couples in the United States is infertile. Half of the time the reason for the infertility is related to the male, and half of the time to conditions present in the female. Uterine infection, physical abnormalities and disorders of the reproductive system, or hormonal imbalance is often the primary reason for infertility. However, many of the causes for infertility aren't yet know.

The link between nutrition and infertility rests primarily in the relationships among diet, weight status, and estrogen levels. Infertility related to nutrition can almost always be corrected.

Some of the first evidence of the influence of nutrition on fertility came from studies undertaken during World War II in Leningrad, Japan, and Holland,[1-3] where famines occurred due to war-induced food shortages. Dietary intakes of people in Leningrad and Japan went from marginally adequate to flatly inadequate during the period of famine, whereas in Holland, people had enjoyed a high standard of living before the food shortages occurred, and were generally well nourished when the famine began. The diets of people in Holland were as poor during the food shortage as those among people in Leningrad and Japan. In each of these areas, the most common effect of the famines was a dramatic drop in fertility. In Holland, half of the women of childbearing age became infertile due to the temporary disappearance of menstrual cycles; the birth rate fell by 53 percent. Normal menstrual cycles were reestablished among most women by six months after the famine ended.

Body-fat content has been related to fertility, and the loss of body fat that accompanied the semistarvation diets during the famines may explain why fertility dropped.

*Body Fat and Infertility*

Both inadequate and excessive levels of body fat have been related to the development of infertility.[4] The effect appears to be due to the influence of body fat on estrogen production. This sex hormone is produced in fat stores as well as in the ovaries. Low levels of body fat tend to reduce the amount of estrogen produced, whereas high body-fat stores increase it. Estrogen plays a leading role in maintaining normal menstrual cycles, and when levels are unusually low or high, these cycles become abnormal or disappear until estrogen levels return to normal. Infertility related to abnormally low levels of body fat may account for 25 to 35 percent of all cases occurring in U.S. women.[5] Weight gain restores menstrual cycles and fertility in most women experiencing body-fat-related infertility.

Females at highest risk of developing body-fat-related infertility are athletes, those with anorexia nervosa, women who become lean while using oral contraceptive pills, and women who lose weight to the point of becoming underweight. Body-fat content among women in these high-risk groups is frequently below the 20 percent level associated with reduced estrogen production and a loss of normal menstrual cycles. The absence of normal menstrual cycles has been reported in up to 50 percent of competitive runners, 44 percent of ballet dancers, 25 percent of noncompetitive runners, and 12 percent of swimmers and cyclists.[6,8] The absence of menstruation is a key characteristic of anorexia nervosa: Nearly all females with anorexia nervosa do not have periods and are infertile. The loss of body fat while "on the pill" increases the likelihood that menstrual cycles will become irregular or stop when the use of the pill is discontinued.[7]

It appears that the loss of menstrual cycles may be a primary motivation for the maintenance of low levels of body fat by some athletes. Gone with the periods is the cramping, swelling, and other bothersome side effects that may interfere with performance. Unfortunately, reduced levels of estrogen affect more than the regular occurrence of menstrual periods. One of the other major functions of estrogen is to increase the deposition of calcium into bones. When estrogen levels are low, less calcium is deposited into bones. This effect can be particularly important if it occurs before the age of thirty, while peak bone mass is accumulating. Bone density and peak bone mass may be decreased in female athletes who have low body-fat content, thereby predisposing them to osteoporosis later in life.[8]

### *Other Relationships between Nutrition and Fertility*

Excessive intake of carotene-rich vegetables has been associated with the development of reversible infertility. In one study, a number of infertile women were found to have the same habit—snacking on carrots or dried green pepper flakes throughout the day. They were all diagnosed as having carotenemia, an otherwise benign condition that results from consuming high levels of carotenes from certain vegetables such as carrots and green peppers. Normal menses returned in each woman when the carotene food habit was broken.[9]

Infertility has also been reported in women who regularly consume megadoses of vitamin C supplements and in some vegans.[10,11] It is not clear why vitamin C produces this effect, but fertility returns after the high-dose supplements are stopped. It has been suggested that infertility reported in vegans may result from the intake of estrogen-containing vegetables, a higher-than-normal excretion of estrogen that may accompany high-fiber diets, or lower levels of body fat in the vegan.

Nutrition may also affect the fertility status of men. Studies involving volunteers who were underfed for a period of months showed that the first sign of impaired fertility among the men was a loss of sex drive. As weight loss progressed, sperm motility decreased and sperm production ceased when weight loss exceeded 25 percent of normal weight. Weight gain restored libido and sperm motility and levels to normal. It appears that body-fat loss in men affects fertility by altering sex hormone levels just as it does in women. Although there is more to learn about nutrition and fertility in men, it is prudent to consider the possibility that malnutrition in men may be responsible for infertility.

Infertility is a problem for one out of five couples. But fertility control may be an issue for the remaining four out of five. Controlling fertility also has implications for nutritional health.

## ORAL CONTRACEPTIVES AND NUTRITION

Oral contraceptives are a popular method of birth control. Approximately 19 percent of females aged fifteen to forty-four years in the United States use them (and that totals 8.7 million females).[12] They are effective in preventing pregnancy primarily because they block the release of an egg from a woman's ovary during the menstrual cycle. Oral contraceptives are one of a few highly effective forms of birth control for people who may want to have a baby in the future. But they do have side effects and some of these unintended effects may influence nutrient needs and health.

The effects of oral contraceptives on nutrient needs and health vary depending on the type of pill used and the duration of use. In general, the side effects of low-dose, estrogen-progestin combination pills include an elevation in blood pressure and weight and increased levels of blood cholesterol, triglycerides, and insulin.[13,14] These effects of oral contraceptives appear to be exacerbated by cigarette smoking. Although the changes produced by the pill are not dramatic, even small changes in the risk-factor status in groups of women have considerable impact in their overall rates of heart disease and diabetes.[13] Women who have elevated blood-cholesterol levels, hypertension, or diabetes, or who are heavy smokers should not take the pill.[15] Blood-cholesterol and glucose levels, and blood pressure, should be periodically monitored in all women who use oral contraceptives.

Pill use also increases a woman's need for vitamin $B_6$ and folic acid. It appears that these effects of the pill are without consequence for women who consume an adequate diet. They may represent problems for women who consume diets that are marginally adequate or inadequate in vitamin $B_6$ or folic acid. (You can get an idea of whether you're getting enough of these two vitamins by referring to the list of food sources of vitamin $B_6$ and folic acid given in chapter 6.) Vitamin $B_6$ deficiency has been identified as a cause of depression that develops among some women during pill use. One group of researchers found that a supplement containing 10 mg of $B_6$ taken for seven days during menstrual cycles by oral contraceptive users brought blood levels of vitamin $B_6$ back to normal and relieved the depression that accompanied the deficiency.[16] The increased need for folic acid during pill use may put some women at risk of developing folic acid deficiency if they become pregnant shortly after their use of the pill stops. It has been recommended that women separate pregnancy from pill use by about six months. This interval gives a woman's body a chance to make up for deficits in vitamin $B_6$ and folic acid that may have occurred while taking the pill.[17]

Although the side effects of pill use pose certain risks to health, oral contraceptives are nonetheless associated with fewer health problems than is pregnancy.[18] Attentive and responsive health care reduces the likelihood that the pill will increase a woman's risk of developing health problems.

## NUTRITION AND PREGNANCY

Women's relatively complex and dynamic reproductive systems affect their nutrient needs and nutritional health continuously. The importance of nutrition, however, takes on new meaning when the reproductive system that has kept a woman geared up for pregnancy is called into service.

Simply stated, the biological changes that occur with pregnancy are profound. How well they proceed largely determines how healthy a woman and infant will be. There are many factors that can affect how smoothly a pregnancy goes and how healthy an infant is at birth, but none is more important than nutrition.

### *Nutrition and the Course and Outcome of Pregnancy: The Evidence*

Remember the World War II studies referred to in the discussion of nutrition and fertility? They also taught us a good deal about how nutrition during pregnancy influences infant health. Total caloric intake among pregnant women in Leningrad and Holland averaged 1,100 calories per day during the food shortage. Average protein intake was about 30 grams per day (an amount that is less than half of the RDA for pregnant women), and it consisted primarily of low-quality proteins such as those found in bread and other grain products. The period of food shortage lasted only eight months in Holland but for two years in Leningrad. Unlike the situation in Holland, the food shortage in Leningrad was imposed on women who were marginally nourished in the first place. The impact of the food shortage on infant health in Leningrad included increased rates of preterm, low-birth-weight, and stillborn infants. In Holland, where women were well nourished prior to the food shortage and experienced a shorter period of poor dietary intake, the primary effect of the food shortage was a drop in birth weight.

Other information about nutrition and reproductive health was generated from studies done in England during World War II. Due to a special food-rationing program, dietary intake of pregnant women improved during the war. The improvement in diets was associated with the births of larger and healthier babies than were born before the war. The rates of preterm birth and infant death declined during the period of special food rationing in England. Birth outcomes worsened, however, after the special food-rationing program ended.

Three major conclusions can be drawn from the results of the World War II studies.

> Nutrition prior to pregnancy affects infant health.
>
> Poor nutrition has a greater negative influence on infant health if it exists *both* before and during pregnancy than if it exists just before *or* just during pregnancy.
>
> Improvement in nutrition during pregnancy has a beneficial effect on infant health.

Many additional studies have examined relationships between diet during pregnancy and the health of mothers and their babies. The results of a number of the studies are incorporated into other parts of this section.

Prepregnant weight-for-height (known as *weight status*) and the amount of weight women gain during pregnancy are strongly related to newborn health, primarily through their effect on fetal growth and birth weight. Infant birth weight is closely related to infant health. Small infants, especially those weighing less than five and one-half pounds, are at least twelve times more likely to die or to have lasting health problems than are infants who weigh around eight pounds at birth.[19] Women who enter pregnancy underweight or who fail to gain enough weight during pregnancy are much more likely to deliver low-birth-weight infants than are women who are of normal weight or above and gain an appropriate amount of weight.[19]

### *What's the Right Amount of Weight to Gain during Pregnancy?*

As far as weight gain during pregnancy goes, there is no one amount that's right for everybody. How much a woman should gain depends on her weight status coming into pregnancy. Normal-weight women tend to deliver infants of optimal birth weight (around eight pounds) if they gain between thirty and thirty-five pounds during pregnancy. On average, underweight women should gain more (thirty-five to forty pounds) and women who enter pregnancy overweight, less (twenty-two to twenty-seven pounds if slightly overweight, and as little as sixteen to twenty pounds if obese).[19] These guidelines are based on rates of maternal weight gain associated with the births of infants of desired weights.

There is another school of thought about weight gain during pregnancy. Rather than basing weight-gain recommendations on infant birth weight, members of this school justify recommendations based on women's weight loss after pregnancy. Women lose an average of twenty-four pounds by six weeks after delivery.[19] Although a twenty-four-pound weight gain does not correspond with optimal infant outcomes in groups of women, it represents a level of gain that is generally lost rather quickly. There is no evidence to suggest, however, that a gain of thirty to thirty-five pounds during pregnancy predisposes women to obesity. It is the range recommended here for normal-weight women because of its beneficial influence on infant health.

Weight gains of over forty-five pounds during pregnancy appear to be counterproductive. Although newborn health does not appear to be jeopardized, women gaining this amount or more are found to experience more cesarean sections and complications during delivery than women who gain less.[20]

Two other factors are important to consider within this topic: the rate of weight gain and the quality of the foods that go into the weight gain. Weight should be gained at a gradual pace during pregnancy and continue an upward movement, even for women who enter pregnancy overweight or obese. The guidelines presented for weight gain during pregnancy assume that it is achieved by eating a high-quality diet.

### WHERE DOES THE WEIGHT GAIN GO?

During the 1700s and 1800s, it was thought that since an infant only weighed about seven pounds at birth, women didn't need to gain much more than that amount. It was assumed that the only tissue that grew during pregnancy was the fetus. But much more than that grows. Fetal growth is accompanied by marked increases in maternal blood volume, fat stores, and breast and uterus size. The accumulation of amniotic fluid (the water that surrounds the fetus in the uterus), the increase in the volume of fluid on the outside of

COMPONENTS OF WEIGHT GAIN DURING PREGNANCY FOR A PREGNANT WOMAN WHO DELIVERS AN EIGHT-POUND INFANT

| *Place* | *Pounds* |
|---|---|
| Fetus | 8 |
| Uterus | 2 |
| Placenta | 1½ |
| Blood | 4½ |
| Amniotic fluid | 2 |
| Breast tissue | 1 |
| Tissue fluid | 2½ |
| Fat stores | 8½ |
| Total | 30 |

*Source: Adapted from Hytten and Leitch,* The Physiology of Human Pregnancy, *2d ed., Oxford: Blackwell Scientific Publications, 1971.*

cells, and the placenta also add to the weight-gain requirement of pregnancy. When broken down into individual components, a weight gain of thirty pounds during pregnancy would be approximately distributed as shown here. By the end of pregnancy, an eight-pound infant accounts for only 28 percent of the total gain. Some of the fat stored during pregnancy is intended for use during breastfeeding.

### *A Pregnant Woman's Need for Calories and Nutrients*

Pregnant women have higher needs for calories and all essential nutrients than women who aren't pregnant. Consuming enough of each is important, but certain ones represent more pressing concern than others. For pregnancy, calories and the nutrients protein, folic acid, vitamin $B_6$, calcium, iron, and zinc capture the spotlight. We'll focus the discussion on these seven.

#### CALORIES

According to the RDAs, pregnant women need 15 percent more calories, but up to 100 percent more nutrients than do nonpregnant women. The relatively high requirement for nutrients means that pregnant women should increase their intake of nutrient-dense foods more than they increase their consumption of calorie-rich foods.

The increased need for calories in pregnancy amounts to about 150 calories per day in the first three months (or the amount of calories in slightly less than half a hamburger with bun) and then by 350 calories per day (or the whole hamburger with bun) in the last six months. These are average figures. Women entering pregnancy underweight will need more calories, and those entering overweight fewer calories, than average. In addition, physically active women require higher caloric intakes to cover their energy needs for pregnancy. It is generally easier and more accurate to monitor the adequacy of caloric intake by tracking weight gain than by counting calories.

### PEAKS AND PLATEAUS IN HUNGER

Hunger and food intake fluctuate widely during pregnancy, and increases in food intake usually don't produce a smooth rate of weight gain. There are spurts in food intake and weight gain. Hunger, food intake, and weight gain generally reach their highest levels between three and six months of pregnancy.

### EFFECTS OF LOW-CALORIE DIETS DURING PREGNANCY

As a ballpark figure, diets during pregnancy that provide fewer than about 1,800 calories per day are considered "low calorie." Such diets present several problems for a growing fetus. The first has to do with the availability of protein for fetal growth and tissue formation. Without enough calories to meet a pregnant woman's need for energy, dietary protein will be diverted from protein tissue construction and used in energy formation. The requirement for energy must be met before protein will be spared from use as a source of energy. This principle applies throughout all phases of life but is particularly relevant to pregnancy, when protein tissue formation is extensive. The second problem is that low calorie intake doesn't supply enough energy to meet the needs for normal fetal growth. This increases the probability that the infant will be born at low birth weight. Third, diets that fail to supply enough calories generally provide inadequate amounts of essential nutrients. This situation can leave the fetus with a short supply of vitamins and minerals and interfere with normal growth and development.

The ill effects of low-calorie diets during pregnancy on fetal growth and development are most pronounced when the restriction lasts throughout pregnancy. Infants born under this circumstance may be permanently delayed in growth and intellectual development.[21] If low calorie intake is the exception rather than the routine, it is not likely that permanent damage to the infant will result. Adaptive mechanisms help the fetus get through the highs and lows of maternal food intake. The best situation is one in which the pregnant woman eats regular meals and snacks and avoids even short periods of fasting and weight loss.

#### PROTEIN

The protein content of a woman's body increases by about two pounds during pregnancy. About half of the increase goes toward the buildup of her uterus, breasts, and blood supply. The other half is deposited in fetal tissues. Protein intake below the 1980 RDA for pregnancy for adult women of 74 grams has been associated with the birth of smaller-than-average infants.[22]

Several studies have shown that infants tend to be healthier when women consume around 90 grams of protein daily during pregnancy than when they consume less.[23,24] Whether U.S. women should be encouraged to consume about 90 grams of protein rather than less is a matter of controversy. Most women in the United States consume between 70 and 90 grams of protein per day during pregnancy.

#### FOLACIN

Folacin has been considered an important nutrient for pregnant women ever since it was discovered that low folacin intake may cause fetal malformations and growth retardation. The link between folacin deficiency and abnormal fetal growth and development is the role of folacin in protein tissue construction. Folacin is a key factor required for the normal production of proteins formed within the body. Dietary deficiencies of folacin during pregnancy have been associated with the development of spinal cord abnormalities such as spina bifida in the fetus.[25]

The increased requirement for folacin is often not met by the diets of pregnant women. Folacin supplements of around 400 mg per day (or 0.4 mg) from the start of pregnancy are recommended.

#### VITAMIN $B_6$

Vitamin $B_6$ is of concern during pregnancy not so much because of the likelihood of a dietary deficiency but because it is often used to treat morning sickness, or nausea and vomiting during pregnancy. Nausea and vomiting occur commonly during the first three months of pregnancy and are related to hormonal changes. For a small proportion of women, it becomes a serious problem because it lasts longer than three months and can produce dehydration, which can threaten the health of mother and baby. The type of morning sickness that most pregnant women experience, however, does not appear to be harmful to pregnancy (although it is a major inconvenience to the women).[26]

Daily doses of vitamin $B_6$ in the range of 5 to 10 mg have been reported to relieve nausea and vomiting in some, but not all, women. Since vitamin $B_6$ deficiency has not been related to the development of this condition, the relief it sometimes provides is due to a "drug effect" rather than the normal functions of $B_6$ in the body. Nausea and vomiting during pregnancy that is severe and lasts beyond three months requires close medical supervision and generally the intravenous administration of fluids to correct dehydration.

#### CALCIUM

Calcium used to support the mineralization of bones in the fetus is supplied by the mother's diet and, if needed, by the calcium in the long bones in her body. But because blood levels of calcium are tightly controlled, calcium will be taken from the mother's bones if needed to maintain a stable level of calcium in the blood. The constant supply of calcium in the blood means that the fetus has regular access to as much calcium as needed, even if the mother's diet contains little calcium. Calcium uptake by the fetus is especially high during the last three months of pregnancy when the bones of a fetus begin to mineralize.

Pregnant women who regularly consume low-calcium diets lose calcium from their bones during pregnancy. Calcium losses, however, come from the long bones and not from the teeth. So the saying that "for every baby a tooth" has no basis in fact. Several studies have shown that teeth do not demineralize as a result of low-calcium diets during pregnancy.[27,28]

#### IRON

Iron deficiency is the most common nutrient deficiency found among pregnant women in the United States.[29] It develops because many women enter pregnancy with low iron stores and fail to consume enough iron during pregnancy. Iron requirements rise during pregnancy due to increases in hemoglobin production and the storage of iron by the fetus.

Short of eating liver twice a day, it is virtually impossible for pregnant women to get the additional iron needed from foods. Consequently, supplemental iron is recommended for the second half of pregnancy. The dose varies depending on a woman's iron status. A daily supplement that provides 18 to 30 mg of iron is appropriate for women who show no signs of developing iron deficiency, such as a hemoglobin level that declines too quickly. (Hemoglobin level normally declines during pregnancy. It's the rate and total amount of decline that is indicative of iron status.) Women who show signs of developing iron deficiency need more iron—30 to 60 mg per day. Women who don't take supplemental iron are more likely to develop iron deficiency and to deliver infants who are small and at increased risk of developing iron deficiency in the first year of life than are women who take them.[30]

Concern has recently developed over the amount of supplemental iron that is usually given to pregnant women. Experts are questioning whether "too much of a good thing" is being passed out. Many health care professionals routinely recommend the use of high amounts of iron (120 mg per day in some cases) throughout pregnancy. Knowledge of the importance of iron to maternal and infant health appears to have led some professionals to overreact and routinely prescribe iron in amounts that are too high. It is not uncommon for pregnant women to be given supplements that provide over 200 mg of iron daily. These high amounts of supplemental iron are poorly absorbed and can produce heartburn and constipation as side effects.[31] High doses of iron (over 100 mg per day) decrease zinc absorption and may lead to zinc deficiency.[32] Rather than cope with the side effects, it is suspected that many women simply quit taking their iron supplement. A panel of experts recently recommended that a dose of 30 mg iron per day is sufficient to meet the needs of most women during pregnancy.[33]

#### ZINC

An additional 5 mg of zinc per day is recommended during pregnancy. This extra amount is primarily used to support protein tissue formation in the mother and fetus.

Since the RDA for nonpregnant women is 15 mg per day, the total recommended daily intake of zinc for pregnant women amounts to 20 mg. On average, however, pregnant women in the United States consume about 8 mg of zinc per day.[34] Although this amount prevents out-and-out signs of zinc deficiency, marginal deficiencies of zinc may be quite common in pregnancy. High-dose iron supplements may contribute to the development of a zinc deficiency, because iron interferes with zinc absorption when too much is present in the gut. Zinc deficiency during pregnancy has been associated with abnormally long labors and the birth of small and malformed infants.[35]

One important route to reducing the possibility of zinc deficiency during pregnancy is the use of 30-mg doses or less of iron supplements. Another is to eat at least three servings of meats and meat alternates per day. Supplementing pregnant women with zinc, however, is not currently recommended. Only folacin and iron are recommended for supplementation during pregnancy.

### *Other Nutrition Issues*

Several other nutrition issues related to salt, dietary fiber, water, alcohol, and vitamin and mineral supplements pertain to the topic of pregnancy.

#### SALT

Should salt restriction be a part of the management of a healthy pregnancy? The answer is no, and you can even make that a *NO*! Although it is no longer recommended, restricting a woman's salt intake during pregnancy was common practice until recently. It used to be believed that reducing salt (or more specifically, sodium) intake during pregnancy would help prevent the development of hypertension.

Results of a number of studies have shown that the hypertension that may develop in pregnancy is not related to high salt intake.[36] In fact, salt-restricted diets tend to aggravate rather than decrease the problem of hypertension during pregnancy.[36] Women should be advised to restrict salt during pregnancy only if they enter pregnancy with a form of hypertension that is lowered by a low-salt diet. It is generally recommended that women salt "to taste" during pregnancy. It is not necessary, however, to encourage the consumption of a high-salt diet. Most women will get all the sodium they need if they consume roughly the same amount of sodium as before pregnancy.

#### DIETARY FIBER

Constipation is a common problem of pregnancy, especially in the last few months, and appears to result from normal hormonal changes. It can be prevented to an extent by including 10 additional grams of dietary fiber in the diet.[37] (Note: food sources of dietary fiber are listed in table 10.) Insoluble fibers, such as those found in whole grains, wheat bran, and seeds, are the type of dietary fiber that add bulk to the intestines and promote normal bowel movements.

Water intake should be increased along with fiber consumption. Fiber doesn't help prevent constipation if fluid intake is low.

Water allows fiber to swell and create the bulk that stimulates the movement of waste products along the intestinal tract.

### WATER

Water requirements increase substantially during pregnancy. A pregnant woman needs more water because of increases in blood volume and the amount of water that is needed for maintaining body temperature. She also needs more water to dilute fetal waste products that flow into her blood and are excreted in her urine. It is widely suspected (although not yet demonstrated) that many pregnant women may fail to drink enough water.

Women are generally advised to stay well hydrated during pregnancy (and to pay special attention to fluid intake if they live in hot climates). For most women, an intake of ten or more cups of water a day (including that in fruit juices, milk, and other beverages) does the job.

### ALCOHOL

Drinking alcohol during pregnancy was said to cause the birth of "sickly" infants as early as the 1800s. The ill effects of alcohol on babies were not, however, fully acknowledged until the 1970s, when several research reports described a condition called *fetal alcohol syndrome.* Women who drank heavily during pregnancy or who "binge drank" were found to be at high risk of delivering infants with specific malformations and retarded growth and mental development. The effects of drinking on the fetus were found to worsen as alcohol intake increased. Heavy drinking in the first half of pregnancy was closely associated with the birth of malformed, small, and mentally impaired infants. When excessive drinking occurred only in the second half of pregnancy, infants were less likely to be malformed but still likely to be small and suffer abnormal mental development. These conditions are lasting—they cannot be corrected with time and special services.

No amount of alcohol has been found to be absolutely safe during pregnancy. Adverse effects of alcohol on fetal development, when only an occasional drink is consumed, appear to be small and rare. To exclude the possibility of even small impairments in fetal growth and development, it is recommended that women do not drink alcohol during pregnancy.

#### VITAMIN AND MINERAL SUPPLEMENTS

Many pregnant women are routinely given a multivitamin and mineral supplement during pregnancy as a precautionary measure. Balanced and adequate diets, however, and not multivitamin and mineral supplements, are recommended for pregnant women. The only nutrients recommended for supplementation during pregnancy are iron and folacin. Other nutrients may be prescribed for women, such as vitamin $B_{12}$ for vegans.

Well-nourished women probably do not need a multivitamin and mineral supplement during pregnancy. If supplements are taken, the dose levels should not exceed 100 percent of the RDA levels for pregnant women. Doses higher than these may increase the risk of adverse reactions in the mother and fetus.

#### SUPPLEMENT OVERUSE: THE CAUTIONS

Broad concern about the effects of excessive levels of individual vitamins and minerals on the fetus has developed only recently. Before the boom in the popularity of supplements, women rarely took high enough amounts of nutrients to cause noticeable problems in babies. Vitamin and mineral supplements were generally thought to be harmless. We now know that they aren't always safe.

Overdose reactions have been observed in pregnant women and newborns for six vitamins and three minerals. They are: vitamins $B_{12}$, C, $B_6$, A, D, and E; and the minerals iron, zinc, and iodine.[38] Amounts taken during pregnancy that have been associated with harmful effects start at two times the RDA; the risk for problem development increases with the dose. A fetus is generally much more susceptible to the ill effects of vitamin and mineral overdoses than is a pregnant woman, primarily because of the small size and rapid growth of the fetus. Overdoses of vitamin and mineral supplements produce the most serious threats to infant health if they occur early in pregnancy, when fetal organs are developing.[38]

#### OVERDOSE REACTIONS FROM VITAMINS

The most common problem observed in infants whose mothers have taken excessive amounts of vitamins $B_{12}$, C, and $B_6$ in pregnancy are *rebound* deficiencies. The excretion mechanisms that rid the body of the high levels of these vitamins are in full swing while the fetus is receiving large amounts of them. The high level of vitamin excretion continues after birth, even though unnecessary because large amounts of the vitamins are no longer being received.

SUMMARY OF THE EFFECTS OF VITAMIN AND MINERAL OVERDOSES ON PREGNANT WOMEN AND INFANTS

| *Vitamins* | *Effect* |
|---|---|
| Vitamin $B_{12}$ | Rebound deficiency in newborn |
| Vitamin C | Rebound deficiency in newborn |
| Vitamin $B_6$ | Rebound deficiency, malformations in newborn |
| Vitamin A | Malformations of central nervous system and bones in infants |
| Vitamin D | Mental retardation, heart abnormalities in infants |
| Vitamin E | Early fetal loss |

| *Minerals* | *Effect* |
|---|---|
| Iron | Gastrointestinal upsets in women |
| Zinc | Preterm delivery |
| Iodine | Goiter and mental retardation in infants |

The newborns end up excreting too much of the vitamins and developing deficiencies within a few days after birth. Infants may be protected from the effects of rebound vitamin deficiencies if given the appropriate vitamin at birth and then gradually weaned from it.[39]

Other, less common problems have also been associated with the overuse of water-soluble vitamins. Very high intakes of vitamin $B_6$, for example, have been related to malformations in infants.[38]

As little as 25,000 IU of vitamin A taken daily in the early months of pregnancy has been associated with central nervous system and bone abnormalities in the newborn.[38] The increasingly popular use of vitamin-A-like compounds for the treatment of acne, wrinkles, and other skin conditions has led to new warnings about their use by women who are, or intend to become, pregnant.

Daily doses of supplemental vitamin D at levels five times the RDA (2,000 IU) have been associated with the birth of infants who are mentally retarded and have heart abnormalities. There is also evidence to indicate that megadoses of vitamin E may result in spontaneous abortions—the early, unexpected loss of a fetus.[38]

#### OVERDOSE REACTIONS FROM MINERALS

Iron overdose primarily affects the pregnant woman by causing gastrointestinal upsets. The fetus does not receive excessive levels of iron because high amounts are not usually absorbed by the mother's intestinal tract. Zinc supplements that deliver about 100 mg per day (or five times the RDA) provide excessive levels of zinc to the fetus. Zinc overdoses in pregnancy have been related to preterm delivery. The consequences of iodine overdose in pregnancy include the development of goiter and mental retardation in infants.

The problems that excessive levels of vitamins and minerals may produce could be prevented if women took no more than the RDA levels for vitamins and minerals during pregnancy. With the exception of folacin and iron, pregnant women can and should get the nutrients they need from a balanced diet and not supplements.

Vitamin and mineral supplements, especially those containing iron, that are not used up during pregnancy should be tossed out or kept in a child-proof container. Iron overdose is a leading cause of accidental poisoning in young children.

### *A Good Diet for Pregnancy*

Good diets for pregnant women contain:

1. sufficient calories to promote an adequate weight gain,
2. a variety of foods from each of the basic food groups,
3. regular meals and snacks,
4. sufficient dietary fiber (about 30 grams per day),
5. 10 or more cups of fluid each day,
6. salt to taste, and
7. no alcohol-containing beverages.

In addition, a good diet for pregnancy is supplemented with iron and folacin. These characteristics hold, no matter if a pregnant female is a vegetarian or a teenager.

Planning diets around the minimum servings of foods from each of the basic groups is the most straightforward approach to meeting nutrient needs for pregnancy. The guidelines shown here are similar to those for nonpregnant women. They include, however, two additional servings of milk and milk products and one additional serving of meat or meat alternates than recommended for nonpregnant women. Consuming only the minimum number of servings from each food group won't provide the needed level of calories. Additional servings of foods within the groups or of miscellaneous foods will be needed to meet caloric needs.

FOOD GROUP RECOMMENDATIONS FOR PREGNANCY[a]

| *Food Group* | *Minimum Number of Servings per Day* |
|---|---|
| Breads and cereals | 4 |
| Vegetables and fruits | (4) |
| Vitamin-A-rich | 1 |
| Vitamin-C-rich | 1 |
| Other | 2 |
| Milk and milk products | 3 |
| Meat or alternates | 3 |
| Miscellaneous | Based on caloric need |

[a]*For additional information on foods contained in the groups and what standard serving sizes are, see Table 7.*

## BREAST-FEEDING

*Food is the first enjoyment of life.*

*Lin Yutang*

A woman's capacity to nourish a growing infant doesn't end at birth—it continues in the form of breast-feeding. Breast milk from healthy and well-nourished women is ideally suited for infant nutrition and health. It provides the calories and nutrients infants need plus regular doses of "preventive medicine." Unlike formula or cow's milk, breast milk contains substances that help protect infants from infectious diseases and allergies. Breast-fed infants are also less likely to develop cancer of the lymph system and diabetes during childhood than infants who are bottle-fed.[40,41]

Breast-feeding provides health benefits to women as well as to infants. Breast-feeding causes the release of oxytocin, a hormone that stimulates the muscles of the uterus to contract. The contraction of the uterus helps stop bleeding caused by the detachment of the placenta from the wall of the uterus during delivery. (This effect of breast-feeding is quite noticeable. During the first few days after delivery, women can feel their uterus contract while breast-feeding.) Breast-feeding appears to reduce the risk of developing breast cancer later in life. The longer women breast-feed, the less likely they are to develop breast cancer. The risk of developing breast cancer also decreases as the number of infants breast-fed increases.[42] An additional and potent advantage is that women who breast-feed find it a great source of satisfaction and enjoyment.[43]

### *How Breast-Feeding Works*

A woman's body begins to prepare for breast-feeding during pregnancy. It prepares by depositing fat in breast tissue and by expanding the network of blood vessels that infiltrate the cells of the breasts. Ducts that channel milk from the milk-producing cells forward to the nipple also mature.

Hormonal changes that occur at delivery signal milk production to begin. Since delivery rather than length of pregnancy initiates milk production, breast milk is available for infants born prematurely.

The milk produced by women during the first few days after delivery is different from milk produced later. The early milk, *colostrum*, contains a higher level of antibodies, protein, and minerals than does the *mature* milk produced when the baby is about three days old. Colostrum is a concentrated source of preventive medicine. It provides infants with a boost of infection-fighting antibodies for their entrance from a germ-free environment into one that is germ-filled. Colostrum doesn't look exactly like mature milk, either; it is thicker and has a yellowish color.

Mature milk comes in two types: ***fore milk*** and ***hind milk***. Fore milk represents about a third of the available milk supply; the rest is hind milk. Present in the ducts that lead from the milk-producing cells to the nipple, fore milk is readily available to the infant. It contains less fat and protein, and therefore fewer calories than hind milk.

Hind milk is stored in the milk-producing cells of the breast. Unlike fore milk, hind milk is not automatically available to the infant, but is released by oxytocin, the same hormone that signals the uterus to contract during the first few days after delivery. Oxytocin causes the milk-producing cells to contract and thereby release the hind milk. This process is commonly referred to as the *letdown reflex*. The milk-releasing effect of oxytocin is so powerful that milk is actually ejected from the breast. If the hind milk is not released, the infant will not get enough milk, will be hungry most of the time, and may grow and develop poorly. A number of conditions can interfere with the release of oxytocin, and therefore with the release of hind milk, during breast-feeding. The failure of the letdown reflex is a major cause of breast-feeding failure.

#### FACTORS AFFECTING THE LETDOWN REFLEX

The letdown reflex is unique among physiological processes in that it can be initiated by either physical or psychological stimuli. Normally, the letdown reflex is signaled by the physical sensation of the infant sucking at the nipple. But it can also occur when a mother hears her infant's cry of hunger or even when the thought "it's time for a feeding" enters her mind. The physical or psychological stimuli signals a part of the brain to release oxytocin into the bloodstream. When it reaches its target, the milk-producing cells, they contract and eject their content of milk.

Oxytocin is normally released within a minute after breast-feeding starts. During the first few weeks of breast-feeding, and sometimes longer than that, the mother can often feel the letdown reflex. It causes a tingling sensation in the nipples.

Certain forms of physical and psychological stimuli can prevent the letdown reflex. Stress, pain, anxiety, and other distractions can block the release of oxytocin. If a woman is distracted by pain or if she is pressured for time, for example, the letdown reflex may not occur when the infant starts to feed, and he or she won't get enough to eat. If this happens often enough, women may think they don't have enough milk and may decide to switch to bottle-feeding. Breast-feeding in comfortable and relaxed surroundings and the uninhibited enjoyment of breast-feeding help foster the letdown reflex.

#### BREAST MILK PRODUCTION

While an infant is consuming one meal, she or he is ordering the next. The pressure produced inside the breast by the infant's suck and the emptying of the breasts during a feed cause the hormone *prolactin* to be released from special cells in the brain. Prolactin stimulates the production of milk; as much milk will be produced as the infant consumes. It generally takes about two hours for the milk-producing cells to make enough milk for the infant's next feeding. An important exception to the two-hour refill time, however, occurs when an infant enters a growth spurt.

Infants, like children and adolescents, grow in spurts, not at a constant rate. In preparation for a growth spurt, hunger increases and the intake of breast milk may double. Growth spurts occur frequently between an infant's third and seventh week of life, but happen less often as an infant gets older. The initial increase in breast milk intake associated with growth spurts increases the time it takes to produce a refill in milk supply. Instead of two hours, it may take up to twenty-four hours for breast milk production to catch up with an infant's need for it. This means that for about a day, the infant will want to feed often and may not have his or her hunger completely satisfied. Although women may spend much of their day breast-feeding an infant who is entering a growth spurt, they may feel they don't have enough milk to satisfy the baby and will give the baby a bottle. Because breast milk production depends on how much and how often an infant feeds, the supplementary bottle feedings lead to a decrease in milk production. Some women stop breast-feeding during the infant's growth spurt because they think they have too little milk to satisfy their infant's need for food. It is very rare that a breast-feeding woman cannot produce enough milk. As long as an infant is allowed to breast-feed as often as desired, production will catch up with the baby's need for milk.

### *How Long Should Breast-Feeding Continue?*

No one knows what the best length of breast-feeding is in terms of infant health. It has been observed over time, however, that women in most cultures generally breast-feed for six months to two years. Milk-producing animals, such as cats, dogs, mice, and rats, tend to breast-feed for about the same length of time as pregnancy. Rats, for example, take about twenty-one days to produce a litter and breast-feed their young for approximately the first twenty-one days after birth. Whether nine months, the length of time it takes for pregnancy in humans, is the best length of time for breast-feeding is debatable. However, it appears that six months to a year may be an appropriate range.[44] It is recommended that breast-feeding exclusively be continued for the first four to six months of life. Between four and six months, infants should be given rice cereal and gradually introduced to vegetables, fruits, meats, juices, and other foods that are specially prepared for infants.

#### SHUTTING OFF BREAST MILK PRODUCTION

Breast milk production will continue as long as an infant feeds at the breast. Milk production decreases when the intervals between feedings lengthen and when the breasts aren't completely emptied during feedings. It ceases altogether when the infant stops breast-feeding.

### *Nutrition for Breast-Feeding Women*

An adequate and balanced diet is needed by breast-feeding women to help them stay healthy during the hectic and tiring times that come with new babies. A good diet will help women replenish their nutrient stores and produce nutritious milk. For breast-feeding women, you "nourish the baby by nourishing the mom."

Women begin breast-feeding after nine months of drawing upon their nutrient stores to support fetal growth. They continue to fully support the energy and nutrient needs of their infants after pregnancy, but the babies are larger and require higher amounts of energy and nutrients than during pregnancy.

### CALORIE AND NUTRIENT NEEDS

The RDA for calories is around 25 percent higher for breast-feeding women than for others. Energy supplied from fat stores that normally accumulate during pregnancy contributes to meeting energy needs for breast-feeding, so not all of the needed energy has to come from a women's diet. In general, a diet that provides about 250 calories more per day than before pregnancy meets a woman's need for energy for breast milk production. It also allows for a loss in weight of approximately one-half pound per week. The nutrient content of breast milk declines when caloric intake during breast-feeding dips below 1,500 calories per day.

The RDAs for nutrients increase between 25 and 67 percent for breast-feeding. As was the case for pregnancy, proportionately higher amounts of nutrients are needed than calories, and that adds up to the need for a nutrient-dense diet. The increases in nutrient allowances for breast-feeding are generally higher than the increases for pregnancy. The RDAs for Vitamins D and C and zinc increase by the most (67 percent). The impressive increases in the RDAs for these nutrients are related to the infant's need for them for bone and tissue formation. Calcium, phosphorus, magnesium, and vitamin A are all involved in bone formation and show 50 percent increases in RDAs.

Concern has been expressed about the possibility that breast-feeding may weaken a woman's bones if she fails to consume enough calcium and other bone-building minerals in her diet. It appears that this concern has a basis in fact. Breast-feeding women, especially those who are under thirty years of age and have not achieved peak bone density, may lose minerals from their bones if they consume a low-calcium diet during breast-feeding.[45] Women who have breast-fed four or more children over time while consuming a low-calcium diet are at increased risk of developing osteoporosis later in life.[46]

With the exception of iron, the RDAs for vitamins and minerals increase by at least 25 percent during breast-feeding. The RDA for iron is not increased because of the savings in iron that occurs with breast-feeding. (However, to rebuild iron stores, it is often recommended that iron supplements started in pregnancy be continued for two to three months after delivery.) Women who breast-feed generally don't resume menstrual periods until the infant consumes most of his or her calories from other foods besides breast milk. The iron saved from the lack of menstrual bleeding counts toward meeting the breast-feeding woman's need for iron.

### EFFECTS OF MATERNAL DIET ON BREAST MILK COMPOSITION

Milk-producing cells in the breast are supplied with the raw materials they need to manufacture milk from the mother's blood. For a number of substances, what ends up in the mother's blood reflects what she has consumed. Consequently, for some substances, the composition of breast milk varies depending on maternal diet. For other substances, the amount that enters breast milk is regulated within the milk-producing cells and the levels remain fairly constant regardless of maternal diet.

Milk-producing cells enforce quality control processes that regulate the amount of carbohydrate, protein, fat, and minerals, including calcium, sodium, potassium, iron, and fluoride, in breast milk. They also regulate the amount of milk produced when maternal caloric intake is too low. Rather than dilute the energy content of milk in response to a low-calorie diet, these cells reduce the volume of milk produced.[47] The amount of carbohydrate, protein, and fat found in breast milk varies only slightly based on maternal diet. However, the *type* of fat present can vary substantially.[48] If a woman consumes more vegetable oils than animal fats, her breast milk will contain a high proportion of unsaturated fats. If she fasts, her milk will contain the type of fat present in her fat stores.

The vitamin content of breast milk corresponds more closely to maternal intake than is the case for the energy nutrients.[49] The amount of thiamin and vitamins C and $B_{12}$ in breast milk, for example, varies based on the types of food and supplements that the mother ingests. Thiamin deficiency (*beriberi*) and vitamin $B_{12}$ deficiency (*pernicious anemia*) have been diagnosed in infants breast-fed by deficient mothers.[50]

The amount of several minerals in breast milk is influenced by what the mother eats. It is clear that the amount of zinc and iodine in breast milk differs depending on the mother's diet.[49] Infants who fail to get enough zinc and iodine grow and develop slowly.

In many respects, a woman's diet and the supplements she takes affect the nutrient content of breast milk and may influence infant growth and development. Consequently, what and how much a woman eats while she is breast-feeding an infant are important to fostering her own as well as her infant's health. Ingestion of an adequate and balanced diet, with reliance on foods rather than supplements to meet vitamin and mineral needs, is the best approach to achieving good nutrition during breast-feeding.

#### EFFECTS OF OTHER SUBSTANCES ON BREAST-MILK COMPOSITION

Foods contain many chemical substances in addition to nutrients, and some chemicals enter a woman's diet through drugs, medications, and other nonfood substances that are ingested. These substances, too, may end up in breast milk.

When a breast-feeding woman drinks coffee, her infant receives a small dose of caffeine. Breast-fed infants of women who are heavy coffee drinkers (10 or more cups per day) may develop "caffeine jitters."[51]

Alcohol is transferred from a woman's diet to breast milk. Oddly enough, however, beer or wine are sometimes recommended to women to "help them relax" before breast-feeding. Although one or two alcohol-containing beverages per day appear to pose no harm to the breast-fed infant, heavy drinking during breast-feeding (six or more drinks per day) can expose infants to dose levels of alcohol that may harm their development. The development of the brain and nervous system of infants born to chronic, heavy drinkers appears to be retarded.[52] If breast-feeding women were to take the advice to relax with a beer before breast-feeding, they would qualify as "heavy drinkers" since during the first few months of breast-feeding, infants eat every three to four hours.

Almost any drug or toxin that enters the mother's blood will end up in her breast milk. Environmental contaminants such as DDT, chlordane, PCB, and PBBs, for example, are transferred into breast milk. Many environmental contaminants are fat soluble and if consumed will be stored in a woman's fat tissue. When her fat stores are broken down for use in breast milk, the contaminants stored in her fat will also enter her milk. The ingestion of fish from the contaminated waters of Lake Ontario and Lake Michigan has been directly related to abnormally high levels of PCB in breast milk.[53,54] Infants exposed to PCB may develop a rash, digestive upsets, and nervous system problems.[55]

Infants are much smaller than women, and it takes a smaller dose of caffeine, alcohol, drugs, or environmental contaminants to have an effect on them than on an adult. Consequently, women may show no adverse effects from these substances while the infant may.

FOOD GROUP RECOMMENDATIONS FOR BREAST-FEEDING WOMEN[a]

| *Food group* | *Minimum Number of Servings per Day* |
| --- | --- |
| Breads and cereals | 4 |
| Vegetables and fruits | (5) |
| Vitamin-A-rich | 1 |
| Vitamin-C-rich | 2 |
| Other | 2 |
| Milk and milk products | 4 |
| Meat or alternates | 3 |
| Miscellaneous | Based on caloric need |

[a]*For additional information on foods contained in the groups and what standard serving sizes are, refer to Table 7.*

Breast-feeding women are advised to limit coffee consumption to four or fewer cups a day, and to keep alcohol consumption to one or two drinks daily. Drugs or medications should only be taken on the advice of a physician, and fish from contaminated lakes should not be eaten.

Vitamins and minerals consumed in supplements also enter breast milk in varying proportions. However, adverse reactions in babies to supplements taken by women who breast-feed have not been reported. Vitamin and mineral doses in supplements should be kept below 100 percent of the RDA for breast-feeding women.

### GOOD DIETS FOR BREAST-FEEDING WOMEN

The calories and nutrients needed by the breast-feeding woman can be obtained from a varied diet that includes foods from each of the basic food groups. Breast-feeding women are advised to consume an additional serving of a vitamin C fruit or vegetable and one more serving of milk or milk products than during pregnancy. Failure to consume enough calories from food can cause milk production to decrease. Weight loss that exceeds one and one-half pounds per week, even in women with a good supply of fat stores, can reduce the amount of milk produced.[56]

Increases in hunger and food intake that go along with breast-feeding generally take care of meeting caloric needs. If the diet includes at least the recommended, minimal number of servings from each food group and enough calories, the breast-feeding woman is providing an adequate diet for herself and her infant.

Nutrition clearly plays a leading role in fostering the health of pregnant women and their infants. But there is more to the story about nutrition and reproduction. The story continues because of the hormonal changes women experience and their effects on physical and emotional health.

PREMENSTRUAL SYNDROME (PMS)

PMS was identified and described over fifty years ago, but has been considered a "medically legitimate" condition for only the past few years. It has likely been endured by women since Eve.

A woman is unlike a man in that during the fertile years, her body undergoes cyclical patterns in hormone levels (principally estrogen and progesterone) that monthly prepare her for conception. A major side effect of the fluctuations in estrogen and progesterone levels ranges from bothersome to debilitating changes in about one out of every three women.[57] A large set of the side effects of hormonal changes is encompassed in the disorder called PMS.

PMS is a complex disorder for which there is no known cure. It is thought to result from hormonal imbalances.[58] Signs of PMS generally occur a week to two weeks before periods and end before menstrual bleeding begins. The syndrome includes a wide variety of problems and symptoms, and the occurrence and severity of each differ greatly from one woman to the next. Hardly any woman experiences all of the characteristic signs of PMS. Rather, individual women tend to experience a specific set of problems. These common sets of problems are shown in table 39.

Between one-third and one-half of women with PMS experience weight gain, swelling, headaches, and tension.[59] Appetite and food intake often increase premenstrually, and changes in food preferences, such as an increased desire for chocolate, sweets, or salty foods, may occur.[60] The development of cravings for specific foods or sweets has been associated with premenstrual feelings of tension or depression.[61] Women with severe signs of PMS tend to experience a greater increase in caloric intake after midcycle than women who experience moderate or mild signs. Overall, the severity of PMS signs increases with age and among women with long and heavy menstrual flows.[59]

There are no physical or laboratory tests that are useful in diagnosing PMS. Consequently, the diagnosis is made by the results of a questionnaire. If a number of the signs of PMS listed in table 39 occur before, and not after, periods on a regular basis, a diagnosis of PMS is usually made.[62] Approaches to the treatment of premenstrual problems vary somewhat depending on the specific signs that occur.

TABLE 39. SYMPTOMS ASSOCIATED WITH THE FOUR MAJOR CATEGORIES OF PMS

| Symptoms | Week before Period | | | | Week after Period | | | |
|---|---|---|---|---|---|---|---|---|
| | NONE | MILD | MODERATE | SEVERE | NONE | MILD | MODERATE | SEVERE |
| *Type 1* | | | | | | | | |
| Nervous tension | ☐ | ☐ | ☐ | ☐ | ☐ | ☐ | ☐ | ☐ |
| Mood swings | ☐ | ☐ | ☐ | ☐ | ☐ | ☐ | ☐ | ☐ |
| Irritability | ☐ | ☐ | ☐ | ☐ | ☐ | ☐ | ☐ | ☐ |
| Anxiety | ☐ | ☐ | ☐ | ☐ | ☐ | ☐ | ☐ | ☐ |
| *Type 2* | | | | | | | | |
| Weight gain | ☐ | ☐ | ☐ | ☐ | ☐ | ☐ | ☐ | ☐ |
| Swelling (arms and legs) | ☐ | ☐ | ☐ | ☐ | ☐ | ☐ | ☐ | ☐ |
| Breast tenderness | ☐ | ☐ | ☐ | ☐ | ☐ | ☐ | ☐ | ☐ |
| Abdominal bloating | ☐ | ☐ | ☐ | ☐ | ☐ | ☐ | ☐ | ☐ |
| *Type 3* | | | | | | | | |
| Headache | ☐ | ☐ | ☐ | ☐ | ☐ | ☐ | ☐ | ☐ |
| Craving for sweets | ☐ | ☐ | ☐ | ☐ | ☐ | ☐ | ☐ | ☐ |
| Increased appetite | ☐ | ☐ | ☐ | ☐ | ☐ | ☐ | ☐ | ☐ |
| Heart pounding | ☐ | ☐ | ☐ | ☐ | ☐ | ☐ | ☐ | ☐ |
| Fatigue | ☐ | ☐ | ☐ | ☐ | ☐ | ☐ | ☐ | ☐ |
| Light headedness | ☐ | ☐ | ☐ | ☐ | ☐ | ☐ | ☐ | ☐ |
| *Type 4* | | | | | | | | |
| Depression | ☐ | ☐ | ☐ | ☐ | ☐ | ☐ | ☐ | ☐ |
| Forgetfulness | ☐ | ☐ | ☐ | ☐ | ☐ | ☐ | ☐ | ☐ |
| Crying | ☐ | ☐ | ☐ | ☐ | ☐ | ☐ | ☐ | ☐ |
| Confusion | ☐ | ☐ | ☐ | ☐ | ☐ | ☐ | ☐ | ☐ |
| Insomnia | ☐ | ☐ | ☐ | ☐ | ☐ | ☐ | ☐ | ☐ |

### *Treatment Approaches*

The lack of a known cure for PMS is perhaps the reason why approaches to treatment are all over the map. Progesterone and other steroid hormones (including oral contraceptives) and dietary modifications represent the most common approaches. Exercise is also recommended, but less often than drugs or dietary changes. No treatment approach is 100 percent effective, and relief from the symptoms may require experimenting with several approaches.

#### DRUGS FOR PMS

Over-the-counter drugs for PMS commonly contain acetaminophen or acetylsalicyclic acid (pain relievers) in combination with caffeine (a mild diuretic) and an antihistamine. These substances have been chosen to relieve the common premenstrual symptoms of headache, joint pain, bloating, and anxiety. They tend to be much more effective in women experiencing mild symptoms. Prescription drugs such as progesterone and oral contraceptives are also used and help relieve symptoms of PMS in some women.[62]

### VITAMIN SUPPLEMENTS

The doses of vitamins used in the treatment of PMS symptoms are high enough to qualify them as drugs. Although many vitamins have been recommended, megadoses of vitamins $B_6$ and E are the most popular. Whether they are effective is unclear. Vitamin $B_6$ acts as a diuretic if taken in large amounts (over 100 mg per day) and may reduce swelling. However, the regular use of more than 50 mg of $B_6$ per day may cause signs of vitamin $B_6$ overdose. Before it became a popular remedy for PMS, vitamin $B_6$ overdose reactions were rarely observed. Now, because so many women have used large doses for the treatment of PMS, it has been learned that vitamin $B_6$ supplements can be hazardous. Some of the first symptoms of vitamin $B_6$ overdose are numbness in the hands and feet and muscle weakness.[63] If vitamin $B_6$ supplements are used, the dose level should probably be kept well below 50 mg per day.

Vitamin E in high doses (400 IU per day and more) has been used to reduce the breast tenderness that may occur prior to periods. Vitamin E overdose reactions are not observed with doses of less than 1,000 IU per day.[64] Although generally safe, large doses of vitamin E appear to be effective for the single symptom of breast tenderness and only among a portion of women who take it.

### DIETARY REMEDIES

An assortment of dietary cures for PMS have been proposed and include: 1) increasing complex carbohydrate (starch) intake; 2) supplementing the diet with primrose oil; 3) decreasing caffeine, sodium, alcohol, and sugar intake; and 4) increasing calcium and magnesium consumption. Of these, the only dietary change that offers a promise of effectiveness so far is reducing caffeine intake. PMS symptoms may increase in severity with high caffeine intake such as can occur when coffee or tea is consumed regularly. "High" means the consumption of four or more caffeine-containing beverages per day.[65] The richest sources of caffeine are coffee and soft drinks with added caffeine. It should be noted that caffeine is also contained in certain medications used to treat asthma and to relieve pain. The ingredient level of medications often reports the amount of caffeine contained in the product.

#### EXERCISE

Can you exercise PMS symptoms away? Maybe. The effect of exercise on PMS symptoms is a new area of investigation. A preliminary report in *Obstetrics and Gynecology News* (vol. 22, 1988) suggests it might help if continued for six months or more. Could it hurt? Probably not; it may be worth a try.

There remain many unanswered questions about the causes of PMS and the reasons why some women experience severe health problems prior to menstruation. The lack of knowledge in these areas is reflected in the current absence of reliable remedies. Until more is known, it is likely that new dietary, vitamin, and mineral "cures" will proliferate. Whether such approaches are worthwhile and do more good than harm will ultimately depend on scientific proof. One shouldn't settle for anything less.

# Chapter 12

## *Diagnosing Nutrition Misinformation*

*True or False:*
*Any food that's white is bad for you.*
*Bread and potatoes are fattening.*
*There are quick and effortless ways to lose weight.*
*High-protein diets build muscles.*
*Grapefruit, vinegar, and lecithin melt away fat.*
*Celery has negative calories.*
*Honey is better for you than sugar.*
*The fetus is a parasite.*
*Pregnant women have "maternal instincts" that draw them to select a good diet during pregnancy.*
*Children, if left alone to choose from an assortment of foods, will select and consume a well-balanced diet.*

▼ Nutrition misinformation: it gets you coming and going. There's probably more of it around (like the preceding false statements) than there is good information. If you have heard of any of these pieces of nutrition "myth-information," then it has been around you too.

Nutrition information and products represent big business in this country and others. For the price of a book, vitamin supplements, "organic" foods, or other products, it is claimed we can nourish our heart, brain, and libido; or we can lengthen our life. Whether you want to lower your weight, raise your child's IQ, or protect yourself from the "poisons" in food, there is information that claims to tell you what foods or dietary supplements can do it. The selling of nutrition information, "health" foods, and other products is a multibillion-dollar business in the United States. The claims made for foods and supplements help keep that business healthy.

There is a lot of nutrition information available, but much of it is nuts. (The word *nuts* just happens to come right after *nutritive* in one edition of the *Random House Dictionary*.) At best, nutrition misinformation may, by coincidence, benefit health. Most often, it is useless but expensive. At worst, nutrition misinformation may damage health. A number of deaths have been directly associated with using liquid-protein diets and potassium supplements.[1,2] Also, lead poisoning has resulted from the use of so-called natural calcium supplements that naturally contain lead.[2] Reports of overdoses of vitamin and mineral supplements are increasingly common.

Why is so much nutrition misinformation available to consumers? It is available because purveyors of nutrition misinformation are not required to tell the truth, the whole truth, and nothing but the truth. The first amendment of the Constitution guarantees free speech and expression, whether or not the ideas expressed are true. As long as there is no direct link to a product, then books, flyers, magazine and tabloid articles, and radio and television talk show personalities can freely promote inaccurate or deceptive nutrition information. Any food can be labeled a "natural" or "health" food. There are no legal definitions for these terms, nor laws that prevent any substance from being labeled a vitamin or dietary supplement. Vitamins and other dietary supplements do not have to contain ingredients that are useful or necessary for health. Sawdust can be sold as a dietary supplement.

Another reason for the proliferation of nutrition misinformation is that there is no regulation for use of the title "nutritionist." Anybody can call themselves a nutritionist or a nutrition expert—even a cat. Dr. Victor Herbert, a well-known and respected scientist, mailed in fifty dollars and an application for nutrition credentials for his cat. The cat received an impressive-looking, frameable certificate from the International Academy of Nutritional Consultants.[3] Only the term *Registered Dietitian* attests that a person has successfully completed approved college courses in nutrition and dietetics, has had work experience, and has passed a national qualifying exam.

Individuals end up being the ones who have to decide if what they read or hear about nutrition is true. But distinguishing nutrition facts from fiction is not always easy. The nutrition misinformation business is sophisticated and has developed very convincing sales techniques. The ploys used, however, have a pattern, and you can often distinguish nutrition fact from fiction by examining how the information is presented.

## CHARACTERISTICS OF NUTRITION MISINFORMATION

### *The Money Motive*

The most common feature of nutrition misinformation is the goal to sell something. Likely being sold is a product, service, or program that offers a "new" or "unique" approach to treating ailments and diseases (otherwise, why would you need it?), so a convincing case is required on why the approach offered actually works. Nutrition misinformation is used liberally to convince customers of the effectiveness of nutrition remedies sold.

To circumvent truth-in-advertising laws, vendors of special foods and dietary supplements may promote their wares in articles that are interspersed with advertisements. Although caution is exhibited on the product label, peddlers of nutrition nonsense can say what they want in articles. The following example is from an article in a popular magazine. Surrounding the article were advertisements for zinc and other supplements.

> Zinc is without a doubt crucial to a healthy sex life. The scientific awareness of zinc's importance grew out of observations made by Dr. Prasad, M.D., Ph.D., in the 1960s. Dr. Prasad and other pioneers conducted studies with undernourished, sexually underdeveloped dwarfs in the Middle East, which showed that the cause of these men's sexual retardation was zinc deficiency. Researchers in this country now use zinc to treat sexual problems.

Here is an excerpt from the results Prasad and his coworkers actually reported regarding zinc deficiency.

> In recent years a syndrome of severe iron deficiency anemia, hepatosplenomegaly,* hypogonadism,* hyperpigmentation,* and dwarfism in Iranian and Egyptian dwarfs has been attributed to primary zinc deficiency. Geophagia* is common in the Iranian dwarfs, and it was suggested that zinc deficiency may have resulted from excessive consumption of a cereal diet containing large amounts of phytate which inhibits zinc absorption. Upon treatment with supplemental zinc salts, a striking response in growth and development of secondary sex characteristics was observed.[4]

(**Hepatosplenomegaly* means enlarged liver and spleen; *hypogonadism* is the term for immature sex glands; *hyperpigmentation* is abnormal skin color; and *geophagia* means the eating of dirt or clay.)

Purveyors of nutrition misinformation are free to misinterpret research results and to draw their own conclusions.

*Connections with the Familiar*

Overweight? Under stress? Losing your hair? Tire easily? Getting wrinkles?

Nutrition misinformation and products are usually aimed at relieving problems that are common but difficult to treat, or are currently untreatable. The "safe, easy, and effective" approaches offered for solving problems are frequently irresistible, although notions may linger that they may be too good to be true. As they say of all huckster pitches, "If it sounds too good to be true, it probably is." If any of the purported cures really worked, why aren't the problems solved and the market for new products gone? Yet, there is always another fad diet book, miracle vitamin or mineral supplement cure, or other nutrition hoax promoted to fix what ails us because the remedies previously sold have failed.

*Filling in the Credibility Gap*

WITH CREDENTIALS

Marketers of nutrition misinformation and products are very aware of the importance of credibility and have developed effective approaches for filling in credibility gaps. One key way to convey credibility is to have an M.D., Ph.D., or a superstar athlete endorse the information or product offered. Unfortunately, nutrition information cannot be taken as credible because of endorsements. Individuals with impeccable credentials, including Nobel Prize–winning scientists, renowned surgeons, and Olympic gold–medal winners have promulgated nutrition schemes. One dietary supplement company that freely promoted nutrition misinformation went as far as to enlist the services of fifteen internationally known scientists and physicians to serve on their "scientific advisory board." All were well respected in their fields of expertise and were employed by such honorable institutions as Harvard Medical School, the University of Washington, the National Institute of Mental Health, and the University of California at Berkeley. None, however, were experts in nutrition. Their affiliation with the company that sold "revolutionary breakthrough" nutrition products for weight loss, protection against cancer and heart disease, and for "sustained energy" sent shock waves through the scientific community. The initial reaction was followed by aftershock when it was learned that many of the members of the "scientific advisory board" were awarded $100,000 research grants by the supplement company.[5] Credibility can be purchased.

WITH TESTIMONIALS

*If it worked for me, it will work for you.*

Testimonials are another common ploy used to make nutrition misinformation credible. Alas, even testimonials need not be based on fact. Testimonials, however, come in very handy when formal tests of a product's effectiveness have not been done or when research results are unlikely to support the case being made. The use of testimonials to support a nutrition claim is a dead giveaway to false or deceptive information.

EXAMINING THE SOURCE

Awareness of the source of nutrition information can help you decide if a grain or a ton of salt needs to be taken along with the information. Some newspapers (particularly tabloids), talk shows, and magazines regularly cover nutrition because their audiences have indicated a strong interest in the topic. The more spectacular or controversial the information, the more likely it is to be covered. (News about how rose-colored glasses will turn off your appetite or how a superstar fought cancer with fish oils, for example, attracts attention.) For these publications and broadcasts, it matters little if the information is from nutrition fantasyland or scientific reports.

Not all of the nutrition information you read or hear is nonsense. Many newspapers, magazines, and broadcasting companies are cautious about the accuracy of information presented. This caution is exercised by investigating the reliability of the sources of the nutrition information, by covering more than one side of controversial topics, and by confirming conclusions with nutrition experts before the information is presented. Some print and broadcasting companies have policies that reject advertisements that make false or deceptive nutrition claims.

RELIABLE SOURCES OF NUTRITION INFORMATION

Sources of nutrition information that earn a seal of approval include:

Government health publications

Information produced by scientifically recognized

professional organizations such as the American Dietetic Association, the American Institute of Nutrition, and the Society for Nutrition Education

Scientific journals that primarily publish research studies

College nutrition textbooks used in nutrition courses

A list of reliable sources of nutrition information and resources available to the public is given in Appendix C.

Other sources of reliable nutrition information exist, but it is impossible to give them blanket approval because the credibility of the information presented varies too much. For example, popular nutrition books written by people with impressive credentials may contain hogwash, or they may be accurate. You can't tell by the credentials of the author alone. Nor can you always trust information relayed in "educational" publications produced by the food and dietary supplement industry. Infant formula companies; organizations representing the meat, wheat, potato, and dairy industries; manufacturers of vitamin and mineral supplements; and a host of other organizations publish nutrition information as a public service. Sometimes the information is accurate, but often it is slanted in favor of the company's products. Advertisements may be included along with the articles on nutrition, and the topics selected for coverage commonly relate only to the types of food, vitamins, or minerals sold by the sponsoring company. It is impossible to group all industry sources of nutrition information as reliable or unreliable. They represent a mixture of both.

## A GUIDE FOR SEPARATING FACTS FROM FICTION: THE CHECKLIST

How do you decide whether to believe questionable nutrition information? A good approach is to check out the information for telltale signs of nutrition nonsense. You can use the "Quick List" shown here to identify the most common characteristics of nutrition misinformation. If the answer to any of these questions is yes, then the accuracy of the information is highly suspect. You can gather additional evidence to confirm your conclusion by answering the questions listed under "Other Considerations."

Much of the information in this chapter relates to stories about nutrition and health that lie outside of what is known to be true. The truth, however, has a lot going for it. It's the stuff you can count on.

CHECKING OUT NUTRITION INFORMATION

| *The Quick List* | *Yes* | *No* |
|---|---|---|
| 1. Is something being sold? | ☐ | ☐ |
| 2. Does the information refer to common dissatisfactions, undesired feelings, or fears? | ☐ | ☐ |
| 3. Are testimonials or success stories included? | ☐ | ☐ |
| 4. Does the information sound too good to be true? | ☐ | ☐ |
| 5. Does the information present a unique or generally unaccepted approach to improving health? | ☐ | ☐ |

| *Other Considerations* | *Yes* | *No* |
|---|---|---|
| 1. Are promises made for quick results that are easily achieved? | ☐ | ☐ |
| 2. Have the words "doctors" or "scientists," or scientific-sounding terms been used to support the credibility of the information presented? | ☐ | ☐ |
| 3. Are the problems addressed those for which there is no common, complete, or easy cure? | ☐ | ☐ |
| 4. Was the information published in a tabloid newspaper, magazine, advertisement, or popular book, or broadcast on a talk show? | ☐ | ☐ |

# Chapter 13

## *Recipes for Good Eating*

▼ What sort of recipes do you keep on file or tucked inside your favorite cookbook? Are they delicious as well as nutritious? If you have an insufficient assortment of such recipes, try these. They have been designed and tested by the nutritionists at Nutrition Plus, Inc., of Minneapolis, Minnesota. Both menus with recipes and single recipes for every course and social occasion are included. Full disclosure about their nutrient contributions is also provided. Your enjoyment of the products of these recipes and your labor need not be lessened by a feeling of guilt about what is in them!

Enjoy.

---

## Country Beef Ragout Dinner

| *Menu* | *Suggested Serving Sizes* |
|---|---|
| Country Beef Ragout | ⅛ of recipe |
| Cooked egg noodles | 1 cup |
| Tossed salad | 1 cup |
| Low-cal dressing | 1 tablespoon |
| Dinner roll | One |
| Margarine | 1 teaspoon |
| Skim milk | 1 cup |
| Frozen yogurt | ½ cup |

## COUNTRY BEEF RAGOUT *(Serves 8)*

**2 lbs. beef stew meat, cut into 1½" cubes**
**3 large onions, each cut into 8 pieces**
**4 large garlic cloves, crushed**
**5 tomatoes, quartered**
**5 T. chopped parsley, divided**
**1 tsp. dried thyme leaves**
**1 tsp. pepper**
**1 c. red Burgundy wine**
**1 c. water**
**8 oz. fresh mushrooms, quartered**
**Wide, flat noodles, cooked**

*Directions*

1. Trim excess fat from stew meat. Spray Dutch oven with vegetable spray; add beef cubes and brown over high heat.
2. Add onions and brown lightly; add garlic.
3. Stir in tomatoes, 3 tablespoons parsley, thyme, pepper, red wine, and water; bring to a boil.
4. Reduce heat; cover and simmer for 1 hour.
5. Add mushrooms; cover and simmer 60 to 90 minutes, until beef is tender.
6. If desired, simmer uncovered last 10 minutes to reduce liquid.
7. Stir in remaining parsley. Serve ragout over hot cooked noodles.

| *Composition of Recipe* | | *Serving Size: ⅛ of Recipe* | |
|---|---|---|---|
| Calories | 244 | Zinc (mg) | 5.7 |
| Protein (g) | 29 | Iron (mg) | 4.7 |
| Total fat (g) | 7 | Vitamin A (IU) | 920 |
| Carbohydrate (g) | 12 | Thiamin (mg) | 0.2 |
| Cholesterol (mg) | 64 | Riboflavin (mg) | 0.4 |
| Fiber (g) | 2 | Niacin (mg) | 7.1 |
| Calcium (mg) | 46 | Vitamin $B_6$ (mg) | 0.5 |
| Magnesium (mg) | 53 | Folacin (mcg) | 32 |
| Sodium (mg) | 79 | Vitamin $B_{12}$ (mcg) | 2.3 |
| Potassium (mg) | 729 | Vitamin C (mg) | 29 |

# Baked Fish Dinner

| *Menu* | *Suggested Serving Sizes* |
|---|---|
| Baked Ocean Perch | ¼ of recipe |
| Asparagus | 4 stalks |
| Margarine | ½ teaspoon |
| Vinaigrette coleslaw | ½ cup |
| Rye bread | One slice |
| Margarine | 1 teaspoon |
| Skim milk | 1 cup |
| Lemon pudding | ½ cup |

**BAKED OCEAN PERCH** *(Serves 4)*

**1 fresh lemon, thinly sliced**
**1 medium onion, thinly sliced**
**1 tsp. salt**
**1 lb. ocean perch fillets**
**1 c. plain low-fat yogurt**
**1 tsp. mustard**
**1 tsp. paprika**

*Directions*

1. Arrange lemon and onion slices in a lightly greased baking dish.
2. Top with fish fillets and season lightly with salt; cover dish with foil.
3. Bake at 400° F for 20 to 25 minutes. Remove foil; turn oven temperature to broil.
4. In a small bowl, blend yogurt, mustard, and paprika; spread over fish.
5. Broil 3 inches from heat for about 5 minutes or until browned.

| *Composition of Recipe* | | *Serving Size: ¼ of Recipe* | |
|---|---|---|---|
| Calories | 186 | Zinc (mg) | 1.8 |
| Protein (g) | 26 | Iron (mg) | 2 |
| Total fat (g) | 2 | Vitamin A (IU) | 368 |
| Carbohydrate (g) | 15 | Thiamin (mg) | 0.1 |
| Cholesterol (mg) | 69 | Riboflavin (mg) | 0.3 |
| Fiber (g) | 0.4 | Niacin (mg) | 2.3 |
| Calcium (mg) | 155 | Vitamin $B_6$ (mg) | 0.3 |
| Magnesium (mg) | 44 | Folacin (mcg) | 15 |

| | | | |
|---|---|---|---|
| Sodium (mg) | 375 | Vitamin $B_{12}$ (mcg) | 1.5 |
| Potassium (mg) | 529 | Vitamin C (mg) | 4 |

## Chicken Cacciatore Dinner

| *Menu* | *Suggested Serving Sizes* |
|---|---|
| Chicken Cacciatore | ⅙ of recipe |
| Hot cooked spaghetti | 1 cup |
| Italian bread | 2 pieces |
| Margarine | 1 teaspoon |
| Skim milk | 1 cup |
| Fruit cocktail | ½ cup |

**CHICKEN CACCIATORE** *(Serves 6)*

**1½ chicken**
**2 T. vegetable oil**
**½ c. flour**
**2 c. thinly sliced onion rings (2 large)**
**½ c. chopped green pepper**
**2 cloves garlic, crushed**
**4 tomatoes, quartered**
**1 can (8 oz.) tomato sauce**
**4 oz. fresh mushrooms, sliced**
**¼ tsp. salt**
**½ tsp. oregano**

*Directions*

1. Wash chicken, pat dry; remove skin and coat chicken with flour.
2. In a Dutch oven or large saucepan, heat oil.
3. Brown chicken in oil; cook over medium heat for 15 to 20 minutes.
4. Remove chicken from saucepan; set aside.
5. Add onion, green pepper, and garlic to saucepan; cook until tender.
6. Add remaining ingredients to saucepan; return chicken to pan.
7. Cover tightly and simmer for 30 to 40 minutes.

| *Composition of Recipe* | | *Serving Size: ⅙ of Recipe* | |
|---|---|---|---|
| Calories | 253 | Zinc (mg) | 2.5 |
| Protein (g) | 31 | Iron (mg) | 2.9 |

| | | | |
|---|---|---|---|
| Total fat (g) | 7 | Vitamin A (IU) | 1,360 |
| Carbohydrate (g) | 21 | Thiamin (mg) | 0.2 |
| Cholesterol (mg) | 81 | Riboflavin (mg) | 0.4 |
| Fiber (g) | 2.8 | Niacin (mg) | 11 |
| Calcium (mg) | 51 | Vitamin $B_6$ (mg) | 0.7 |
| Magnesium (mg) | 57 | Folacin (mcg) | 39 |
| Sodium (mg) | 378 | Vitamin $B_{12}$ (mcg) | 0.3 |
| Potassium (mg) | 762 | Vitamin C (mg) | 49 |

## Taco Salad Supper

| *Menu* | *Suggested Serving Sizes* |
|---|---|
| Taco Salad | ⅙ of recipe |
| Skim milk | 1 cup |
| Sherbet | 1 cup |

**TACO SALAD** *(Serves 6)*

**1 lb. extra-lean ground beef**
**½ clove garlic, crushed**
**1 can (4 oz.) chopped, mild green chiles**
**1 can (16 oz.) tomatoes, undrained**
**¼ tsp. salt**
**⅛ tsp. pepper**
**1 head iceberg lettuce, torn into bite-size pieces**
**⅔ c. grated cheddar cheese (3 oz.)**
**3 oz. tortilla chips, crushed**
**½ c. chopped green onion**
**1 tomato, sliced**

*Directions*

1. Sauté beef and garlic until beef is browned. Drain.
2. Add green chiles, canned tomatoes, salt, and pepper and mix well. Cook uncovered over low heat for 30 minutes.
3. Just before serving, arrange lettuce, cheese, chips, and green onion in a salad bowl. Add meat mixture and toss lightly. Garnish with sliced tomato and serve immediately.

This is also a good main-course luncheon salad.

| *Composition of Recipe* | | *Serving Size: ⅙ of Recipe* | |
|---|---|---|---|
| Calories | 220 | Zinc (mg) | 4.6 |
| Protein (g) | 23 | Iron (mg) | 3.5 |
| Total fat (g) | 7 | Vitamin A (IU) | 1,560 |

| | | | |
|---|---|---|---|
| Carbohydrate (g) | 17 | Thiamin (mg) | 0.2 |
| Cholesterol (mg) | 49 | Riboflavin (mg) | 0.3 |
| Fiber (g) | 2.7 | Niacin (mg) | 4.6 |
| Calcium (mg) | 287 | Vitamin $B_6$ (mg) | 0.5 |
| Magnesium (mg) | 53 | Folacin (mcg) | 38 |
| Sodium (mg) | 372 | Vitamin $B_{12}$ (mcg) | 1.2 |
| Potassium (mg) | 589 | Vitamin C (mg) | 47 |

## Spinach-Cheese Frittata Dinner

| *Menu* | *Suggested Serving Sizes* |
|---|---|
| Tomato soup | ¾ cup |
| Crackers | Two |
| Spinach-Cheese Frittata | ⅙ of recipe |
| Three-bean salad | ½ cup |
| Skim milk | 1 cup |
| Molasses cookie | One |

**SPINACH-CHEESE FRITTATA** *(Serves 6)*

**⅓ c. chopped onion**
**1 T. margarine**
**3 eggs**
**1 pkg. (10½ oz.) chopped spinach, thawed and drained**
**12 oz. low-fat cottage cheese**
**1 T. flour**
**½ tsp. thyme**
**1 tomato, sliced**
**¼ c. fine bread crumbs**
**¼ c. Parmesan cheese**

*Directions*

1. In a 10'', ovenproof skillet, melt margarine and sauté onion until limp.
2. In mixing bowl, beat eggs; then add drained spinach, cottage cheese, flour, and thyme.
3. Pour spinach mixture into skillet and stir with onions.
4. Place skillet in oven and bake at 350° F for 35 minutes.
5. Add sliced tomato to top, sprinkle with bread crumbs and Parmesan cheese.

6. Turn oven to broil, broil 1 to 2 minutes until brown.

| *Composition of Recipe* | | *Serving Size: ⅙ of Recipe* | |
|---|---|---|---|
| Calories | 155 | Zinc (mg) | 1.0 |
| Protein (g) | 14 | Iron (mg) | 2.2 |
| Total fat (g) | 7 | Vitamin A (IU) | 4,560 |
| Carbohydrate (g) | 9 | Thiamin (mg) | 0.1 |
| Cholesterol (mg) | 136 | Riboflavin (mg) | 0.3 |
| Fiber (g) | 1.3 | Niacin (mg) | 0.7 |
| Calcium (mg) | 165 | Vitamin $B_6$ (mg) | 0.3 |
| Magnesium (mg) | 47 | Folacin (mcg) | 59 |
| Sodium (mg) | 382 | Vitamin $B_{12}$ (mcg) | 0.7 |
| Potassium (mg) | 321 | Vitamin C (mg) | 17 |

## Appetizers

### MIDDLE EASTERN HUMMUS *(Makes 2 cups)*

**½ c. sesame seeds**
**1 large onion, chopped**
**3 garlic cloves, minced**
**1 T. olive oil**
**1 can (16 oz.) chickpeas or garbanzo beans, drained and rinsed**
**1½ tsp. lemon juice**
**1 T. soy sauce**
**¼ c. tahini paste**
**Pita bread**

*Directions*

1. Place sesame seeds on a cookie sheet; toast at 300° F for 10 to 15 minutes, or until lightly browned.
2. In a skillet, sauté onion and garlic in olive oil until limp.
3. Place toasted sesame seeds in a blender or food processor; blend into a paste.
4. Add sautéd mixture and remaining ingredients and blend until smooth.
5. Serve by dipping pieces of pita bread into the hummus.

| *Composition of Recipe* | | *Serving Size: 2 T. hummus and 1 pita bread* | |
|---|---|---|---|
| Calories | 176 | Zinc (mg) | 1.6 |
| Protein (g) | 6 | Iron (mg) | 1.8 |
| Total fat (g) | 6 | Vitamin A (IU) | 10 |
| Carbohydrate (g) | 23 | Thiamin (mg) | 0.1 |

| | | | |
|---|---|---|---|
| Cholesterol (mg) | 1 | Riboflavin (mg) | 0.1 |
| Fiber (g) | 5.4 | Niacin (mg) | 1.2 |
| Calcium (mg) | 51 | Vitamin $B_6$ (mg) | 0.1 |
| Magnesium (mg) | 27 | Folacin (mcg) | 11 |
| Sodium (mg) | 219 | Vitamin $B_{12}$ (mcg) | 0 |
| Potassium (mg) | 149 | Vitamin C (mg) | 1 |

---

**SOY CHICKEN WINGS** *(Makes 16 appetizers)*

**⅔ c. sugar**
**⅔ c. water**
**½ c. reduced-sodium soy sauce**
**16 raw chicken wings**
**¼ tsp. black pepper**
**½ tsp. garlic powder**

*Directions*

1. In a blender, combine sugar, water, and soy sauce.
2. Marinate wings in this mixture for 6 hours (or overnight) in the refrigerator.
3. Remove wings and place into a 9" × 13" baking dish. Season wings with pepper and garlic powder.
4. Bake, covered, for 1½ hours at 375° F.
5. Uncover and bake 30 minutes longer until wings are brown.

| *Composition of Recipe* | | *Serving Size: 1 chicken wing* | |
|---|---|---|---|
| Calories | 79 | Zinc (mg) | 0.4 |
| Protein (g) | 7 | Iron (mg) | 0.7 |
| Total fat (g) | 2 | Vitamin A (IU) | 12 |
| Carbohydrate (g) | 9 | Thiamin (mg) | 0 |
| Cholesterol (mg) | 17 | Riboflavin (mg) | 0.1 |
| Fiber (g) | 0 | Niacin (mg) | 1.5 |
| Calcium (mg) | 11 | Vitamin $B_6$ (mg) | 0.1 |
| Magnesium (mg) | 36 | Folacin (mcg) | 3 |
| Sodium (mg) | 410 | Vitamin $B_{12}$ (mcg) | 0.1 |
| Potassium (mg) | 77 | Vitamin C (mg) | 0 |

---

**TANGY PORKBALLS** *(Makes 48 small meatballs)*

**1 lb. fresh ground low-fat pork**
**3 bread slices, torn**
**2 T. brown sugar**
**½ tsp. dry mustard**
**1 T. soy sauce**
**¼ c. water**

*Sauce for dipping:*

**⅔ c. apricot jam**
**3 T. horseradish**

*Directions*

1. Mix ground pork and torn bread crumbs; shape into 1'' balls.
2. Spray heavy skillet with vegetable spray; brown meatballs over medium heat.
3. Remove meatballs from skillet and set aside; remove fat from skillet.
4. In the skillet, combine sugar, mustard, soy sauce, and water; bring to a boil.
5. Return meatballs to skillet and cook, turning frequently; cook until liquid is reduced.
6. Serve meatballs hot with mixture of apricot jam and horseradish for dipping sauce.

*Composition of Recipe* — *Serving Size: 2 meatballs and sauce*

| | | | |
|---|---|---|---|
| Calories | 90 | Zinc (mg) | 0.4 |
| Protein (g) | 4 | Iron (mg) | 0.4 |
| Total fat (g) | 4 | Vitamin A (IU) | 1 |
| Carbohydrate (g) | 9 | Thiamin (mg) | 0.1 |
| Cholesterol (mg) | 14 | Riboflavin (mg) | 0.1 |
| Fiber (g) | 0.1 | Niacin (mg) | 0.9 |
| Calcium (mg) | 7 | Vitamin $B_6$ (mg) | 0.1 |
| Magnesium (mg) | 8 | Folacin (mcg) | 2 |
| Sodium (mg) | 83 | Vitamin $B_{12}$ (mcg) | 0.1 |
| Potassium (mg) | 72 | Vitamin C (mg) | 0 |

---

**TINY TOSTADAS** *(Makes 24 appetizers)*

**1 c. canned refried beans**
**¼ c. taco sauce**
**24 round tortilla chips**
**½ c. shredded cheddar cheese**
**10-12 cherry tomatoes, each cut into 3 to 4 slices**

*Directions*

1. Mix refried beans with taco sauce.
2. Spread 1 teaspoon of mixture on each chip.
2. Top each with small amount of shredded cheese.
3. Place 6 to 8 tostadas on a microwave-safe plate lined with paper towel.

4. Microwave, uncovered, at medium power for 1 to 3 minutes.
5. Top each with tomato slice.

Note: This recipe is best when *not* made ahead of time.

| *Composition of Recipe* | | *Serving Size: 1 appetizer* | |
|---|---|---|---|
| Calories | 48 | Zinc (mg) | 0.2 |
| Protein (g) | 2 | Iron (mg) | 0.3 |
| Total fat (g) | 3 | Vitamin A (IU) | 236 |
| Carbohydrate (g) | 5 | Thiamin (mg) | 0 |
| Cholesterol (mg) | 2 | Riboflavin (mg) | 0 |
| Fiber (g) | 0.8 | Niacin (mg) | 0.3 |
| Calcium (mg) | 27 | Vitamin $B_6$ (mg) | 0 |
| Magnesium (mg) | 69 | Folacin (mcg) | 7 |
| Sodium (mg) | 91 | Vitamin $B_{12}$ (mcg) | 0 |
| Potassium (mg) | 84 | Vitamin C (mg) | 4 |

# Salads

## CREAMY LO-CAL COLESLAW *(Serves 8)*

**4 cups shredded raw cabbage**
**½ c. red or green pepper, chopped**
**¼ c. milk**
**2 T. cider vinegar**
**½ c. low-calorie mayonnaise**
**2 T. sugar**

*Directions*

1. In a large bowl, combine cabbage and chopped pepper.
2. In a small bowl, blend milk, vinegar, mayonnaise, and sugar.
3. Pour dressing over cabbage mixture; stir to mix.

| *Composition of Recipe* | | *Serving Size: ½ cup* | |
|---|---|---|---|
| Calories | 81 | Zinc (mg) | 0.3 |
| Protein (g) | 1 | Iron (mg) | 0.3 |
| Total fat (g) | 5 | Vitamin A (IU) | 152 |
| Carbohydrate (g) | 7 | Thiamin (mg) | 0 |
| Cholesterol (mg) | 2 | Riboflavin (mg) | 0 |
| Fiber (g) | 0.7 | Niacin (mg) | 0.2 |
| Calcium (mg) | 35 | Vitamin $B_6$ (mg) | 0.1 |
| Magnesium (mg) | 12 | Folacin (mcg) | 16 |
| Sodium (mg) | 116 | Vitamin $B_{12}$ (mcg) | 0 |
| Potassium (mg) | 158 | Vitamin C (mg) | 37 |

## CUCUMBERS WITH ROSEMARY AND THYME
*(Serves 8)*

**4 c. cucumber slices (2 cucumbers, unpared and scored)**
**½ small onion, thinly sliced**
**½ tsp. salt**
**1½ T. water**
**1½ T. olive oil**
**2 T. red wine vinegar**
**1 T. Dijon-style mustard**
**1 tsp. sugar**
**1 tsp. dried rosemary**
**1 tsp. thyme leaves, crushed**
**⅛ tsp. black pepper**

*Directions*

1. Place cucumbers and onion in a small bowl with lid.
2. Combine all remaining ingredients; pour over cucumbers and onions.
3. Refrigerate. Toss to coat every few hours.

| *Composition of Recipe* | | *Serving Size:* ⅛ of Recipe | |
|---|---|---|---|
| Calories | 41 | Zinc (mg) | 0.1 |
| Protein (g) | 1 | Iron (mg) | 0.4 |
| Total fat (g) | 3 | Vitamin A (IU) | 2 |
| Carbohydrate (g) | 3 | Thiamin (mg) | 0 |
| Cholesterol (mg) | 0 | Riboflavin (mg) | 0 |
| Fiber (g) | 0.4 | Niacin (mg) | 0.2 |
| Calcium (mg) | 20 | Vitamin $B_6$ (mg) | 0 |
| Magnesium (mg) | 7 | Folacin (mcg) | 9 |
| Sodium (mg) | 162 | Vitamin $B_{12}$ (mcg) | 0 |
| Potassium (mg) | 131 | Vitamin C (mg) | 8 |

---

## ORANGE-ONION SALAD *(Serves 4)*

**2 T. oil**
**2 tsp. tarragon vinegar**
**1 tsp. sugar**
**⅛ tsp. salt**
**3 drops hot sauce**
**⅛ tsp. pepper**
**2 large oranges**
**¼ red onion, cut into rings**
**Lettuce leaves**

*Directions*

1. In a small bowl or jar, combine oil, vinegar, sugar, salt, hot sauce, and pepper. Stir or shake thoroughly and set aside.
2. Line salad plates with lettuce leaves. Peel oranges with a knife, removing membrane. Cut each orange into 6 round slices.
3. Arrange orange slices and onion rings on lettuce leaves.
4. Before serving, pour oil and vinegar mixture over salad.

| *Composition of Recipe* | | *Serving Size: ¼ of Recipe* | |
|---|---|---|---|
| Calories | 114 | Zinc (mg) | 0.4 |
| Protein (g) | 2 | Iron (mg) | 0.7 |
| Total fat (g) | 7 | Vitamin A (IU) | 336 |
| Carbohydrate (g) | 13 | Thiamin (mg) | 0.1 |
| Cholesterol (mg) | 0 | Riboflavin (mg) | 0.1 |
| Fiber (g) | 1.9 | Niacin (mg) | 0.5 |
| Calcium (mg) | 46 | Vitamin $B_6$ (mg) | 0.1 |
| Magnesium (mg) | 22 | Folacin (mcg) | 4.2 |
| Sodium (mg) | 75 | Vitamin $B_{12}$ (mcg) | 0 |
| Potassium (mg) | 254 | Vitamin C (mg) | 47 |

---

## Soups

### GREEK LEMON SOUP *(Serves 6)*

**2 cans (10¾ oz. each) condensed chicken broth**
**2 cans (10¾ oz. each) water**
**½ c. uncooked rice**
**2 egg yolks**
**¼ c. lemon juice**
**1 peeled lemon, cut into paper-thin slices, if desired**
**Snipped fresh chives, if desired**

*Directions*

1. Heat chicken broth and water in large saucepan over medium heat to boiling; stir in rice.
2. Cook uncovered, stirring occasionally, until rice is soft, about 15 minutes.
3. In a small bowl, whisk egg yolks and lemon juice until light and lemon-colored.

4. Whisk 1 cup of the hot broth gradually into egg yolk mixture.
5. Remove the saucepan from heat; slowly stir egg yolk mixture into broth.
6. Garnish soup with lemon slices and chopped chives.

| *Composition of Recipe* | | *Serving Size: 1/6 of Recipe* | |
|---|---|---|---|
| Calories | 113 | Zinc (mg) | 0.6 |
| Protein (g) | 7 | Iron (mg) | 1.2 |
| Total fat (g) | 3 | Vitamin A (IU) | 170 |
| Carbohydrate (g) | 15 | Thiamin (mg) | 0.1 |
| Cholesterol (mg) | 85 | Riboflavin (mg) | 0.1 |
| Fiber (g) | 2.6 | Niacin (mg) | 2.8 |
| Calcium (mg) | 20 | Vitamin $B_6$ (mg) | 0.1 |
| Magnesium (mg) | 7 | Folacin (mcg) | 9 |
| Sodium (mg) | 832 | Vitamin $B_{12}$ (mcg) | 0.2 |
| Potassium (mg) | 206 | Vitamin C (mg) | 5 |

---

## SPRING VEGETABLE SOUP *(Serves 8)*

**1 T. olive oil**
**1 onion, thinly sliced**
**2 cloves garlic, finely chopped**
**1 small eggplant, peeled and cubed (about 1½ cups)**
**1 medium-size zucchini, sliced**
**½ green pepper, seeded and diced**
**2 fresh tomatoes, chopped**
**5 c. water**
**1¼ tsp. basil**
**½ tsp. ground coriander**
**¾ tsp. oregano**
**1 tsp. salt**
**¼ tsp. pepper**
**½ c. small shell macaroni, uncooked**

*Directions*

1. Heat olive oil in a heavy kettle; sauté onions and garlic until tender but not browned.
2. Add eggplant, zucchini, and green pepper; cook, stirring, over medium heat until lightly browned, about 8 to 10 minutes.
3. Add remaining ingredients except for macaroni. Bring to a boil, cover, and simmer 10 minutes or until vegetables are barely tender.

4. Add macaroni, cover; allow to rest for 10 minutes.

| *Composition of Recipe* | | *Serving Size: 1 cup* | |
|---|---|---|---|
| Calories | 80 | Zinc (mg) | 0.3 |
| Protein (g) | 3 | Iron (mg) | 1.1 |
| Total fat (g) | 2 | Vitamin A (IU) | 451 |
| Carbohydrate (g) | 14 | Thiamin (mg) | 0.1 |
| Cholesterol (mg) | 0 | Riboflavin (mg) | 0.1 |
| Fiber (g) | 1.2 | Niacin (mg) | 1.1 |
| Calcium (mg) | 32 | Vitamin $B_6$ (mg) | 0.1 |
| Magnesium (mg) | 23 | Folacin (mcg) | 10 |
| Sodium (mg) | 271 | Vitamin $B_{12}$ (mcg) | 0 |
| Potassium (mg) | 254 | Vitamin C (mg) | 25 |

---

## TURKEY BARLEY SOUP *(Serves 8)*

**1 turkey carcass**
**8 c. water**
**⅓ c. barley**
**1½ c. chopped onion**
**¼ c. chopped fresh parsley**
**1 bay leaf**
**1 tsp. poultry seasoning**
**1 c. sliced carrots**
**½ c. sliced celery**
**1 can (16 oz.) tomatoes**
**1 tsp. salt-free Creole seasoning**
**1 tsp. salt**

*Directions*

1. Place turkey carcass in large kettle or stock pot and cover with water. Bring to a boil, then simmer for 1½ hours, covered. Turn turkey, if necessary, during cooking.
2. Remove carcass. Strip meat from bones and add to broth.
3. Add barley; bring to a boil and simmer 15 minutes.
4. Add remaining ingredients and seasonings. Cook until vegetables are tender, about 15 minutes.

| *Composition of Recipe* | | *Serving Size: 1 cup* | |
|---|---|---|---|
| Calories | 70 | Zinc (mg) | 0.7 |
| Protein (g) | 8 | Iron (mg) | 2.3 |
| Total fat (g) | 1 | Vitamin A (IU) | 2,650 |
| Carbohydrate (g) | 9 | Thiamin (mg) | 0.1 |
| Cholesterol (mg) | 13 | Riboflavin (mg) | 0.1 |
| Fiber (g) | 1.3 | Niacin (mg) | 3.1 |
| Calcium (mg) | 45 | Vitamin $B_6$ (mg) | 0.2 |

| | | | |
|---|---|---|---|
| Magnesium (mg) | 25 | Folacin (mcg) | 18 |
| Sodium (mg) | 304 | Vitamin $B_{12}$ (mcg) | 0.1 |
| Potassium (mg) | 347 | Vitamin C (mg) | 21 |

# Entrées

## SLIMMING SEAFOOD SALAD *(Serves 3)*

**1 lb. skinned fish fillets, fresh or frozen**
**1 c. boiling water**
**2 T. lemon juice**
**½ small onion, thinly sliced**
**½ tsp. salt**
**2 peppercorns or dash of pepper**
**1 medium sprig of parsley**
**½ bay leaf**
**Salad greens**
**Tomato, cucumber, and celery**
**Low-calorie dressing**

*Directions*

1. Place fillets into lightly oiled, 10'' skillet. Add remaining ingredients except salad greens and fresh vegetables.
2. Cover and simmer 5 to 10 minutes, or just until fish flakes easily when tested with a fork. Carefully remove, drain, and place in a covered dish. Chill in refrigerator.
3. Arrange salad greens in bowl or plate with chilled poached fish and fresh vegetables.
4. Serve with 1 to 2 tablespoons of low-calorie dressing.

| *Composition of Recipe* | | *Serving Size: ⅓ of Recipe* | |
|---|---|---|---|
| Calories | 145 | Zinc (mg) | 0.9 |
| Protein (g) | 22 | Iron (mg) | 1.8 |
| Total fat (g) | 2 | Vitamin A (IU) | 870 |
| Carbohydrate (g) | 11 | Thiamin (mg) | 0.1 |
| Cholesterol (mg) | 35 | Riboflavin (mg) | 0.1 |
| Fiber (g) | 1.2 | Niacin (mg) | 2.3 |
| Calcium (mg) | 93 | Vitamin $B_6$ (mg) | 0.2 |
| Magnesium (mg) | 50 | Folacin (mcg) | 33 |
| Sodium (mg) | 717 | Vitamin $B_{12}$ (mcg) | 0.8 |
| Potassium (mg) | 708 | Vitamin C (mg) | 29 |

**VERMICELLI SALAD** *(Serves 6)*

**1 pkg. (7 oz.) vermicelli coils (about 3 cups cooked)**
**½ c. chopped red onion**
**½ chopped green pepper**
**1 T. chopped parsley**
**1 tsp. celery seed**
**½ tsp. oregano**
**½ tsp. chopped chives**
**¼ c. low-calorie mayonnaise**
**¼ c. plain low-fat yogurt**
**12 oz. cooked shrimp or crabmeat, marinated in:**
**½ c. lemon juice (optional)**

*Directions*

1. Cook vermicelli in boiling water, stirring constantly; drain and blanch with cold water.
2. Add onion, green pepper, parsley, celery seed, chives, oregano, and Italian dressing.
3. Combine mayonnaise with yogurt and add to salad mixture.

| *Composition of Recipe* | | *Serving Size: ⅙ of Recipe* | |
|---|---|---|---|
| Calories | 218 | Zinc (mg) | 1.6 |
| Protein (g) | 18 | Iron (mg) | 3.0 |
| Total fat (g) | 5 | Vitamin A (IU) | 193 |
| Carbohydrate (g) | 25 | Thiamin (mg) | 0.1 |
| Cholesterol (mg) | 81 | Riboflavin (mg) | 0.1 |
| Fiber (g) | 0.6 | Niacin (mg) | 2.1 |
| Calcium (mg) | 106 | Vitamin $B_6$ (mg) | 0.1 |
| Magnesium (mg) | 53 | Folacin (mcg) | 10 |
| Sodium (mg) | 244 | Vitamin $B_{12}$ (mcg) | 0.5 |
| Potassium (mg) | 232 | Vitamin C (mg) | 28 |

**SHANGHAI CHICKEN SALAD** *(Serves 4)*

**2 c. cooked skinless chicken, diced and refrigerated until cool**
**2 T. sesame tahini sauce**
**2 T. reduced-sodium soy sauce**
**2 tsp. white vinegar**
**⅛ tsp. red pepper (cayenne)**
**1 green onion, chopped**
**1 T. fresh cilantro (coriander), chopped**

**1 T. water**
**½ head lettuce, shredded**
**2 T. peanuts, chopped**

*Directions*

1. In a small bowl, combine tahini sauce, soy sauce, and vinegar.
2. Blend in red pepper, green onion, and cilantro. Whisk until thoroughly blended. Mix in water.
3. Gently combine chicken with sauce.
4. Mound lettuce on a platter or individual plates; arrange chicken salad on lettuce and sprinkle with chopped peanuts.

| *Composition of Recipe* | | *Serving Size: ¼ of Recipe* | |
|---|---|---|---|
| Calories | 200 | Zinc (mg) | 2.0 |
| Protein (g) | 23 | Iron (mg) | 1.6 |
| Total fat (g) | 10 | Vitamin A (IU) | 243 |
| Carbohydrate (g) | 4 | Thiamin (mg) | 0.1 |
| Cholesterol (mg) | 64 | Riboflavin (mg) | 0.2 |
| Fiber (g) | 1.0 | Niacin (mg) | 7.8 |
| Calcium (mg) | 34 | Vitamin $B_6$ (mg) | 0.4 |
| Magnesium (mg) | 48 | Folacin (mcg) | 23 |
| Sodium (mg) | 419 | Vitamin $B_{12}$ (mcg) | 0.2 |
| Potassium (mg) | 305 | Vitamin C (mg) | 3 |

---

**TURKEY PASTA SALAD** *(Serves 5)*

**2 c. smoked cooked turkey, cut in ½" cubes**
**4 c. cooked pasta (8 oz. dry)**
**¼ c. chopped green or red pepper**
**¼ c. chopped green onion**
**1 c. cherry tomatoes, cut in half**
**⅓ c. plain low-fat yogurt**
**⅓ c. buttermilk**
**3 T. olive oil**
**3 T. red wine vinegar**
**1 T. lemon juice**
**½ tsp. celery seed**
**4 drops hot sauce**
**⅛ tsp. black pepper**
**¼ tsp. garlic powder**
**Lettuce leaves**

*Directions*

1. In a large bowl, combine cubed turkey, cooked pasta, green pepper, green onion, and tomatoes.
2. Make dressing by combining all of the remaining ingredients in a container, covering tightly, and shaking until thoroughly mixed.
3. Pour dressing over turkey mixture and stir gently to blend.
4. Serve turkey pasta on lettuce leaves.

| *Composition of Recipe* | | *Serving Size: ⅕ of Recipe* | |
|---|---|---|---|
| Calories | 363 | Zinc (mg) | 1.9 |
| Protein (g) | 26 | Iron (mg) | 2.2 |
| Total fat (g) | 13 | Vitamin A (IU) | 685 |
| Carbohydrate (g) | 38 | Thiamin (mg) | 0.2 |
| Cholesterol (mg) | 45 | Riboflavin (mg) | 0.2 |
| Fiber (g) | 0.8 | Niacin (mg) | 8.4 |
| Calcium (mg) | 65 | Vitamin $B_6$ (mg) | 0.3 |
| Magnesium (mg) | 48 | Folacin (mcg) | 20 |
| Sodium (mg) | 78 | Vitamin $B_{12}$ (mcg) | 0.4 |
| Potassium (mg) | 526 | Vitamin C (mg) | 25 |

---

**CREOLE RED SNAPPER** *(Serves 8)*

**2 lbs. fresh red snapper fillets, cut into 3" pieces**
**1 pkg. (10 oz.) okra**
**1 can (29 oz.) tomatoes, crushed**
**1 large onion, chopped**
**¼ tsp. tabasco sauce**
**½ tsp. filé powder**
**½ tsp. salt**
**2 T. olive oil**

*Directions*

1. In a casserole dish, mix olive oil and chopped onion. Dash with tabasco sauce.
2. Layer with ½ package of okra, then add layer of *1* pound of fish; cover with ½ can of tomatoes.
3. Sprinkle tomatoes with ½ tsp. filé; repeat layering of okra, fish, then tomatoes. On top layer of tomatoes, sprinkle chopped onion.
4. Bake at 350° F for 45 minutes.

Suggestion: Serve in large soup bowl with crusty bread and tabasco sauce.

| *Composition of Recipe* | | *Serving Size: ⅛ of Recipe* | |
|---|---|---|---|
| Calories | 199 | Zinc (mg) | 1.5 |
| Protein (g) | 30 | Iron (mg) | 1.9 |
| Total fat (g) | 5 | Vitamin A (IU) | 1,020 |
| Carbohydrate (g) | 8 | Thiamin (mg) | 0.5 |
| Cholesterol (mg) | 76 | Riboflavin (mg) | 0.1 |
| Fiber (g) | 1.9 | Niacin (mg) | 5 |
| Calcium (mg) | 74 | Vitamin $B_6$ (mg) | 1.1 |
| Magnesium (mg) | 70 | Folacin (mcg) | 38 |
| Sodium (mg) | 232 | Vitamin $B_{12}$ (mcg) | 1.2 |
| Potassium (mg) | 767 | Vitamin C (mg) | 32 |

## CREOLE SHRIMP CASSEROLE *(Serves 4)*

**8 oz. fresh mushrooms, sliced**
**1 T. margarine**
**1 c. shrimp, cooked and cleaned**
**1 c. cooked rice**
**½ c. diced green pepper**
**½ c. chopped onion**
**¼ c. chopped celery**
**¼ c. chopped red pepper**
**1 tomato, finely chopped**
**¼ tsp. salt**
**¼ tsp. chili powder**
**¼ tsp. garlic powder**
**¾ tsp. thyme**
**1 tsp. filé powder**
**1 tsp. basil**
**1 tomato, thinly sliced**

*Directions*

1. In a skillet, heat margarine and sauté mushrooms until tender.
2. In a large bowl, combine the cooked rice, green pepper, onion, celery, red pepper, chopped tomato, and all of the seasonings. Add the sautéed mushrooms and mix.
3. Place into a 2-qt. microwave casserole and cover with wax paper.
4. Microwave on High for 6 minutes; stir, then microwave another 6 minutes.
5. Stir in cooked shrimp. Top with thinly sliced tomato and cover.
6. Microwave an additional 3 minutes on High.

| *Composition of Recipe* | | *Serving Size: ¼ of Recipe* | |
|---|---|---|---|
| Calories | 166 | Zinc (mg) | 1.2 |
| Protein (g) | 12 | Iron (mg) | 2.9 |
| Total fat (g) | 4 | Vitamin A (IU) | 933 |
| Carbohydrate (g) | 24 | Thiamin (mg) | 0.2 |
| Cholesterol (mg) | 44 | Riboflavin (mg) | 0.4 |
| Fiber (g) | 4.8 | Niacin (mg) | 4.2 |
| Calcium (mg) | 72 | Vitamin $B_6$ (mg) | 0.3 |
| Magnesium (mg) | 50 | Folacin (mcg) | 31 |
| Sodium (mg) | 483 | Vitamin $B_{12}$ (mcg) | 0.2 |
| Potassium (mg) | 570 | Vitamin C (mg) | 55 |

## MICROWAVE FISH FILLETS ALMANDINE

*(Serves 6)*

**⅓ c. slivered almonds**
**2 T. margarine**
**1½ lbs. fish fillets**
**½ tsp. seasoned salt**
**1½ T. fresh lemon juice**
**6 lemon wedges**
**1 tsp. seasoned pepper**

*Directions*

1. In microwave oven, toast slivered almonds for 5 to 7 minutes.
2. Melt margarine and blend with seasoned salt and seasoned pepper.
3. Lightly cover fillets with margarine and arrange around the outside of a 2-qt. glass dish.
4. Sprinkle fillets with lemon juice and cover dish with wax paper.
5. Microwave for 6 to 8 minutes, rotating dish ¼ turn halfway through the cooking time.
6. Rest fillets for 5 minutes. Top with toasted almonds and serve with lemon wedges.

| *Composition of Recipe* | | *Serving Size: ⅙ of Recipe* | |
|---|---|---|---|
| Calories | 206 | Zinc (mg) | 0.7 |
| Protein (g) | 23 | Iron (mg) | 1 |
| Total fat (g) | 12 | Vitamin A (IU) | 304 |
| Carbohydrate (g) | 2 | Thiamin (mg) | 0.1 |
| Cholesterol (mg) | 40 | Riboflavin (mg) | 0.1 |
| Fiber (g) | 0.2 | Niacin (mg) | 2.4 |
| Calcium (mg) | 39 | Vitamin $B_6$ (mg) | 0.2 |
| Magnesium (mg) | 40 | Folacin (mcg) | 9 |
| Sodium (mg) | 234 | Vitamin $B_{12}$ (mcg) | 0.6 |
| Potassium (mg) | 360 | Vitamin C (mg) | 2 |

**RED SNAPPER SUPREME** *(Serves 4)*

**1¼ lbs. red snapper steaks**
**2 T. margarine**
**1 T. chopped fresh parsley**
**¼ tsp. basil**
**½ carrot, minced**
**1 celery stalk, minced**
**1 c. white or rosé wine**
**¼ tsp. salt**
**¼ tsp. pepper**
**Lemon slices**

*Directions*

1. Melt margarine in baking dish.
2. Arrange fish in dish and cover with parsley, carrots, and celery. Sprinkle basil over top and pour the wine over.
3. Bake uncovered at 350° F for 20 to 25 minutes.
4. Arrange snapper on hot platter and pour sauce over it. Garnish with lemon slices. Serve immediately.

*Microwave Directions*

Use microwave baking dish; cover fish and vegetables; microwave on High for 6 to 8 minutes, turning the dish once; let rest 2 to 3 minutes before serving.

| *Composition of Recipe* | | *Serving Size: ¼ of Recipe* | |
|---|---|---|---|
| Calories | 231 | Zinc (mg) | 1.5 |
| Protein (g) | 28 | Iron (mg) | 1.5 |
| Total fat (g) | 7 | Vitamin A (IU) | 1,340 |
| Carbohydrate (g) | 4 | Thiamin (mg) | 0.2 |
| Cholesterol (mg) | 76 | Riboflavin (mg) | 0 |
| Fiber (g) | 0.3 | Niacin (mg) | 4.1 |
| Calcium (mg) | 40 | Vitamin $B_6$ (mg) | 1 |
| Magnesium (mg) | 49 | Folacin (mcg) | 16 |
| Sodium (mg) | 324 | Vitamin $B_{12}$ (mcg) | 1.2 |
| Potassium (mg) | 578 | Vitamin C (mg) | 4 |

## SOLE FILLET WITH SHRIMP SAUCE *(Serves 6)*

**2 pkgs. (12 oz. each) frozen sole fillets, partially thawed**
**¼ tsp. pepper**
**2 T. finely chopped onion**
**¾ c. dry white wine**
**2 T. margarine**
**1½ T. flour**
**1 c. skim milk**
**5 oz. frozen, medium-size cooked shrimp, thawed**
**3 T. chopped fresh parsley**

*Directions*

1. Separate sole fillets; arrange in single layer in lightly greased oven-to-table baking dish (9" × 13").
2. Sprinkle with pepper and onion. Pour wine over fish.
3. Bake uncovered at 325° F for 10 to 15 minutes, until fish flakes evenly.
4. While fish is baking, melt margarine in saucepan. Blend in flour and stir to form smooth paste. Gradually add milk, stirring constantly until sauce is thick and smooth, about 5 minutes.
5. When fish is done, pour fish juices into a saucepan and heat over medium until juices are reduced to ⅓ cup. Stir into white sauce.
6. Add thawed cooked shrimp to white sauce.
7. Spoon sauce over fish and garnish with parsley.

| *Composition of Recipe* | | *Serving Size: ⅙ of Recipe* | |
|---|---|---|---|
| Calories | 188 | Zinc (mg) | 1.3 |
| Protein (g) | 24 | Iron (mg) | 1.9 |
| Total fat (g) | 5 | Vitamin A (IU) | 375 |
| Carbohydrate (g) | 5 | Thiamin (mg) | 0.1 |
| Cholesterol (mg) | 63 | Riboflavin (mg) | 0.1 |
| Fiber (g) | 0.3 | Niacin (mg) | 2 |
| Calcium (mg) | 137 | Vitamin $B_6$ (mg) | 0.2 |
| Magnesium (mg) | 47 | Folacin (mcg) | 11 |
| Sodium (mg) | 319 | Vitamin $B_{12}$ (mcg) | 1 |
| Potassium (mg) | 473 | Vitamin C (mg) | 5 |

**ARMENIAN SHISH KABOBS** *(Serves 6)*

**2 lbs. boneless lamb, cut into 1" cubes**
**½ tsp. salt**
**¼ tsp. pepper**
**½ tsp. celery salt**
**½ tsp. paprika**
**1 tsp. Worcestershire sauce**
**2 garlic cloves, crushed**
**½ tsp. thyme**
**¼ c. fresh lemon juice**
**1 c. plain low-fat yogurt**
**3 lemons, cut into quarters**
**6 long skewers**

*Directions*

1. Combine all ingredients, except lemon quarters.
2. Place into a resealable, plastic food bag. Refrigerate overnight or 24 hours.
3. Before broiling, thread a lemon quarter on each of the 6 skewers; then thread on the cubes of marinated lamb. End each skewer with another lemon quarter.
4. Broil 3 to 4 inches from heat source for 5 to 6 minutes; turn, then broil additional 5 minutes. (Can also be grilled over charcoal for about 20 minutes or until lamb is tender but still pink inside.)

*Note*: The yogurt makes basting unnecessary, but kabobs may be basted with any barbecue sauce during the last 5 minutes for more color and flavor.

| *Composition of Recipe* | | *Serving Size: ⅙ of Recipe* | |
|---|---|---|---|
| Calories | 275 | Zinc (mg) | 5.5 |
| Protein (g) | 36 | Iron (mg) | 4 |
| Total fat (g) | 10 | Vitamin A (IU) | 156 |
| Carbohydrate (g) | 6 | Thiamin (mg) | 0.2 |
| Cholesterol (mg) | 90 | Riboflavin (mg) | 0.5 |
| Fiber (g) | 0.1 | Niacin (mg) | 8 |
| Calcium (mg) | 67 | Vitamin $B_6$ (mg) | 0.3 |
| Magnesium (mg) | 31 | Folacin (mcg) | 5 |
| Sodium (mg) | 291 | Vitamin $B_{12}$ (mcg) | 2.7 |
| Potassium (mg) | 544 | Vitamin C (mg) | 25 |

## SMOKED TURKEY WILD RICE CASSEROLE
*(Serves 8)*

**3 c. cooked wild rice**
**½ lb. fresh mushrooms, sliced**
**4 T. margarine**
**2 c. diced smoked turkey**
**1 can (12½ oz.) evaporated skim milk**
**1½ c. water**
**2 T. chopped chives**
**1¾ c. Parmesan cheese, divided**

*Directions*

1. In a large saucepan, melt butter; sauté sliced mushrooms.
2. Add cooked wild rice, diced smoked turkey, evaporated skim milk, water, and chives; mix thoroughly.
3. Pour mixture into a buttered 2½-qt. casserole dish. Sprinkle with *1 cup* Parmesan cheese.
4. Bake, covered, at 350° F for 1 hour.
5. At mealtime, sprinkle each serving with *2 tablespoons* Parmesan cheese.

| *Composition of Recipe* | | *Serving Size: ⅛ of Recipe* | |
|---|---|---|---|
| Calories | 319 | Zinc (mg) | 2.9 |
| Protein (g) | 28 | Iron (mg) | 2 |
| Total fat (g) | 11 | Vitamin A (IU) | 459 |
| Carbohydrate (g) | 27 | Thiamin (mg) | 0.2 |
| Cholesterol (mg) | 49 | Riboflavin (mg) | 0.6 |
| Fiber (g) | 0.8 | Niacin (mg) | 6.9 |
| Calcium (mg) | 407 | Vitamin $B_6$ (mg) | 0.3 |
| Magnesium (mg) | 69 | Folacin (mcg) | 14 |
| Sodium (mg) | 299 | Vitamin $B_{12}$ (mcg) | 0.6 |
| Potassium (mg) | 476 | Vitamin C (mg) | 2 |

---

## STIR-FRY CHICKEN AND BROCCOLI WITH RICE
*(Serves 4)*

**2 chicken breasts, skinned, boned, and thinly sliced**
**3 T. cornstarch**
**4 T. low-sodium soy sauce**
**2 T. peanut oil**
**½ lb. broccoli, broken into small pieces**
**1 medium onion, sliced or chopped**
**2 c. fresh bean sprouts**

**1 c. chicken broth**
**4 c. hot cooked rice**

*Directions*

1. In a medium bowl, blend cornstarch with soy sauce; add chicken slices and stir until chicken is thoroughly coated. Let stand 15 minutes.
2. Heat oil in wok over high heat. Add chicken and stir-fry until browned.
3. Remove chicken from wok; add broccoli and onion to wok and stir-fry 2 minutes.
4. Add mushrooms, bean sprouts, and chicken to wok; stir in chicken broth.
5. Cover and cook gently for 5 minutes or until vegetables are crisp-tender. Serve with rice.

| *Composition of Recipe* | | *Serving Size: ¼ of Recipe* | |
|---|---|---|---|
| Calories | 506 | Zinc (mg) | 3.3 |
| Protein (g) | 31 | Iron (mg) | 4.9 |
| Total fat (g) | 13 | Vitamin A (IU) | 1,950 |
| Carbohydrate (g) | 69 | Thiamin (mg) | 0.4 |
| Cholesterol (mg) | 59 | Riboflavin (mg) | 0.4 |
| Fiber (g) | 14 | Niacin (mg) | 8.7 |
| Calcium (mg) | 132 | Vitamin $B_6$ (mg) | 0.4 |
| Magnesium (mg) | 112 | Folacin (mcg) | 27 |
| Sodium (mg) | 1,536 | Vitamin $B_{12}$ (mcg) | 0.2 |
| Potassium (mg) | 666 | Vitamin C (mg) | 78 |

---

## TURKEY DIVAN *(Serves 4)*

**1 pkg. (10 oz.) broccoli spears, thawed**
**½ lb. sliced cooked turkey breast**
**3 T. flour**
**1 can (10½ oz.) ready-to-serve low-sodium chicken broth**
**⅓ c. cheddar cheese, shredded**
**⅛ tsp. pepper**
**⅛ tsp. salt**

*Directions*

1. Arrange broccoli in bottom of 8" × 8" microwave-safe dish.
2. Layer turkey slices on top of broccoli.
3. Mix flour, salt, and pepper with broth in saucepan or glass measuring cup.

4. Cook, stirring constantly, until thickened; add shredded cheese.
5. Stir until cheese is melted; pour sauce over turkey and broccoli.
6. *Microwave Method*: Cover dish and microwave on High for 9 minutes or until broccoli is done. *Conventional Method*: Bake covered at 375° F for 20–25 minutes.

| *Composition of Recipe* | | *Serving Size: ¼ of Recipe* | |
|---|---|---|---|
| Calories | 197 | Zinc (mg) | 1.9 |
| Protein (g) | 27 | Iron (mg) | 1.7 |
| Total fat (g) | 7 | Vitamin A (IU) | 1,790 |
| Carbohydrate (g) | 8 | Thiamin (mg) | 0.1 |
| Cholesterol (mg) | 53 | Riboflavin (mg) | 0.3 |
| Fiber (g) | 2.8 | Niacin (mg) | 8.4 |
| Calcium (mg) | 141 | Vitamin $B_6$ (mg) | 0.3 |
| Magnesium (mg) | 32 | Folacin (mcg) | 20 |
| Sodium (mg) | 572 | Vitamin $B_{12}$ (mcg) | 0.3 |
| Potassium (mg) | 528 | Vitamin C (mg) | 58 |

## LINGUINE WITH TOMATOES AND ZUCCHINI

*(Serves 6)*

**4 oz. linguine, cooked and drained (about 2 cups)**
**1 T. margarine**
**⅓ c. chopped onion**
**1 green pepper, seeded and cut into strips**
**2½ c. sliced zucchini**
**4 medium tomatoes, peeled, seeded, and cut into strips**
**¼ c. chopped parsley**
**¼ c. freshly grated Parmesan cheese**
**2 oz. low-fat cheese**

*Directions*

1. Melt margarine in a skillet and sauté onion for about 5 minutes. Add green pepper and cook a few minutes more.
2. Combine with all remaining ingredients, reserving 2 T. Parmesan cheese for top.
3. Place in a greased 2-qt. casserole, and sprinkle with remaining Parmesan cheese.
4. Bake covered at 350° F for 30 to 40 minutes, or until cheese is bubbling. Do not overcook.

| *Composition of Recipe* | | *Serving Size: 1/6 of Recipe* | |
|---|---|---|---|
| Calories | 169 | Zinc (mg) | 0.9 |
| Protein (g) | 10 | Iron (mg) | 2.0 |
| Total fat (g) | 5 | Vitamin A (IU) | 2,130 |
| Carbohydrate (g) | 26 | Thiamin (mg) | 0.2 |
| Cholesterol (mg) | 6 | Riboflavin (mg) | 0.2 |
| Fiber (g) | 2.6 | Niacin (mg) | 2.6 |
| Calcium (mg) | 169 | Vitamin $B_6$ (mg) | 0.3 |
| Magnesium (mg) | 53 | Folacin (mcg) | 40 |
| Sodium (mg) | 276 | Vitamin $B_{12}$ (mcg) | 0.1 |
| Potassium (mg) | 659 | Vitamin C (mg) | 83 |

# Vegetables

## THREE-CHEESE SCALLOPED POTATOES

*(Serves 6)*

**4 large baking potatoes, peeled and cut into slices**
**1/8 tsp. dried thyme**
**2 oz. crumbled blue cheese**
**2 oz. shredded low-fat cheese (e.g., Monterey Jack)**
**Salt and pepper**
**1 can (12 oz.) evaporated skim milk**
**1 tsp. cornstarch**
**1/4 c. Parmesan cheese**

*Directions*

1. Place the potatoe slices in a saucepan. Add thyme and cover with boiling water.
2. Bring to a boil, cover, lower heat, and simmer 3 minutes. Do not overcook.
3. Drain thoroughly and carefully; layer half of potato slices on bottom of greased, shallow baking dish.
4. Blend blue cheese and shredded Monterey Jack cheese to form a paste.
5. Spread paste over the potato slices in baking pan; sprinkle with salt and pepper.
6. Layer remaining potato slices on top.
7. Dissolve cornstarch in milk, then pour over layered potatoes.
8. Sprinkle with Parmesan cheese.
9. Bake at 350° F for 1 hour, or until top is golden brown, potatoes are tender, and the liquid has been absorbed.

| *Composition of Recipe* | | *Serving Size: 1/6 of Recipe* | |
|---|---|---|---|
| Calories | 182 | Zinc (mg) | 1.1 |
| Protein (g) | 10 | Iron (mg) | 0.7 |
| Total fat (g) | 6 | Vitamin A (IU) | 227 |
| Carbohydrate (g) | 22 | Thiamin (mg) | 0.1 |
| Cholesterol (mg) | 33 | Riboflavin (mg) | 0.3 |
| Fiber (g) | 0.9 | Niacin (mg) | 1.4 |
| Calcium (mg) | 259 | Vitamin $B_6$ (mg) | 0.4 |
| Magnesium (mg) | 45 | Folacin (mcg) | 16 |
| Sodium (mg) | 221 | Vitamin $B_{12}$ (mcg) | 0.3 |
| Potassium (mg) | 497 | Vitamin C (mg) | 16 |

## MARINATED CARROTS *(Serves 10)*

**2 lbs. carrots, scraped and cut into chunks**
**1 large sliced onion**
**1 green pepper, cut in slices**
**1 can (10½ oz.) low-sodium tomato soup**
**½ c. sugar**
**¼ c. oil**
**½ tsp. pepper**
**6 T. vinegar**
**½ tsp. dill weed**

*Directions*

1. Cook carrots in water until tender; drain.
2. Add sliced onion and green pepper to cooked carrots.
3. In a saucepan, combine soup (do not dilute) and remaining ingredients; heat until sugar is dissolved.
4. Pour mixture over carrots, onion, and pepper and cover. Refrigerate.

Note: If desired, onion and pepper may be omitted.

| *Composition of Recipe* | | *Serving Size: 1/10 of Recipe* | |
|---|---|---|---|
| Calories | 149 | Zinc (mg) | 0.5 |
| Protein (g) | 2 | Iron (mg) | 0.1 |
| Total fat (g) | 6 | Vitamin A (IU) | 8,710 |
| Carbohydrate (g) | 24 | Thiamin (mg) | 0.1 |
| Cholesterol (mg) | 1 | Riboflavin (mg) | 0.1 |
| Fiber (g) | 1.7 | Niacin (mg) | 0.7 |
| Calcium (mg) | 38 | Vitamin $B_6$ (mg) | 0.2 |
| Magnesium (mg) | 25 | Folacin (mcg) | 14 |
| Sodium (mg) | 277 | Vitamin $B_{12}$ (mcg) | 0 |
| Potassium (mg) | 383 | Vitamin C (mg) | 29 |

## ORIENTAL ZUCCHINI *(Serves 6)*

**1 lb. zucchini (3–4 small)**
**1 T. reduced-sodium soy sauce**
**½ tsp. salt**
**¼ tsp. pepper**
**Vegetable oil spray**

*Directions*

1. Wash zucchini and slice ⅛'' thick.
2. Lightly spray skillet with vegetable oil spray; add sliced zucchini and cook about 2 minutes.
3. Season with soy sauce, salt, and pepper. Serve hot.

| *Composition of Recipe* | | *Serving Size: ⅙ of Recipe* | |
|---|---|---|---|
| Calories | 12 | Zinc (mg) | 0.1 |
| Protein (g) | 1 | Iron (mg) | 0.5 |
| Total fat (g) | 0 | Vitamin A (IU) | 227 |
| Carbohydrate (g) | 2 | Thiamin (mg) | 0 |
| Cholesterol (mg) | 0 | Riboflavin (mg) | 0.1 |
| Fiber (g) | 0.5 | Niacin (mg) | 0.6 |
| Calcium (mg) | 22 | Vitamin $B_6$ (mg) | 0.1 |
| Magnesium (mg) | 17 | Folacin (mcg) | 1 |
| Sodium (mg) | 223 | Vitamin $B_{12}$ (mcg) | 0 |
| Potassium (mg) | 119 | Vitamin C (mg) | 7 |

---

## RED CABBAGE AND APPLES *(Serves 4)*

**4 c. shredded red cabbage**
**3 T. water**
**2 medium-size cooking apples, pared, cored, and sliced**
**1 T. margarine**
**1 tsp. flour**
**2 T. brown sugar**
**2 T. vinegar**
**1 tsp. salt**
**⅛ tsp. pepper**

*Directions*

1. Place shredded cabbage, sliced apples, and water in saucepan.
2. Cook, covered over medium heat for about 10 minutes.
3. Combine remaining ingredients, add to cabbage and apples, and heat thoroughly.

*Microwave Directions*

1. Place shredded cabbage, sliced apples, and water in 2½-qt. casserole. Cover and microwave for 5 to 6 minutes.
2. Stir, then microwave for 5 to 6 more minutes, until apples are tender.
3. Combine remaining ingredients, add to cabbage and apples, and microwave for 1 minute.
4. Let stand, covered, for about 2 minutes before serving.

| *Composition of Recipe* | | *Serving Size: ¼ of Recipe* | |
|---|---|---|---|
| Calories | 119 | Zinc (mg) | 0.5 |
| Protein (g) | 2 | Iron (mg) | 0.9 |
| Total fat (g) | 4 | Vitamin A (IU) | 299 |
| Carbohydrate (g) | 23 | Thiamin (mg) | 0.1 |
| Cholesterol (mg) | 0 | Riboflavin (mg) | 0.1 |
| Fiber (g) | 2.7 | Niacin (mg) | 0.4 |
| Calcium (mg) | 66 | Vitamin $B_6$ (mg) | 0.2 |
| Magnesium (mg) | 23 | Folacin (mcg) | 31 |
| Sodium (mg) | 595 | Vitamin $B_{12}$ (mcg) | 0 |
| Potassium (mg) | 345 | Vitamin C (mg) | 53 |

# Breads

**BANANA BRAN MUFFINS** *(Makes 12 muffins)*

**3 T. margarine**
**6 T. sugar**
**2 eggs**
**1½ c. whole bran cereal (e.g., dry oatmeal, All Bran)**
**⅓ c. buttermilk**
**⅔ c. whole wheat flour**
**½ tsp. salt**
**1 tsp. baking soda**
**¼ tsp. allspice**
**2 ripe bananas, mashed**

*Directions*

1. Cream margarine and sugar; beat in eggs, one at a time.
2. Add cereal and buttermilk.
3. Blend in flour, salt, soda, and allspice.
4. Fold in mashed bananas.
5. Spoon into 12 muffin cups, filling each ¾ full.

6. Bake at 375° F for 15 minutes.
Serve with honey.

*Composition of Recipe* — *Serving Size: 1 muffin*

| | | | |
|---|---|---|---|
| Calories | 129 | Zinc (mg) | 1.7 |
| Protein (g) | 4 | Iron (mg) | 2.1 |
| Total fat (g) | 4 | Vitamin A (IU) | 653 |
| Carbohydrate (g) | 23 | Thiamin (mg) | 0.2 |
| Cholesterol (mg) | 42 | Riboflavin (mg) | 0.2 |
| Fiber (g) | 3.9 | Niacin (mg) | 2.2 |
| Calcium (mg) | 27 | Vitamin $B_6$ (mg) | 0.3 |
| Magnesium (mg) | 57 | Folacin (mcg) | 46 |
| Sodium (mg) | 328 | Vitamin $B_{12}$ (mcg) | 0.1 |
| Potassium (mg) | 244 | Vitamin C (mg) | 7 |

---

**BREAKFAST BRAN MUFFINS** *(Makes 30 muffins)*

**1 c. boiling water**
**1 c. dry oatmeal**
**½ c. plus 1 T. vegetable shortening**
**1¼ c. sugar**
**2 eggs, beaten**
**2 c. buttermilk**
**2 c. all bran cereal**
**2½ c. whole wheat flour**
**2½ tsp. baking soda**
**½ tsp. salt**

*Directions*

1. In a separate bowl, pour the boiling water over the dry oatmeal.
2. In a large mixing bowl, cream the shortening and sugar; add the beaten eggs and buttermilk.
3. Add the all bran cereal, flour, baking soda, and salt; mix.
4. Fold in the soaked oatmeal.

*Note*: At this point, the batter may be refrigerated in a tightly covered container for up to 6 weeks. If desired, spoon out into greased muffin tins before breakfast and bake.

5. Fill greased muffin tins about ¾ full. Bake at 400° F for 15 to 18 minutes.

*Composition of Recipe* — *Serving Size: 1 muffin*

| | | | |
|---|---|---|---|
| Calories | 128 | Zinc (mg) | 1.4 |
| Protein (g) | 3 | Iron (mg) | 1.7 |
| Total fat (g) | 4 | Vitamin A (IU) | 373 |

| | | | |
|---|---|---|---|
| Carbohydrate (g) | 22 | Thiamin (mg) | 0.2 |
| Cholesterol (mg) | 17 | Riboflavin (mg) | 0.2 |
| Fiber (g) | 3.4 | Niacin (mg) | 1.8 |
| Calcium (mg) | 33 | Vitamin $B_6$ (mg) | 0.2 |
| Magnesium (mg) | 44 | Folacin (mcg) | 34 |
| Sodium (mg) | 221 | Vitamin $B_{12}$ (mcg) | 0.1 |
| Potassium (mg) | 164 | Vitamin C (mg) | 4 |

## RAISIN SCONES *(Makes 8 scones)*

**1¾ c. flour**
**2 tsp. baking powder**
**1 T. sugar**
**½ tsp. salt**
**¼ c. shortening**
**1 egg, beaten**
**½ c. milk**
**⅓ c. raisins**
**1 tsp. sugar**

*Directions*

1. Combine the flour, baking powder, 1 T. sugar, and salt.
2. Cut the shortening into the mixture until it is coarse.
3. Add the beaten egg, milk, and raisins to the flour mixture. Combine with a few strokes until the dough leaves the side of the bowl. Handle as little as possible.
4. Place dough on a lightly greased baking pan; pat (with lightly floured hands) into a round shape about ¾''. Sprinkle with 1 tsp. sugar and cut into 8 wedges.
5. Bake at 425° F for 12 to 15 minutes. Serve at once with jam.

| *Composition of Recipe* | | *Serving Size: 1 scone* | |
|---|---|---|---|
| Calories | 192 | Zinc (mg) | 0.4 |
| Protein (g) | 4 | Iron (mg) | 1.1 |
| Total fat (g) | 7 | Vitamin A (IU) | 61 |
| Carbohydrate (g) | 28 | Thiamin (mg) | 0.1 |
| Cholesterol (mg) | 34 | Riboflavin (mg) | 0.1 |
| Fiber (g) | 1.2 | Niacin (mg) | 0.9 |
| Calcium (mg) | 44 | Vitamin $B_6$ (mg) | 0 |
| Magnesium (mg) | 11 | Folacin (mcg) | 9 |
| Sodium (mg) | 262 | Vitamin $B_{12}$ (mcg) | 0.1 |
| Potassium (mg) | 102 | Vitamin C (mg) | 0 |

**WHOLE WHEAT NUT BREAD**
*(Makes about 22 slices)*

**1 c. flour**
**2 c. whole wheat flour**
**½ c. sugar**
**1 tsp. salt**
**1½ T. baking powder**
**3 eggs, beaten**
**3 T. oil**
**1½ c. milk**
**1 c. chopped nuts**

*Directions*

1. Combine flours, sugar, salt, and baking powder. Mix to blend.
2. Make a well in the center of the flour mixture; add beaten eggs, oil, and milk.
3. Stir gently until the mixture is blended, but allowing lumps to remain.
4. Stir in chopped nuts.
5. Pour batter into a greased loaf pan (8½" × 4½"). Bake at 350° F for 55 to 60 minutes. After cooling, remove from bread pan and cut into slices.

| *Composition of Recipe* | | *Serving Size: 1 slice* | |
|---|---|---|---|
| Calories | 151 | Zinc (mg) | 0.6 |
| Protein (g) | 5 | Iron (mg) | 0.8 |
| Total fat (g) | 7 | Vitamin A (IU) | 65 |
| Carbohydrate (g) | 19 | Thiamin (mg) | 0.1 |
| Cholesterol (mg) | 37 | Riboflavin (mg) | 0.1 |
| Fiber (g) | 1.6 | Niacin (mg) | 1.8 |
| Calcium (mg) | 47 | Vitamin $B_6$ (mg) | 0.1 |
| Magnesium (mg) | 24 | Folacin (mcg) | 10 |
| Sodium (mg) | 419 | Vitamin $B_{12}$ (mcg) | 0.1 |
| Potassium (mg) | 111 | Vitamin C (mg) | 0 |

---

## Beverages

**BANANA BREAKFAST SHAKE** *(Makes 1 serving)*

**1 banana**
**¼ c. orange juice**
**¼ c. plain low-fat yogurt**
**1 tsp. orange marmalade**
**¼ tsp. cinnamon**
**1 tsp. nonfat dry milk**

*Directions*

Blend all ingredients in a blender or food processor.

| *Composition of Recipe* | | *Serving Size: Full Recipe* | |
|---|---|---|---|
| Calories | 192 | Zinc (mg) | 0.9 |
| Protein (g) | 6 | Iron (mg) | 1.2 |
| Total fat (g) | 1 | Vitamin A (IU) | 447 |
| Carbohydrate (g) | 42 | Thiamin (mg) | 0.2 |
| Cholesterol (mg) | 4 | Riboflavin (mg) | 0.3 |
| Fiber (g) | 1.9 | Niacin (mg) | 1.2 |
| Calcium (mg) | 161 | Vitamin $B_6$ (mg) | 0.7 |
| Magnesium (mg) | 75 | Folacin (mcg) | 34 |
| Sodium (mg) | 56 | Vitamin $B_{12}$ (mcg) | 0.4 |
| Potassium (mg) | 746 | Vitamin C (mg) | 43 |

---

**HOT CRANBERRY PUNCH** *(Makes 10 servings)*

**1 can (16 oz.) jellied cranberry sauce**
**3 T. light-brown sugar**
**¼ tsp. ground cinnamon**
**¼ tsp. ground allspice**
**⅛ tsp. ground cloves**
**⅛ tsp. ground nutmeg**
**2 c. water**
**2 c. unsweetened pineapple juice**
**⅛ tsp. butter flavoring**

*Directions*

1. In a large saucepan, crush the cranberry sauce with a fork.
2. Mix with brown sugar, cinnamon, allspice, cloves, and nutmeg.
3. Add water and pineapple juice. Cover and simmer 2 hours.
4. Just before serving, add the butter flavoring and ladle into mugs.

| *Composition of Recipe* | | *Serving Size: 5 oz.* | |
|---|---|---|---|
| Calories | 110 | Zinc (mg) | 0.1 |
| Protein (g) | 0 | Iron (mg) | 0.4 |
| Total fat (g) | 0 | Vitamin A (IU) | 15 |
| Carbohydrate (g) | 28 | Thiamin (mg) | 0 |
| Cholesterol (mg) | 0 | Riboflavin (mg) | 0 |
| Fiber (g) | 0.3 | Niacin (mg) | 0.1 |
| Calcium (mg) | 16 | Vitamin $B_6$ (mg) | 0.1 |
| Magnesium (mg) | 7 | Folacin (mcg) | 1 |

| | | | |
|---|---|---|---|
| Sodium (mg) | 28 | Vitamin $B_{12}$ (mcg) | 0 |
| Potassium (mg) | 104 | Vitamin C (mg) | 7 |

**PEACHY DRINK** *(Makes 12 servings)*

**1 pkg. (16 oz.) frozen peach slices, partially thawed**
**1 can (6 oz.) frozen orange concentrate, partially thawed**
**1 pt. (2 cups) frozen vanilla yogurt, softened**
**3½ c. low-calorie ginger ale, chilled**

*Directions*

1. In a blender or food processor, combine peaches, orange concentrate, softened yogurt and *half* the ginger ale. Cover.
2. Blend at medium-low speed until smooth; add remainder of ginger ale.
3. To serve, pour mixture into beverage glasses. If desired, serve after dinner as a dessert.

| *Composition of Recipe* | | *Serving Size: 5 oz.* | |
|---|---|---|---|
| Calories | 75 | Zinc (mg) | 0.3 |
| Protein (g) | 2 | Iron (mg) | 0.3 |
| Total fat (g) | 0 | Vitamin A (IU) | 550 |
| Carbohydrate (g) | 16 | Thiamin (mg) | 0.1 |
| Cholesterol (mg) | 0 | Riboflavin (mg) | 0.1 |
| Fiber (g) | 0.5 | Niacin (mg) | 0.6 |
| Calcium (mg) | 50 | Vitamin $B_6$ (mg) | 0 |
| Magnesium (mg) | 14 | Folacin (mcg) | 2 |
| Sodium (mg) | 12 | Vitamin $B_{12}$ (mcg) | 0 |
| Potassium (mg) | 179 | Vitamin C (mg) | 31 |

**STRAWBERRY BREAKFAST SHAKE**
*(Makes 1 serving)*

**½ c. strawberries**
**¼ c. orange juice**
**¼ c. plain low-fat yogurt**
**1 tsp. orange marmalade**
**¼ tsp. ginger**
**1 tsp. nonfat dry milk**

*Directions*

Blend all ingredients in a blender or food processor.

| *Composition of Recipe* | | *Serving Size: Full Recipe* | |
|---|---|---|---|
| Calories | 119 | Zinc (mg) | 0.7 |
| Protein (g) | 5 | Iron (mg) | 1 |
| Total fat (g) | 1 | Vitamin A (IU) | 241 |
| Carbohydrate (g) | 23 | Thiamin (mg) | 0.1 |
| Cholesterol (mg) | 4 | Riboflavin (mg) | 0.2 |
| Fiber (g) | 1.5 | Niacin (mg) | 0.8 |
| Calcium (mg) | 160 | Vitamin $B_6$ (mg) | 0.1 |
| Magnesium (mg) | 29 | Folacin (mcg) | 20 |
| Sodium (mg) | 56 | Vitamin $B_{12}$ (mcg) | 0.4 |
| Potassium (mg) | 433 | Vitamin C (mg) | 78 |

## Desserts

**APPLE BROWN BETTY** *(Makes 6 servings)*

**7 slices dry bread, cubed (2 cups)**
**4 T. melted margarine**
**5 c. tart apples (about 3 Granny Smith apples), pared, cored, and sliced**
**½ c. brown sugar**
**1½ T. lemon juice**
**1 tsp. grated lemon peel**
**½ tsp. cinnamon**
**⅔ c. hot water**

*Directions*

1. Mix bread cubes and margarine in a small bowl.
2. Combine apples, brown sugar, lemon juice and peel, and cinnamon in large bowl; toss well.
3. Spread ⅓ of the bread mixture in bottom of greased 2-qt. baking dish. Top with *half* of the apple mixture. Repeat layers.
4. Top with remaining bread mixture. Pour water over all.
5. Bake covered at 350° F for 30 minutes; remove cover. Bake until apples are tender and top is golden brown and crisp, about 30 minutes. Cool slightly.

| *Composition of Recipe* | | *Serving Size: ⅙ of Recipe* | |
|---|---|---|---|
| Calories | 273 | Zinc (mg) | 0.3 |
| Protein (g) | 3 | Iron (mg) | 1.7 |
| Total fat (g) | 9 | Vitamin A (IU) | 385 |
| Carbohydrate (g) | 46 | Thiamin (mg) | 0.1 |
| Cholesterol (mg) | 1 | Riboflavin (mg) | 0.1 |
| Fiber (g) | 3 | Niacin (mg) | 0.8 |
| Calcium (mg) | 50 | Vitamin $B_6$ (mg) | 0 |

| | | | |
|---|---|---|---|
| Magnesium (mg) | 21 | Folacin (mcg) | 7 |
| Sodium (mg) | 258 | Vitamin $B_{12}$ (mcg) | 0 |
| Potassium (mg) | 196 | Vitamin C (mg) | 6 |

## BLUEBERRIES AND LEMON SHERBET

*(Makes 4 servings)*

**1 pt. lemon sherbet**
**1 pt. fresh blueberries, washed**
**4 sprigs fresh mint (optional)**

*Directions*

1. In tall parfait glasses, place spoonful of blueberries; add a scoop of lemon sherbet.
2. Continue alternating small scoops of lemon sherbet with fresh blueberries; top with blueberries.
3. If desired, garnish with mint sprig. Serve with long-handled spoons.

| *Composition of Recipe* | | *Serving Size: ¼ of Recipe* | |
|---|---|---|---|
| Calories | 179 | Zinc (mg) | 0.2 |
| Protein (g) | 1 | Iron (mg) | 0.8 |
| Total fat (g) | 2 | Vitamin A (IU) | 138 |
| Carbohydrate (g) | 41 | Thiamin (mg) | 0 |
| Cholesterol (mg) | 0 | Riboflavin (mg) | 0.1 |
| Fiber (g) | 2.1 | Niacin (mg) | 0.4 |
| Calcium (mg) | 26 | Vitamin $B_6$ (mg) | 0.1 |
| Magnesium (mg) | 13 | Folacin (mcg) | 5 |
| Sodium (mg) | 11 | Vitamin $B_{12}$ (mcg) | 0 |
| Potassium (mg) | 81 | Vitamin C (mg) | 12 |

## FROSTED FRUIT IN COINTREAU

*(Makes 16 servings)*

**1 can (20 oz.) pineapple chunks, in own juices**
**1 pkg. (16 oz.) frozen sliced peaches**
**1 pkg. (16 oz.) frozen mixed fruit**
**1 pkg. (12 oz.) frozen raspberries**
**2 fresh lemons**
**½ c. Cointreau**

*Directions*

1. Remove fruit from packages before it is thawed; place in large bowl.
2. Squeeze juice of 2 lemons over fruit; pour Cointreau over all.

3. Stir until fruit separates and is well coated. Allow 30 to 60 minutes for fruit to thaw with intermittent stirring. Keeps well in refrigerator.

| *Composition of Recipe* | | *Serving Size: ½ cup* | |
|---|---|---|---|
| Calories | 83 | Zinc (mg) | 0.1 |
| Protein (g) | 1 | Iron (mg) | 0.6 |
| Total fat (g) | 0 | Vitamin A (IU) | 411 |
| Carbohydrate (g) | 16 | Thiamin (mg) | 0 |
| Cholesterol (mg) | 0 | Riboflavin (mg) | 0 |
| Fiber (g) | 2.2 | Niacin (mg) | 0.5 |
| Calcium (mg) | 19 | Vitamin $B_6$ (mg) | 0.1 |
| Magnesium (mg) | 23 | Folacin (mcg) | 5 |
| Sodium (mg) | 2 | Vitamin $B_{12}$ (mcg) | 0 |
| Potassium (mg) | 197 | Vitamin C (mg) | 16 |

---

**FRUIT KABOBS** *(Makes 8 servings)*

**½ c. sugar**
**¼ c. lemon juice**
**¼ c. water**
**3 T. orange liqueur**
**2 c. fresh pineapple chunks**
**1 can (11 oz.) mandarin oranges, drained**
**3 medium bananas**
**1 pt. fresh strawberries**
**16 wooden skewers**

*Directions*

1. Combine sugar, juice, water, and liqueur.
2. Pour marinade over pineapple and oranges; cover and refrigerate overnight.
3. Shortly before serving, cut bananas into thick slices; add to fruit in marinade; stir gently to coat. Drain.
4. Alternate chunks of pineapple, orange, and banana on skewer; place strawberry on end of each skewer.
5. Serve on a plate or stick skewers into whole fresh pineapple.

*Variation*: Fresh peach or nectarine wedges may be used for mandarin oranges. Canned pineapple chunks may be used for fresh.

| *Composition of Recipe* | | *Serving Size: 2 kabobs* | |
|---|---|---|---|
| Calories | 143 | Zinc (mg) | 0.3 |
| Protein (g) | 1 | Iron (mg) | 1.0 |

| | | | |
|---|---|---|---|
| Total fat (g) | 0 | Vitamin A (IU) | 246 |
| Carbohydrate (g) | 33 | Thiamin (mg) | 0.1 |
| Cholesterol (mg) | 0 | Riboflavin (mg) | 0.1 |
| Fiber (g) | 2.1 | Niacin (mg) | 0.6 |
| Calcium (mg) | 28 | Vitamin $B_6$ (mg) | 0.3 |
| Magnesium (mg) | 34 | Folacin (mcg) | 20 |
| Sodium (mg) | 2 | Vitamin $B_{12}$ (mcg) | 0 |
| Potassium (mg) | 325 | Vitamin C (mg) | 44 |

---

## OLD ENGLISH TRIFLE *(Makes 12 servings)*

***Custard***

**¼ c. sugar**
**1 c. skim milk**
**4 tsp. cornstarch**
**1 tsp. vanilla**
**1 egg**

***Cake***

**1 (12 oz.) custard-flavored angel food cake**
**1 c. sherry**

***Filling***

**1 pkg. (12 oz.) frozen raspberries, thawed**
**¼ c. raspberry jam**
**1 pkg. (2.6 oz.) Amarettini Di Saroonna almond-flavored macaroons**
**1 c. whipping cream, whipped**
**1 can (8 oz.) sliced cling peaches, drained**

*Directions*

1. In a saucepan, mix sugar and cornstarch; add milk. Bring to a boil. Remove from heat and cool 5 minutes. Add vanilla and egg; beat thoroughly with a whisk.
2. Cut cake *vertically* into 2 rings. Crumble the inner cake ring into the bottom of a 3-qt. trifle bowl or straight-sided bowl. Cut the outer cake ring into long pieces and press them against the sides of the bowl. Pour the sherry over the cake.
3. Reserve 8 macaroons for the topping.
4. Spread the jam over the bottom cake crumbs. Layer *half* of the raspberries, followed by *half* of the remaining macaroons. Repeat layering with the rest of the raspberries and macaroons.

5. Pour the custard over the fruit and macaroons. Cover and refrigerate overnight.
6. Top with whipped cream; garnish with peach slices and reserved macaroons.

| *Composition of Recipe* | | *Serving Size: 1/12 of recipe* | |
|---|---|---|---|
| Calories | 350 | Zinc (mg) | 0.5 |
| Protein (g) | 6 | Iron (mg) | 0.7 |
| Total fat (g) | 10 | Vitamin A (IU) | 433 |
| Carbohydrate (g) | 59 | Thiamin (mg) | 0 |
| Cholesterol (mg) | 53 | Riboflavin (mg) | 0.2 |
| Fiber (g) | 1.6 | Niacin (mg) | 0.5 |
| Calcium (mg) | 62 | Vitamin $B_6$ (mg) | 0.1 |
| Magnesium (mg) | 29 | Folacin (mcg) | 6 |
| Sodium (mg) | 108 | Vitamin $B_{12}$ (mcg) | 0.2 |
| Potassium (mg) | 214 | Vitamin C (mg) | 4 |

---

**PEACH MELBA** *(Makes 4 servings)*

**2 large peaches**
**2 c. fresh raspberries**
**1/4 c. sugar**
**1 pt. vanilla frozen yogurt**

*Directions*

1. Put the peaches in a bowl and cover with boiling water. Leave for no more than 1 minute, then drain and peel them.
2. Cut the peaches in half, carefully remove the pits, and set the fruit aside.
3. Rub the raspberries through a fine sieve into a mixing bowl; sweeten the resulting puree with the sugar.
4. Assemble the dessert by placing 2 scoops of vanilla yogurt in each individual serving glass; place one peach half on top, rounded side up, and spoon over part of the raspberry puree. Serve at once.

| *Composition of Recipe* | | *Serving Size: 1/4 of Recipe* | |
|---|---|---|---|
| Calories | 213 | Zinc (mg) | 0.7 |
| Protein (g) | 5 | Iron (mg) | 0.8 |
| Total fat (g) | 2 | Vitamin A (IU) | 730 |
| Carbohydrate (g) | 47 | Thiamin (mg) | 0 |
| Cholesterol (mg) | 0 | Riboflavin (mg) | 0.2 |
| Fiber (g) | 4 | Niacin (mg) | 0.8 |
| Calcium (mg) | 130 | Vitamin $B_6$ (mg) | 0.1 |
| Magnesium (mg) | 38 | Folacin (mcg) | 3 |

| | | | |
|---|---|---|---|
| Sodium (mg) | 2 | Vitamin $B_{12}$ (mcg) | 0 |
| Potassium (mg) | 220 | Vitamin C (mg) | 13 |

---

**SPARKLING FRUIT CUP** *(Makes 10 servings)*

**1 pkg. (16 oz.) frozen fruit medley**
**1 lb. seedless grapes**
**2 oranges, peeled and cut up**
**1 tsp. grated orange rind**
**2½ tsp. honey**
**1 c. flavored sparkling soda such as black cherry, blueberry, or nonalcoholic ginger beer or ginger ale**

*Directions*

1. Before cutting up fresh orange, grate 1 tsp. of rind for recipe.
2. In a large bowl, combine fruit medley, grapes, and cut-up orange.
3. Stir in grated orange rind and honey.
4. Just before serving, gently add sparkling soda. Serve in individual fruit cups.

| *Composition of Recipe* | | *Serving Size: 1/10 of Recipe* | |
|---|---|---|---|
| Calories | 107 | Zinc (mg) | 0.2 |
| Protein (g) | 1.6 | Iron (mg) | 0.4 |
| Total fat (g) | 1 | Vitamin A (IU) | 244 |
| Carbohydrate (g) | 26 | Thiamin (mg) | 0.1 |
| Cholesterol (mg) | 0 | Riboflavin (mg) | 0 |
| Fiber (g) | 1.5 | Niacin (mg) | 0.4 |
| Calcium (mg) | 20 | Vitamin $B_6$ (mg) | 0.1 |
| Magnesium (mg) | 11 | Folacin (mcg) | 12 |
| Sodium (mg) | 5 | Vitamin $B_{12}$ (mcg) | 0 |
| Potassium (mg) | 192 | Vitamin C (mg) | 52 |

# Postscript

▼ It is far easier to start a book on nutrition than to end one. Results of new research on diet and health relationships are reported daily. The constant flow of information makes it difficult to call a halt to writing so the book can be sent to press. Although the nutrition principles presented aren't likely to change much, some of the conclusions about diet and health will, and new, important relationships will be identified. Holding on to all of the conclusions presented will guarantee that your knowledge about nutrition and health will become outdated. To stay informed, stay tuned and scrutinize your sources of nutrition information carefully. Most of all, keep up your healthy interest in nutrition.

# Appendixes

## *Appendix A: Glossary*

**Absorption:** The process by which nutrients and other substances are transported from the gastrointestinal tract into the body proper.

**Adaptive mechanisms:** In the context of nutrition, adaptive mechanisms are body processes that act to maintain a constant and balanced supply of nutrients to cells.

**Adequate diet:** One that supplies approximately the RDAs for essential nutrients and enough calories to meet a person's need for energy.

**Aerobic:** With oxygen. The pathway of energy formation that requires oxygen is the citric acid cycle.

**Albumin:** One of the most common types of protein found in blood. It is a relatively small polypeptide that is used as a carrier of certain nutrients in blood and serves as a source of amino acids for cells.

**Alcohol:** A chemical substance primarily derived from carbohydrates.

**Alcohol sugar:** Monosaccharides that contain an alcohol group within their chemical structure.

**Allergy:** When applied to food or a specific component of food, it means the development of immune system reactions in response to the presence of an offending food protein in the body. True allergies can be diagnosed by the presence of antibodies in the blood following ingestion and absorption of an antigen—or the offending protein substance. Gluten in wheat, egg white protein, and cow's milk protein are examples of substances that cause allergic responses in some individuals.

**Amniotic fluid:** Fluid that surrounds the fetus in the uterus. Amniotic fluid is contained in a thick membrane called the amniotic sac.

**Anaerobic:** Without oxygen. The anaerobic pathway of energy formation is glycolysis.

**Anemia:** A condition in which the body's content of red blood cells, or the amount of hemoglobin within the cells, is lower than normal. (There are many types of anemia, including the genetically determined sickle cell anemia and those caused by vitamin $B_{12}$ or folic acid deficiency. Iron deficiency is the most common cause of anemia.)

**Anorexia nervosa** [*an* = not, *orexis* = appetite, *nervosa* = assumed to have psychological origins]**:** A condition in which a person appears to have no appetite. The definition represents a misnomer, however. People with anorexia nervosa do have appetite, but they don't eat in response to it and they deny that they are too thin. Thought to be due to psychological factors, a person with anorexia nervosa looks like a starving person. The physical effects closely correspond to those of starvation.

**Antibodies:** Substances secreted in response to the presence of a foreign protein or *antigen*. Antibodies act to neutralize the harmful effects of bacteria, viruses, and other sources of foreign proteins that enter the body.

**Antigens:** Foreign proteins that enter the body through food, bacteria, viruses, and other substances. The presence of antigens prompts the body to produce antibodies that attempt to destroy them.

**Appetite:** The desire to eat. Appetite may develop for reasons not related to hunger, such as the availability of food or thoughts about eating.

**Ariboflavinosis:** The name for the riboflavin deficiency disease. The *a* in *ariboflavinosis* means without, *osis* means an abnormal condition.

**Associations:** Relationships identified by scientific studies between the presence of specific conditions and an outcome. Associations do not show cause-and-effect relationships; they indicate that a relationship may exist between one or more conditions and a particular outcome. High-fat diets, high blood pressure, and smoking are all *associated* with the development of heart disease, for example, but it is not yet clear that any of these conditions actually *causes* heart disease.

**Atherosclerosis:** A type of "hardening of the arteries" in which cholesterol and other blood components build up in the walls of arteries. The substance formed in the artery is called *plaque*. As atherosclerosis progresses, the arteries narrow and the supply of blood to the heart, brain, muscles, and other organs and tissues is reduced.

**Balanced diet:** A diet that consists of a variety of foods that together provide calories and nutrients in amounts that promote health. A balanced diet is balanced in both directions, neither containing too little nor too much energy (calories), fat, protein, vitamins, minerals, and other substances such as fat, alcohol, and fiber.

**Basal Metabolic Rate (BMR):** The amount of energy used for basal metabolic processes over a twenty-four-hour period. Basal metabolic rate is very similar to *Resting Metabolic Rate* (RMR). RMR is measured when a person is resting quietly at various times during the day. It is not significantly different from BMR if measured three to four hours after a meal.

**Basal metabolism:** Energy used to support the body's ongoing metabolic processes while the body is in a state of complete physical, digestive, and emotional rest. Basal metabolism represents the energy the body expends to keep the heart beating, the lungs working, body temperature normal, and that spent in a variety of other ongoing processes.

**Beriberi:** The name for the thiamin deficiency disease.

**Binge:** Eating of excessive quantities of food, usually in secret.

**Bioavailability:** The percentage of the total amount of a mineral consumed that is absorbed.

**Biological value:** The percentage of absorbed protein retained by the body for use in growth and tissue maintenance.

**Bulimia:** Literally, the word means *ox hunger*—or a huge appetite. It is also referred to as *bulimia nervosa*. People with bulimia generally undertake repeated episodes of dieting and binging on food. Food binges may be followed by *purging* the body, by either self-induced vomiting or the use of laxatives.

**Calorie:** In nutrition, refers to the kilocalorie (Kcal), the amount of energy needed to raise the temperature of one kilogram of water from 15° to 16° C. (In scientific writing, the nutrition Calorie is capitalized to distinguish it from the calorie that is a unit of measure in physics.)

**Carotenemia:** Yellowish discoloration of the skin caused by excessive intake of carotene. Also called *hypercarotenemia*.

**Cause-and-effect relationship:** A conclusion drawn by scientific studies that show a condition produces a particular outcome. For example, bacteria *cause* a wound to become infected, and vitamin C deficiency *causes* the disease scurvy.

**Chemical bonds:** Energy in the form of electrons that hold together atoms within a molecule.

**Cholesterol:** A fat-soluble, colorless liquid found in animals but not in plants. Cholesterol is used by the body to form steroid hormones such as testosterone and estrogen and is a component of animal cell membranes.

**Chylomicrons:** Tiny droplets containing triglycerides, phospholipids, cholesterol, and protein that are manufactured in the cells lining the small intestines. They serve to transport some of the end products of fat digestion to the heart and general circulation by way of the lymph system. They are just barely soluble in water.

**Citric acid cycle:** A complex series of chemical reactions that lead to the formation of energy from fatty acids, certain amino acids, and the glucose fragments left at the end of glycolysis. The citric acid cycle is the *aerobic* or oxygen-requiring phase of energy formation. (Also called the *Krebs cycle* and the *tricarboxylic acid cycle*.)

**Collagen:** Protein found in connective tissue in bones, skin, ligaments, and cartilage. Collagen represents about 30 percent of total body protein.

**Colostrum:** The name given to milk produced during the first few days following delivery. Colostrum is thicker and contains more antibodies, protein, and certain minerals than *mature milk*, milk that is produced later.

**Complementary proteins:** Combinations of incomplete sources of protein that produce a complete protein. Specifically, it means combining protein sources so that the limiting amino acid is complemented by the presence of that same amino acid in another.

**Complete proteins:** Proteins that contain all of the essential aminio acids in the amount needed to support growth and tissue maintenance.

**Cretinism:** A condition in which the thyroid fails to function normally in the fetus and infant. Cretinism is characterized by small stature and mental retardation. When related to iodine deficiency, it is referred to as *endemic cretinism*.

**Critical period:** A specific interval of time when the cells of a tissue or organ are programmed to multiply. Growth by cell division can take place only during the preset intervals. Without an adequate supply of nutrients during the critical periods of growth, cell multiplication does not occur and the affected tissues or organs will remain smaller than nature intended.

**Dehydration:** A condition that occurs when water losses from the body exceed water intake. Dehydration may result from a failure to consume enough water to equal losses, from impaired thirst mechanisms, or from high concentrations of minerals, alcohol, or protein in body fluids.

**Dementia:** From the Latin *dementare*, to make insane. A deteriorative mental state.

**Dermatitis:** [*dermis*=skin, *itis*=inflammation]: Inflammation of the skin.

**Development:** The processes involved in bringing out the capabilities or possibilities of a human; the maturation of humans to more advanced and complex stages of functioning. (The brain *grows* in size, but the ability to reason *develops*.)

**Diabetes:** A disorder of carbohydrate metabolism that is characterized by high blood-glucose levels. It results from the inadequate production of insulin by the body or, more commonly, from abnormal cellular utilization of insulin. Two major types of diabetes are recognized: insulin-dependent and non-insulin-dependent.

**Diet:** Foods and fluids regularly consumed in the course of living.

**Dietary fiber:** Polysaccharides and carbohydratelike substances that, because of their chemical structure, cannot be digested by enzymes produced by humans.

**Differentiation:** The development of cells whose functions are different from those of the parent cell.

**Digestion:** The process by which ingested food is prepared for use by the body. Digestion takes place in the gastrointestinal tract and involves multiple mechanical processes and thousands of chemical reactions.

**Digestive tract:** The portion of the digestive system that consists of the stomach and intestines. Although the mouth and esophagus are also involved in digestion, the vast majority of digestive processes take place in the stomach and intestines. (The gastrointestinal tract is sometimes referred to as the *gut*.)

**Disaccharides:** Sugars consisting of two (*di*) molecules of monosaccharides.

**Dopamine:** A neurotransmitter formed from the amino acid tyrosine. It is thought to be involved with emotions, motor functions, and hormone release.

**Double bonds:** The common sharing of four electrons between adjacent atoms.

**Edema:** A condition in which fluid accumulates in the spaces between cells. Also called *swelling*.

**Elastin:** A protein found in elastic connective tissue such as blood vessels and ligaments.

**Electrolytes:** Chemical substances that form charged particles and conduct an electrical current when in solution. The chief electrolytes in body fluids are sodium, potassium, and chloride.

**Empty-calorie foods:** Foods that provide an excess of calories in relation to nutrients. Soft drinks, candy, sugar, alcohol, and fats such as butter, margarine, and oil are considered empty-calorie foods.

**Endemic:** A disease or condition that recurs among a significant number of people within a population. Protein-calorie malnutrition and goiter are examples of endemic problems in some countries. Iron deficiency and obesity are endemic problems in the United States.

**Energy balance:** A state in which the amount of energy consumed in foods equals the amount used by the body.

**Enrichment:** The replacement of thiamin, riboflavin, niacin, and iron lost during the refining of flour and other grains. Enrichment applies only to grain products. The levels of nutrients used to enrich refined grains are regulated.

**Environment:** Factors that exist outside the body that affect what happens inside the body. It includes physical, economic, psychosocial, and dietary factors that compose the circumstances under which people live.

**Enzymes:** Complex protein substances that increase the rate of chemical reactions without being permanently changed themselves in the process. Enzymes are sometimes referred to as catalysts. The body contains hundreds of enzymes. They are found in particularly high amounts in the gastrointestinal tract. Enzymes are specific in their action, only acting upon a particular chemical substance. The ending *-ase* is commonly used on enzyme names: amyl*ase* and sucr*ase* are examples. They may also end in *-in*, as in tryps*in* and peps*in*.

**Epidemic:** The appearance of a disease or condition that occurs among many people within a population at the same time. Outbreaks of polio in the early 1900s and the recent spread of acquired immune deficiency syndrome (AIDS) are examples of epidemics in the United States.

**Epinephrine:** A chemical messenger derived from the amino acid tyrosine. It increases blood pressure, the force of the contractions of the heart, and pulse rate. Epinephrine is the *fight-or-flight* chemical that is secreted into the bloodstream in response to physical threats or serious emotional stressors. (Also called adrenalin.)

**Epithelial tissue:** The outermost layer of cells that form the surface of the skin and eyes, and the lining of the respiratory, reproductive, and gastrointestinal tracts.

**Essential amino acids:** Amino acids that cannot be produced, or cannot be produced in adequate amounts, by humans and therefore must be obtained from the diet.

**Essential fatty acid:** A fatty acid that is required but cannot be produced by the body. It must be provided in the diet. (See *linoleic acid*.)

**Essential hypertension:** Hypertension of no known cause. It is also called *primary* or *idiopathic* hypertension, and accounts for about 95 percent of all cases of hypertension.

**Essential nutrient:** Specific chemical substances found in food that are required by the body for normal growth and health. Essential nutrients cannot be manufactured or produced in sufficient amounts by the body. They are unique from other nutrients in that they must be obtained in the diet.

**Fatty acids:** Fat-soluble molecules containing carbon, hydrogen, and an acid group (COOH). When combined with glycerol, they make a *fat*. Fatty acids come in many forms. They may be short-, medium-, or long-chained; and saturated, monounsaturated, or polyunsaturated.

**Ferritin:** The storage form of iron. The liver contains most of our supply of ferritin.

**Fertility:** The biological ability to conceive and maintain a pregnancy.

**Fetus:** The baby in the womb from the eighth week of pregnancy until birth. Before that time, it is called the *embryo*.

**Fluorosis:** Fluoride overdose characterized by discolored or mottled teeth in children. Fluorosis generally results from water supplies that naturally contain a high level of fluoride.

**Food additives:** Any substance put in foods that becomes part of the food and/or affects the characteristics of the food. The term applies both to substances intentionally added to foods and to substances added inadvertently, such as particles from packaging materials.

**Food intolerance:** Any adverse reaction caused by the consumption of food or a particular component of food that does not involve the body's immune system. Lactose intolerance and adverse reactions to MSG (monosodium glutamate) are examples of food intolerance.

**Food poisoning:** An imprecise term indicating an illness resulting from ingestion of foods containing a harmful substance such as bacteria, bacterial toxins, poisonous insecticides, or toxic materials such as mercury or lead.

**Fore milk:** Breast milk that accumulates in the ducts of the breast. It makes up about one-third of the total amount of milk consumed by an infant during a normal feeding.

**Fortification:** The addition of nutrients to foods. Nutrients used in fortification may or may not have been present in the original food. Any type of food product can be fortified, and there are no regulations governing the type of nutrients that can be employed.

**Free radical:** An unpaired electron in a molecule; the presence of a single electron in a molecule that requires a pair of electrons for stability. Free radicals are highly reactive. (Daffinition: a 1960s hippie who has found peace.)

**Fruitarian:** Persons who consume fruits as their dietary staple.

**Globulins:** Polypeptides found as a component of blood such as gamma globulin. Globulins help protect the body from infectious diseases.

**Glucagon:** A hormone secreted by the pancreas that acts to raise blood-glucose levels. Glucagon stimulates the breakdown of glycogen and the release of glucose by the liver, thereby increasing blood-glucose levels. It helps to maintain normal blood-glucose levels between meals or during periods of fasting.

**Glycerol:** The water-soluble, glucoselike component of fats. Glycerol accounts for about 16 percent of the weight of a fat molecule.

**Glycolysis:** The *lysis* or splitting of glucose to yield energy. Glucose, which as six carbon atoms, is split by a series of enzymes into two smaller molecules having three carbons each. The process releases energy that is made available for body processes. Unlike energy formation from fatty acids and certain types of amino acids, glycolysis does not require oxygen. Glycolysis is the *anaerobic*—or non-oxygen-requiring phase of energy production.

**Goiter:** Enlargement of the thyroid gland. When specifically related to a dietary lack of iodine, the disease is referred to as iodine deficiency goiter.

**Growth:** An increase in size due to an expansion of cell numbers and the size of cells.

**Heme iron:** Iron attached to hemoglobin and myoglobin in animal tissues. About 40 percent of the total amount of iron found in meats is in the heme form.

**Hemoglobin:** The iron containing protein of red blood cells.

**Hind milk:** Milk that is stored in the milk-producing cells in the breast. Hind milk is released by hormonal stimulation about one minute after sucking begins. About two-thirds of the infant's total feed is from hind milk.

**Homeostasis:** The state of equilibrium of the internal environment of the body. Homeostatic mechanisms act to maintain a constant balance among fluid, nutrients, and other substances in the body.

**Hormones:** Chemical substances produced by specific glands in the body that affect the functions of *target* cells, cells that chemically recognize them.

**Hunger:** Physical sensations that result from the lack of food. Hunger is usually accompanied by weakness, an overwhelming desire to eat, and "hunger pangs" in the lower part of the chest that coincide with powerful contractions of the stomach.

**Hydrogenation:** The addition of hydrogen to one or more atoms within a molecule.

**Hypercalcemia:** Above-normal levels of calcium in the blood.

**Hypertension:** A condition in which blood pressure is higher than normal. Hypertension is generally defined by blood pressure levels that exceed 140/90 mm of mercury.

**Hypervitaminosis A:** The name for the vitamin A toxicity disease.

**Hypoglycemia** [*hypo*=low, *glyc*=glucose, *emia*=in the blood]**:** A condition in which blood-glucose levels are abnormally low. It can be caused by certain tumors that lead to an excessive level of insulin secretion or by other processes that interfere with the body's normal utilization of glucose or insulin.

**Hypothesis:** An educated guess about what the result of an experiment will be. Hypotheses are formed during the planning stage of a study to focus the research undertaken on the specific issue addressed. They are tested by the research implemented and may be proven or disproven.

**Immunity:** Resistance to a disease. Immunity is generally conferred by the presence of specific antibodies in the blood that destroy bacteria and viruses.

**Incomplete proteins:** Proteins that are missing or contain low levels of one or more essential amino acids. Incomplete proteins do not support normal growth or tissue maintenance.

**Infertility:** Biological inability to conceive, or an inability to maintain a pregnancy.

**Inorganic:** Chemical substances occurring in nature that cannot be produced by living matter.

**Insoluble fiber:** Dietary fiber that is not soluble in water. Whole grains and seeds are good sources of insoluble fiber.

**Insulin:** A hormone secreted by the pancreas that acts to lower blood-glucose levels. Insulin helps to transport glucose into cells and to return blood-glucose levels back to normal after a meal. Inadequate secretion, or a lack of cell sensitivity to the presence of insulin, results in an inadequate cell supply of glucose and an overutilization of fatty acids for energy.

**Ions:** Atoms that carry an electrical charge.

**Keratins:** Proteins that provide external protection. Keratins are found in skin, hair, and nails.

**Ketone bodies:** A group of chemical by-products formed by the incomplete utilization of fat for energy.

**Ketosis:** A condition in which *ketone bodies*, or breakdown products from fats used in energy formation, accumulate in the blood and urine. Ketosis results when people primarily depend on dietary fat or body fat stores for energy.

**Kwashiorkor:** A deficiency disease primarily caused by a lack of complete protein in the diet. It usually occurs after children are taken off breast milk and given solid foods that contain protein of low biologic value.

**Lacto-ovo vegetarian:** Diets that include plants, milk, and eggs.

**Lacto vegetarian:** Diets that include plants and milk.

**Letdown reflex:** The letdown or release of hind milk in the breast. The letdown reflex is stimulated by the release of oxytocin during breast-feeding. The release of oxytocin can be initiated by the physical sensations produced by breast-feeding or by psychological stimuli within the mother.

**Limiting amino acid:** The essential amino acid found in the lowest concentration in a food.

**Linoleic acid:** A fatty acid that is required by humans. Because it is not produced in the body, humans need a dietary source of linoleic acid. For healthy adults, linoleic acid is the only known essential fatty acid.

**Lipoproteins** [*lipo/lipid* = fat]: Water-soluble substances containing fat and protein molecules. The vast majority of lipids found in blood are lipoproteins.

**Low birth weight:** Infants who weigh less than five and one-half pounds at birth.

**Lymph vessels:** A network of vessels that absorb and transport some of the breakdown products of fat digestion. Lymph vessels transport these products to the heart, where they are mixed with blood and enter the general circulation.

**Macrobiotics:** Persons who consume vegan diets restricted to the use of unprocessed, unrefined foods and foods that are believed to be endowed with special health properties.

**Malnutrition:** Poor nutrition caused by an inadequate or excessive intake of calories of one or more nutrients. Protein-calorie malnutrition is caused by a lack of protein and calories. Obesity is also a form of malnutrition, but it is related to an excessive intake of calories.

**Maximal oxygen consumption:** The largest amount of oxygen we can make available to cells for use in the citric acid cycle of energy formation. It is also referred to as $VO_2max$.

**Megaloblasts:** Large and irregularly shaped red blood cells. This type of cell is found in cases of folacin and vitamin $B_{12}$ deficiency.

**Menopause:** The period of life for women when the ability to reproduce stops. Menopause generally occurs around the age of fifty and is accompanied by changes in the level of sex hormones produced.

**Menses:** Periodic uterine bleeding accompanied by a shedding of the endometrium, or lining of the uterus. It occurs, on average, every twenty-seven to twenty-eight days, and lasts an average of four to five days. (Also called *menstruation*.) *Menses* is Latin for monthly.

**Menstrual cycle:** The interval between one menses (or menstrual period) and the next.

**Metabolism:** The chemical changes that take place within the body.

**Micelles** \'mī-selz\: Loosely bound molecules containing long-chain fatty acids, monoglycerides, phospholipids, and cholesterol. They are soluble in water.

**Minimum Daily Requirements (MDRs):** Standards of nutrient intake levels based on amounts of nutrients needed to prevent deficiency disease. These standards are no longer recognized as appropriate for labeling purposes.

**Molecule:** Chemical substances formed from the union of two or more atoms. For example, oxygen and hydrogen are elements, but if bonded together they yield $H_2O$, or molecules of water.

**Monosaccharides** [*mono*=one, *saccharide*=sugar]: Carbohydrates containing one sugar molecule. Monosaccharides are the basic chemical units from which all sugars are built.

**Monounsaturated fatty acids:** Fatty acids that contain one double bond between carbons.

**Muscular dystrophy:** A condition characterized by a wasting away and weakening of muscles.

**Myoglobin:** The iron-containing protein in muscle cells.

**Myosin:** A protein present in muscle. Myosin constitutes about 65 percent of total muscle protein and is responsible for the elastic property of muscles, or their ability to expand and contract.

**Naturally occurring toxicants:** Substances that are a natural part of foods that can have a harmful effect on health if consumed in excessive quantities.

**Negative energy balance:** The situation that exists when energy intake is less than energy output, so the body's energy stores must be used to make up the difference.

**Neurotransmitters:** Small molecules most often formed from amino acids that direct cells to perform specific chemical reactions. Epinephrine (adrenalin) and serotonin are two examples of neurotransmitters made from amino acids.

**Nitrogen balance:** Nitrogen intake minus nitrogen excretion.

**Nonessential amino acids:** Amino acids that can be readily produced by humans from components of the diet. Because we can produce them, there are no dietary requirements nor deficiency diseases associated with inadequate intakes of nonessential amino acids.

**Nonheme:** Iron in foods that is not bound to hemoglobin or myoglobin.

**Norepinephrine:** A neurotransmitter, formed from tyrosine, involved in motor function and hormone release.

**Nutrient-dense foods:** Foods that contain relatively high amounts of nutrients compared to their content of calories. Broccoli, collards, bread, and cantaloupe are examples of nutrient-dense foods.

**Nutrients:** Chemical substances found in food that are used by the body to maintain health. There are six categories of nutrients—carbohydrates, proteins, fats, vitamins, minerals, and water.

**Nutrition:** The study of how the substances in food affect the body and health.

**Organic:** Chemical substances that arise from living matter. Organic chemicals contain the element *carbon*.

**Osteoblasts** [*osteo*=bones, *blasts*=germinating or growing cells]: Bone cells that cause bone formation.

**Osteoclasts** [*clasts*=breaking or destroying]: Bone cells that cause the breakdown of bone.

**Osteomalacia:** The vitamin D deficiency disease in adults.

**Osteoporosis** [*osteo*=bones, *poro*=porous, *osis*=abnormal condition]: A condition characterized by porous bones. It is due to the loss of mineral content of bones.

**Ovo vegetarian:** Diets that include plants and eggs.

**Oxidation:** The addition of oxygen to, or the removal of electrons from, a molecule.

**Oxytocin:** A hormone that causes the release of hind milk stored in the milk-producing cells in the breast. Oxytocin release is stimulated by a baby's sucking and can also be stimulated by a baby's cry or, for some women, by thoughts about breast-feeding.

**Pellagra** [*pelle*=skin, *agra*=rash]: The niacin deficiency disease. The title *pellagra* was given to niacin deficiency because of the characteristic rash that occurs with the disease.

**Percentiles:** Growth standards that represent the normal distribution of weight for length, weight for age, or length for age in children. For example, 15 percent of children will have growth measurements that place them between the 75th and 90th growth percentile curves. If a child is assessed to be at the 50th percentile curve, that means that 50 percent of children will be smaller, and 50 percent bigger.

**Pernicious anemia** [*pernicious*=destructive, fatal]: A severe form of anemia characterized by an increase in the size and a decrease in the number of red blood cells. Pernicious anemia is accompanied by degenerative changes in nerve cells and impaired nervous system functions.

**pH:** A measure of how acidic or basic (*alkaline*) a solution is. The point where a solution is neither acidic nor basic is pH 7. Acidity increases as pH drops from 7 to 0, and how basic a solution is increases as pH moves from 7 to 14. As reference points, lemon juice has a pH of 2.2, tomato juice 4.2, milk 6.6, water 7.0 (neutral), and ammonia 11.1.

**Phospholipids** [*phospho*=phosphorus]**:** Substances that contain fatty acids and phosphorus, and sometimes nitrogen. They are soluble in both water and fat. Lecithin is a common type of phospholipid found in the body.

**Pica:** The regular ingestion of nonfood items, most commonly laundry starch, clay, and dirt. Pica most often occurs during pregnancy and childhood.

**Placebo:** A substance having no medical properties that is given as a control in tests of the effects of a biologically active substance. Placebo also means a sugar pill, or a substance that has no medicinal effects but is given merely to satisfy a patient who supposes it to be medicine.

**Placebo effect:** An improvement in physical health associated with the use of a placebo. Some people who receive a placebo will report feeling better than before because they expect the placebo will work.

**Placenta:** An organ that connects the fetus with the mother's blood supply. Within a week after conception, the placenta starts to form and becomes the nutrient supply line from the mother to the fetus. It is a complex organ that performs many functions related to fetal nutrition.

**Plaque:** A soft and sticky material that forms on the surface of teeth and contains a dense collection of bacteria.

**Polysaccharides** [*poly*=many]**:** Complex carbohydrates (starches, dietary fibers, and glycogen) consisting of three or more monosaccharides or monosaccharidelike substances.

**Polyunsaturated fatty acid:** One that contains two or more double bonds between carbons.

**Positive energy balance:** The situation that occurs when energy intake exceeds energy output and results in energy being stored in the body.

**Preterm:** Infants born at or before thirty-seven weeks of pregnancy. Infants born between thirty-eight and forty-two weeks of pregnancy are considered *term*.

**Primary malnutrition:** Malnutrition that directly results from inadequate or excessive dietary intake. Vitamin A deficiency and toxicity are examples of primary malnutrition.

**Prolactin:** A hormone that initiates milk production. It is stimulated by an infant's sucking and the emptying of milk from the breasts.

**Prostaglandins:** Hormonelike substances derived from specific types of fatty acids. Over ninety different types of prostaglandins are found in the human body.

**Protein-efficiency ratio**: A measure of the growth-promoting effect of sources of dietary protein. It measures the relative efficiency of protein sources to produce growth in laboratory animals.

**Provitamin:** A vitaminlike substance that is converted into the active vitamin by metabolic reactions in the body.

**Puberty:** The stage in life during which humans become biologically capable of reproduction.

**Purge:** Self-induced vomiting or laxative use intended to prevent weight gain due to a binge.

**Radioactive particles:** Substances that emit rays of energy from their center (or nucleus). Iodine-131 ($^{131}I$), strontium-90 ($^{90}Sr$), and uranium are examples of radioactive particles. The energy emitted by the nuclei of these atoms can damage human cells.

**Recommended Dietary Allowances (RDAs):** Specified intake levels of essential nutrients considered, on the basis of available scientific evidence, to be adequate to meet the known nutritional needs of practically all healthy people.

**Remodeling:** The breakdown and buildup of bone tissues. The process serves the purpose of maintaining healthy bone.

**Rhodopsin:** The light-sensitive component of rods contained in the retina. It is made from retinal, a form of vitamin A, and opsin. It is also called *visual purple.*

**Rickets:** The vitamin D deficiency disease in children.

**Risk factors:** Conditions that increase the likelihood that a particular disease or condition will develop. For example, high-saturated-fat diets increase the likelihood of developing heart disease, so they are said to be a risk factor for heart disease.

**Rooting reflex:** The instinctive movement of an infant's mouth to the nipple when his or her face touches a breast.

**Satiety:** Having eaten to the point of satisfaction. Satiety occurs when a person no longers feels a need for food, and interest in eating is lost.

**Saturated fatty acids:** Fatty acids that contain only single bonds between adjacent carbons. They are saturated with hydrogens, or contain as many hydrogen-carbon bonds as possible.

**Secondary malnutrition:** Malnutrition that results from disorders not directly related to dietary intake. Weight loss related to a gastrointestinal tract infection is an example of secondary malnutrition.

**Selenosis:** The name for the selenium toxicity disease.

**Semivegetarian:** Diets that include some types of meat, such as poultry and fish, in addition to plants. These diets generally exclude red meat.

**Serotonin:** A neurotransmitter formed from the amino acid tryptophan. It is involved in the processes of sleep, pain, appetite, and perception of well-being.

**Single bonds:** Bonds formed by the common sharing of two electrons from adjacent atoms within a molecule.

**Singlet oxygen:** A high-energy, highly reactive form of oxygen. Singlet oxygen participates in reactions that cause free-radical formation.

**Soluble fiber:** Dietary fibers that are soluble in water and turn the water into gel. Soluble fibers are mainly found in the pulp part of fruits and vegetables. Pectin, a substance found in fruits and used to make jelly gel, is an example of soluble fiber.

**Starch:** A polysaccharide produced by plants from glucose. It is the plant-storage form of glucose.

**Steroid hormones:** Hormones such as estrogen and testosterone that are synthesized from cholesterol.

**Stillborn infants:** Infants who are not alive when delivered.

**Substrate:** The substance being acted upon by enzymes. Food particles are substrates of digestive enzymes.

**Tetany:** A condition in which muscles contract but fail to relax.

**Thermogenesis** [*thermo* = heat, *genesis* = producing]**:** Related to total caloric need, thermogenesis is the rise in metabolic rate that occurs as a result of eating. It represents the energy the body expends in the digestion of foods and the absorption and processing of nutrients. The elevation in metabolism due to thermogenesis is greatest two hours after a meal and lasts for three to four hours. Thermogenesis is also referred to as *dietary thermogenesis* and *specific dynamic action*.

**Thyroxine:** A hormone secreted by the thyroid gland that increases the rate at which energy is formed in the body. Thyroxine plays a major role in stimulating energy formation during times of growth. Adults who produce too little or too much thyroxine have trouble maintaining a constant body weight because of disruptions in energy metabolism.

**Toxemia:** A term commonly used in the past to denote the condition in pregnancy in which blood pressure becomes abnormally high and when swelling is extensive. Women who develop toxemia during pregnancy are at high risk of delivering a small infant early. The condition called *pregnancy-induced hypertension* is now used in preference to the diagnosis of toxemia.

**Toxic:** Poisonous; harmful to the body.

**Unsaturated fatty acids:** Fatty acids that contain one or more double bonds between adjacent carbons.

**U.S. RDAs:** The United States Recommended Dietary Allowances were developed to serve as standard levels by which the nutrient composition of food products could be assessed and reported on food labels. They are based on the 1968 RDA table.

**Uterus:** The womb. A pear-shaped, muscular tissue that is the home of the fetus during pregnancy.

**Vegan:** Diets that exclude all animal products.

**Water balance:** The appropriate distribution of water between the outside and inside of cells. A balanced supply of water in the outside and inside of cells is needed for normal cell functioning.

**Water intoxication:** A condition that occurs when water intake exceeds water losses. Water intoxication may result from consuming too much water or from drugs and diseases that decrease the concentration of minerals in body fluids. Although uncommon, the dilution of minerals caused by excessive water can produce giddiness, nausea, convulsions, coma, and death.

**Waxes:** Fat-soluble substances made from long-chain fatty acids and alcohol.

**Xerophthalmia:** *Dry eyes*—A condition caused by vitamin A deficiency. If not corrected in its early stages, xerophthalmia can produce permanent blindness. Xerophthalmia is generally accompanied by chronic infections of the eye.

## *Appendix B: Reliable Sources of Nutrition Information*

Many sources of nutrition information are available to consumers, but the quality of the information varies widely. Attention is directed here to sources that provide scientifically based information. Although it is not all encompassing, you can use the list to help identify nutrition information you can trust.

### PROFESSIONALS

Registered dietitians (hospitals)
Public health nutritionists (public health departments)
College nutrition instructors/professors (universities)
Home extension service agency (state and county departments of agriculture)
Consumer affairs staff of the Food and Drug Administration (national, regional, and state FDA offices)

### PROFESSIONAL ASSOCIATIONS (NATIONAL AND STATE LEVELS)

American Dental Association
American Diabetes Association
American Dietetic Association
American Heart Association
American Home Economics Association
American Institute of Nutrition
American Medical Association
American National Red Cross
American Public Health Association
March of Dimes
Nutrition Foundation
Society of Nutrition Education

### OTHER SOURCES OF NUTRITION INFORMATION

American Diabetes Association
18 East 48th Street
New York, NY 10017

American Dietetics Association
216 West Jackson Boulevard, Suite 800
Chicago, IL 60606-6995

American Heart Association
7320 Greenville Avenue
Dallas, TX 75231

American Medical Association
Council on Food and Nutrition
535 North Dearborn
Chicago, IL 60610

Food Safety
Consumer Inquiry Section
Food and Drug Administration
5600 Fishers Lane
Rockville, MD 20857
Call toll free: 1-800-426-3758

Food Stamps
Food and Nutrition Service
U.S. Department of Agriculture
Washington, DC 20250

Food and Drug Administration
Consumer Inquiries
Parklawn Building
5600 Fishers Lane
Rockville, MD 20857

Food and Nutrition Information Center
National Agriculture Library, Room 304
10301 Baltimore Boulevard
Beltsville, MD 20705

La Leche League International
9616 Minneapolis Avenue
Franklin Park, IL 60131
(Breast-feeding)

March of Dimes Birth Defects Foundation
1275 Mamaroneck Avenue
White Plains, NY 10605

National Cancer Institute
Call toll free: 1-800-422-6237

National Cholesterol Education Program
National High Blood Pressure Education Program
NHLBI Smoking Education Program
Information Center
4733 Bethesda Avenue, Suite 530
Bethesda, MD 20814

National Dairy Council
6300 North River Road
Rosemont, IL 60019-9922

National Health Information Clearing House
Call toll free: 1-800-336-4797

National Maternal and Child Health Clearing House
3520 Prospect Street NW, Suite 1
Washington, DC 20057

Nutrition Foundation
1122 16th Street NW
Washington, DC 20036

Office of Disease Prevention and Health Promotion
Mary E. Switze Bldg., Room 2132
330 C Street SW
Washington, DC 20201

School Lunch Program
Child Nutrition Programs
Food and Nutrition Service
U.S. Department of Agriculture
Washington, DC 20250

Special Supplemental Food Program for Women,
Infants, and Children (WIC)
Supplemental Food Programs
U.S. Department of Agriculture
Washington, DC 20250

Many of the organizations listed also have state affiliates that you can contact for nutrition information.

## *Appendix C: Shopping for a Balanced Diet*

You can only prepare and serve the foods you have available. Shop with this list to increase your chances of having the right foods on hand when it's time to cook or eat.

*Breads and Cereals.*

BREADS AND CRACKERS

- ☐ Bagels
- ☐ Bread sticks[s]
- ☐ Buns
- ☐ Crackers[s]
- ☐ Croutons
- ☐ English muffins
- ☐ Raisin bread
- ☐ Rice wafers
- ☐ Whole grain bread
- ☐ Whole grain rolls
- ☐ Tortillas
- ☐ Other: ____________

CEREALS (READY-TO-EAT)

- ☐ All-Bran
- ☐ Bran buds
- ☐ Grape-Nuts
- ☐ Raisin bran
- ☐ Shredded wheat
- ☐ Other: ____________

CEREALS (COOKED)

- ☐ Cream of Wheat
- ☐ Grits
- ☐ Malt-O-Meal
- ☐ Oatmeal
- ☐ Other: ____________

OTHER GRAIN PRODUCTS (INCLUDES WHOLE GRAIN PRODUCTS)

- ☐ Macaroni
- ☐ Noodles
- ☐ Popcorn
- ☐ Rice
- ☐ Spaghetti
- ☐ Wild rice
- ☐ Other: ____________

---

[s]means high in salt unless "low-salt" product used.

*Vegetables and Fruits* (fresh or frozen)

VITAMIN-A- AND BETA-CAROTENE-RICH

- ☐ Apricots
- ☐ Asparagus
- ☐ Broccoli
- ☐ Cantaloupe
- ☐ Carrots
- ☐ Collard greens
- ☐ Green peppers
- ☐ Mixed vegetables
- ☐ Nectarines
- ☐ Papayas
- ☐ Peas and carrots
- ☐ Pumpkin
- ☐ Spinach
- ☐ Sweet potatoes
- ☐ Watermelon
- ☐ Winter squash

VITAMIN-C-RICH

- ☐ Brussels sprouts
- ☐ Cantaloupe
- ☐ Grapefruit
- ☐ Grapefruit juice
- ☐ Green peppers
- ☐ Honeydew melon
- ☐ Kiwi fruit
- ☐ Mangos
- ☐ Orange juice
- ☐ Orange-grapefruit juice
- ☐ Orange-pineapple juice
- ☐ Oranges
- ☐ Strawberries
- ☐ Tangerines
- ☐ Tomatoes

OTHER FRUITS AND VEGETABLES

- ☐ Apple juice
- ☐ Apples
- ☐ Applesauce
- ☐ Bananas
- ☐ Bean sprouts
- ☐ Beets
- ☐ Blueberries
- ☐ Brussels sprouts
- ☐ Cabbage
- ☐ Cauliflower
- ☐ Cherries
- ☐ Corn
- ☐ Cranberry juice
- ☐ Cucumber
- ☐ Eggplant
- ☐ Figs
- ☐ Grape juice
- ☐ Grapes
- ☐ Green beans
- ☐ Green onions
- ☐ Lettuce
- ☐ Lima beans

*Vegetables and Fruits continued*

OTHER FRUITS AND VEGETABLES

- ☐ Mushrooms
- ☐ Okra
- ☐ Onions
- ☐ Parsnips
- ☐ Peaches
- ☐ Pears
- ☐ Pineapple
- ☐ Pineapple juice
- ☐ Plums
- ☐ Potatoes
- ☐ Prune juice
- ☐ Prunes
- ☐ Radishes
- ☐ Raisins
- ☐ Raspberries
- ☐ Romaine
- ☐ Summer squash
- ☐ Vegetable juice[s]
- ☐ Water chestnuts
- ☐ Other: ____________

*Milk and milk products*
(includes low-fat products)

- ☐ Milk (type ____________)
- ☐ Soy milk
- ☐ Cheese[f]
- ☐ Cottage cheese
- ☐ Ice cream[f]
- ☐ Ice milk
- ☐ Yogurt
- ☐ Other: ____________

*Meats and meat alternates*
(includes lean meats)

- ☐ Beef [c,f]
- ☐ Black-eyed peas
- ☐ Canadian bacon[s]
- ☐ Chicken
- ☐ Chuck roast
- ☐ Crab*
- ☐ Cube steak
- ☐ Eggs[c]
- ☐ Egg substitute
- ☐ Fish
- ☐ Flank steak
- ☐ Ham[s]
- ☐ Hamburger, lean[c,f]
- ☐ Lamb
- ☐ Liver[c]

---

[s]*means high in salt unless "low-salt" product used.*

[c]*means high in cholesterol.*

[f]*means high in fat*

**Crab and shrimp are no longer considered to be high in cholesterol. They are low in fat and contribute omega-3 fatty acids (the type of fat that appears to protect against heart disease) to the diet.*

*Meats and meat alternates continued*

- ☐ Peanut butter
- ☐ Pork, lean
- ☐ Round steak
- ☐ Scallops
- ☐ Shrimp*
- ☐ Tofu
- ☐ Turkey
- ☐ Turkey ham
- ☐ Veal
- ☐ Nuts, seeds[s,f]
- ☐ Other: ____________

*Miscellaneous (optional)*

- ☐ Butter[f]
- ☐ Cream[f]
- ☐ Oil[f]
- ☐ Margarine[f]
- ☐ Mayonnaise[f]
- ☐ Salad dressings[f]
- ☐ Other: ____________

---

[s]*means high in salt unless "low-salt" product used.*

[f]*means high in fat.*

**Crab and shrimp are no longer considered to be high in cholesterol. They are low in fat and contribute omega-3-fatty acids (the type of fat that appears to protect against heart disease) to the diet.*

## *Appendix D: Weight and Measure Equivalents*

| WEIGHT | EQUIVALENTS |
|---|---|
| Ton | 2,000 pounds |
| Kilogram (kg) | 2.2 pounds, 1,000 grams, 4.4 liquid cups |
| Pound (lb) | 16 ounces, 454 grams, 2 liquid cups |
| Ounce (oz) | 28.35 grams, 2 liquid tablespoons, ⅛ liquid cup |
| Gram (g, gm) | 0.04 ounce, 1,000 milligrams |
| Milligram (mg) | 0.00004 ounce, 1,000 micrograms |
| Microgram (mcg) | 0.0000004 ounce |
| VOLUME | |
| Bushel | 4 pecks |
| Peck | 8 quarts, 2 gallons |
| Gallon (gal)* | 4 quarts, 3.799 liters |
| Quart (qt) | 2 pints, 4 cups, 0.95 liter |
| Liter (L) | 1.06 quarts, 4.23 cups, 1,000 milliliters |
| Pint (pt) | 2 cups, 16 liquid ounces |
| Cup (c) | ½ pint, 16 tablespoons, 48 teaspoons |
| Tablespoon (Tbls, T) | 8 liquid ounces |
| Teaspoon (tsp.) | ⅓ tablespoon, ⅙ fluid ounce, 5 liquid grams |
| Milliliter (ml) | ⅕ teaspoon, 1 liquid gram |
| LENGTH | |
| Kilometer (Km) | 0.62 mile |
| Meter (M) | 1.09 yards, 39.37 inches |
| Yard (yd) | 3 feet, 0.91 meters |
| Foot (ft) | 12 inches, 30.48 centimeters, 300 millimeters |

| | |
|---|---|
| Inch (in) | 2.54 centimeters, 25 millimeters |
| Centimeter (cm) | 0.39 inch |
| Millimeter (mm) | 0.04 inch |

*Memory hint: The 2-2-4 interchange: 2 cups in a pint, 2 pints in a quart, 4 quarts in a gallon.

# References

# *References*

## *Preface: The "Healthier Sex"*

1. National Center for Health Statistics. Life tables. Vital statistics of the United States 1985. Hyattsville, MD: National Center for Health Statistics, 1988. (DHHS Publication (PHS) 88–1104)
2. Public Health Service. Women's Health, Vol. II. Washington, DC: Public Health Service, 1985. (DHHS Publication (PHS) 85–50206)
3. McMillen MM, Haynes SG. Changes in the sex differential in mortality: United States, 1900–80. Abstract No. 2172. American Public Health Association Annual Meeting, October 21, 1987.
4. Fallon A, Rozin P. Sex differences in perception of desirable body shape. Journal of Abnormal Psychology 1985;94:102–5.
5. Update on diet and premenstrual syndrome. Tufts University Diet and Nutrition Letter 1985;3:1.

## *Chapter 1: Health and the U.S. Diet*

1. Califano A Jr. America's health care revolution: health promotion and disease prevention. Journal of the American Dietetic Association 1987;87:437–40.
2. Health expenditures. The Nation's Health, March 1986:4.
3. National Center for Health Statistics. Charting the nation's health trends since 1960. Washington, DC: U.S. Government Printing Office, 1985. (DHHS Publication (PHS) 85–125)
4. Roemer MI. The value of medical care for health promotion. American Journal of Public Health 1984;74:243–8.
5. World Health Organization. WHO Health Statistics Annual for 1985. Geneva: WHO, 1988.
6. McGinnis M. Prevention—today's dietary challenges. Journal of the American Dietetic Association 1980;77:129–32.
7. Naughton JM, O'Dea K, et al. Animal foods in traditional Australian aboriginal diets: polyunsaturated and low in fat. Lipids 1986;21: 684–90.
8. Eason RJ, Pada J, et al. Changing patterns of hypertension, diabetes, obesity and diet among Melanesians and Micronesians in the Solomon Islands. Medical Journal of Australia 1987;146:465–9, 473.
9. Bilderbeck N, Holdsworth MD, et al. Changing food habits among 100 elderly men and women in the United Kingdom. Journal of Human Nutrition 1981;35:448–55.

10. Slattery ML, Randell DE. Trends in coronary heart disease mortality and food consumption in the United States between 1909 and 1980. American Journal of Clinical Nutrition 1988;47:1060–7.
11. Berleson DM, Stambler J. Epidemiology of the killer chronic disease. In: Winick M, ed. Nutrition and the killer diseases. New York: John Wiley and Sons, 1981:17–55.
12. Friend B. Changes in nutrients in the US diet caused by alterations in food intake patterns. Paper presented to the Changing Food Supply in America Conference, Washington, DC, May 1974.
13. Forbes, A. Government regulations and nutrition alternatives. Proceedings from a conference in "Balancing the Balanced Diet." Port St. Lucie, FL: Vitamin Nutrition Information Service, 1981:24–32.

## *Chapter 2: The Nutrition Test*

1. Nutrition for physical fitness and athletic peformance for adults: technical support paper. Journal of the American Dietetic Association 1987;87:934–9.
2. White CC, Powell KE, et al. The behavioral risk factor surveys: IV, The descriptive epidemiology of exercise. American Journal of Preventive Medicine 1987;3:304–10.
3. Thornberry RW, Wilson RW, et al. Health promotion data for the 1990 objectives. Advance Data from Vital and Health Statistics, No. 126. Hyattsville, MD: Public Health Service, 1986. (DHHS Publication (PHS) 86–1250)
4. Wing RR, Epstein LH, et al. Psychologic stress and blood glucose in nondiabetic subjects. Psychosomatic Medicine 1985;47:558–64.
5. Holmes S. Stress and nutrition. Nursing Times 1984;80:53–5.

## *Chapter 3: The Inside Story of Nutrition*

1. Food and Nutrition Board, National Research Council. Recommended Dietary Allowances, 9th ed. Washington, DC: National Academy of Sciences, 1980.
2. Hodges RE. Vitamin C. In: Human nutrition, a comprehensive treatise. 3B. Nutrition and the adult. New York: Plenum, 1980:73–96.
3. Mertz W. The essential trace elements. Science 1981;213:1332–8.
4. Underwood BA, Stekel A. In: Sahn OE, Lockwood R, et al, eds. Methods for the evaluation of the impact of food and nutrition programs. Toyko: United Nations University Press, 1984:65–93.
5. Goodman DS. Vitamin A and retinoids in health and disease. New England Journal of Medicine 1984;310:1023–31.
6. Michelsen O, Yang NG, et al. Naturally occurring toxic foods. In: Goodhart RS, Shils ME, eds. Modern nutrition in health and disease. Philadelphia: Lea and Febiger, 1973:412–33.
7. Comar CL, Thompson JC Jr. Radioactivity in foods. In: Goodhart RS, Shils ME, eds. Modern nutrition in health and disease. Philadelphia: Lea and Febiger, 1973:442–54.

8. Robinson D. Irradiation of foods. Institute of Food Science and Technology (U.K.) 1986;19:165–8.
9. Aspartame. Community Nutrition Institute Newsletter, December 19, 1985:3.
10. Yokogoshi H, Roberts CH, et al. Effects of aspartame and glucose administration on brain and plasma levels of large neutral amino acids and brain 5-hydroxyindoles. American Journal of Clinical Nutrition 1984;40:1–7.
11. Wurtman RJ. Letter to the editor. Lancet 1985;2:1060; and Lipton RB, Newman LC, et al. Aspartame and headache. New England Journal of Medicine 1988;318:1200–01.
12. Finer N. Sugar substitutes in the treatment of obesity and diabetes mellitus. Clinical Nutrition 1985;4:207–14.
13. Stellman SD, Garfinkel L. Artificial sweeteners use and one-year weight change among women. Preventive Medicine 1986;15:195–202.
14. Shaw JH. Diet and dental health. American Journal of Clinical Nutrition 1985;41:1117–31.
15. Artificial fats. Nutrition Week, Community Nutrition Institute Newsletter, May 21, 1987:6.
16. Caballero B. Food additives in the pediatric diet. Clinical Nutrition 1985;4:200–6.

## *Chapter 5: A Look at Carbohydrates, Proteins, and Fats*

1. Lieberman HR. Sugars and behavior. Clinical Nutrition 1985;4:195–9.
2. USDA, Economic Research Service. Sugar and sweetener outlook and situation reports. Washington, DC: USDA, 1984:28.
3. Sugar: How sweet it is—and isn't. FDA Consumer, February 1980:21–24.
4. Kruesi MJP, et al. Effects of sugar and aspartame on aggression and activity in children. American Journal of Psychiatry 1987;144:1487–90.
5. Eason RJ, Pada J, et al. Changing patterns of hypertension, diabetes, obesity and diet among Melanesians and Micronesians in the Solomon Islands. Medical Journal of Australia 1987;146:465–9, 473.
6. Forster ES. The works of Aristotle. In: Problemata, UN VII. London: Oxford University Press, 1927:931.
7. Shaw JH. Diet and dental health. American Journal of Clinical Nutrition 1985;41:1117–31.
8. Ismail A. Food cariogenicity in Americans aged from 9 to 29 years accessed in a national cross-sectional study, 1971–74. Journal of Dental Research 1986;65:1435–40.
9. Ismail A, Burt BA, et al. The cariogenicity of soft drinks in the United States. Journal of the American Dental Association 1984;109:241–5.
10. Glass RL. Effects of dental caries incidence of frequent ingestion of small amounts of sugars and stannous EDTA in chewing gums. Caries Research 1981;15:256–62.
11. Schachtele CF, Harlander SK. Will the diets of the future be less cariogenic? Journal of the Canadian Dental Association 1984;3:213–19.

12. Leverett OH. Fluorides and the changing prevalence of dental caries. Science 1982;217:26–30.
13. Dietary Guidelines for Americans. Washington, DC: USDA, Human Nutrition Information Service, Home and Garden Bulletin No. 232, 1986.
14. Shorey RL, Day PJ, et al. Effect of soybean polysaccharide on plasma lipids. Journal of the American Dietetic Association 1985;85:1461–5.
15. Jenkins DJ, Jenkins AL. Dietary fiber and the glycemic response. Proceedings of the Society of Experimental Biology and Medicine 1985;180:422–31.
16. Stevens J, Vansoesf PJ, et al. Effect of psyllium gum and wheat bran on spontaneous energy intake. American Journal of Clinical Nutrition 1987;46:812–7.
17. Diet, nutrition and cancer prevention: a guide to food choices. U.S. Dept. of HHS, November 1984. (NIH Publication 85–2711)
18. Committee on Diet, Nutrition, and Cancer, National Research Council. Diet, nutrition, and cancer. National Academy Press, 1982.
19. Office of Disease Prevention and Health Promotion, Public Health Service. Prevention '82. Washington, DC: U.S. Dept. of HHS, 1982. (DHHS Publication (PHS) 82–50157)
20. Klatsky AL, Armstrong MA, et al. Relations of alcoholic beverage use to subsequent coronary artery disease hospitalization. American Journal of Cardiology 1986;58:710–14.
21. Eisenstein AB. Nutritional and metabolic effects of alcohol. Journal of the American Dietetic Association 1982;81:247–52.
22. Roper Poll results. In: Freeland-Graves JH, Greninger SA, et al. A demographic and social profile of age and sex matched vegetarians and non-vegetarians. Journal of the American Dietetic Association 1986;86:913–8.
23. Position paper on the vegetarian approach to eating. Journal of the American Dietetic Association 1980;77:61–8.
24. Lithell H, Bruce A. Changes in lipoprotein metabolism during a supplemented fast and an ensuing vegetarian diet period. Upsala Journal of Medical Science 1985;90:73–83.
25. Truswell AS. ABC of nutrition. Some principals. British Medical Journal 1985;291:1486–90.
26. Food and Nutrition Board, National Research Council. Recommended Dietary Allowances, 9th ed. Washington, DC: National Academy of Sciences, 1980.
27. Chanarin I, Malkowska V, et al. Megaloblastic anemia in vegetarian Hindu community. Lancet 1985;2:1168–72.
28. Lovenberg WM. Biochemical regulation of brain function. Nutrition Reviews (Suppl) 1986;44:6–11.
29. Lieberman HR, Wurtman JJ, et al. Changes in mood after carbohydrate consumption among obese individuals. American Journal of Clinical Nutrition 1986;44:772–8.

30. Welsh SO, Marston RM. Review of trends in food use in the United States, 1909 to 1980. Journal of the American Dietetic Association 1982;81:120–5.

## *Chapter 6: Basic Truths about Vitamins and Minerals*

1. Prasad AS. Discovery and importance of zinc in human nutrition. Federation Proceedings 1984;43:2829–34.
2. Monsen ER, Balintfy JL. Calculating dietary iron bioavailability: refinement and computerization. Journal of the American Dietetic Association 1982;80:307–11.
3. Linden MC. Food quality and its determinants, from field to table. In: Linden MC, ed. Nutritional biochemistry and metabolism. New York: Elsevier, 1985:239–54.
4. Head, MK. Nutrient losses in institutional food handling. Journal of the American Dietetic Association 1974;65:423–7.
5. Conserving the nutrient values in foods. Washington, DC: USDA, Home and Garden Bulletin No. 90, 1980.
6. Scrimshaw NS. Nutrition and preventive medicine. In: Last JM, ed. Public health and preventive medicine, 12th ed. Norwalk, CT: Appleton-Century-Crofts, 1986:1515–42.
7. Horwitt MK. Niacin. In: Goodhart RS, Shils ME, eds. Modern nutrition in health and disease. Philadelphia: Lea and Febiger, 1973:198.
8. Knopp RH, Ginsberg J, et al. Contrasting effects of unmodified and time-release forms of niacin on lipoproteins in hyperlipidemic subjects. Metabolism 1985;34:642–50.
9. Food and Nutrition Board, National Research Council. Recommended Dietary Allowances, 9th ed. Washington, DC: National Academy of Sciences, 1980.
10. Miller DR, Hayes KC. Vitamin excess and toxicity. In: Hathcock JN, ed. Nutritional toxicology. New York: Academic Press, 1982:81–133.
11. Dalton K, Dalton MJT. Characteristics of pyridoxine overdose neuropathy syndrome. Acta Neurological Scandinavica 1987;76:8–11.
12. Butterworth CE Jr, Santini R Jr, et al. The pteroylglutamate composition of American diets as determined by chromatographic fractionation. Journal of Clinical Investigation 1963;42:1929–39.
13. Herbert V. Folic acid and vitamin $B_{12}$. In: Goodhart RS, Shils ME, eds. Modern nutrition in health and disease. Philadelphia: Lea and Febiger, 1973:221–44.
14. Bailey LB, Mahan CS, et al. Folacin and iron status in low-income pregnant adolescents and mature women. American Journal of Clinical Nutrition 1980;33:1997–2001.
15. Hodges RE, Baker EM. Ascorbic acid. In: Goodhart RS, Shils ME, eds. Modern nutrition in health and disease. Philadelphia: Lea and Febiger, 1973:245–55.
16. Newberne PM, Suphakarin V. Nutrition and cancer: a review, with emphasis on the role of Vitamins C and E and selenium. Nutrition and Cancer 1983;5:107–119.

17. Welsh SO, Marston RM. Review of trends in food use in the United States, 1909 to 1980. Journal of the American Dietetic Association 1982;81:120–5.
18. Visagie ME, DuPlessis JP, et al. Effect of vitamin C supplementation on black mine-workers. South African Medical Journal 1975;49:889–92.
19. Effects of isotrentinoin on plasma lipids and lipoproteins. Nutrition Reviews 1986;44:196–8.
20. Perisse J, Polacchi W. Geographical distribution and recent changes in world supply of vitamin A. Food and Nutrition (Roma) 1980;6:21–7.
21. Micozzi MS, et al. Carotenodermia in men with elevated carotenid intake from foods and beta-carotene supplements. American Journal of Clinical Nutrition 1988;48:1061–4.
22. Kemmann E, Pasquale SA, et al. Amenorrhea associated with carotenemia. Journal of the American Medical Association 1983;249:926–9.
23. Some facts and myths of vitamins. FDA Consumer. Rockville, MD: Food and Drug Administration, Government Printing Office, 1981. (DHHS Publication (FDA) 79–2117)
24. Edidin DV, Levitsky LL, et al. Resurgence of nutritional rickets associated with breast feeding and special dietary practices. Pediatrics 1980;65:232–35.
25. Chow CK. Nutritional influences on cellular antioxidant defense systems. American Journal of Clinical Nutrition 1979;32:1066–81.
26. Machlin LJ, Brin M. Vitamin E. In: Alfin–Slater RB, Kritchevsky D. Nutrition and the adult. New York: Plenum, 1980:245–60.
27. Krasinski SD, Russell RM, et al. The prevalence of vitamin K deficiency in chronic gastrointestinal disorders. American Journal of Clinical Nutrition 1985;41:639–43.
28. Consensus Development Conference. Osteoporosis. Journal of the American Medical Association 1984;252:799–802.
29. Forster J. Kemps unveils high-calcium yogurt. Minnesota Daily, April 30, 1986;87:4.
30. Albanese AA. Effects of dietary calcium: phosphorus ratios on utilization of dietary calcium for bone synthesis in women 20–75 years of age. Nutrition Reports International 1986;33:879–91.
31. Data are from the National Health and Nutrition Examination Survey II, 1976–1980. Hyattsville, MD: National Center for Health Statistics, 1985.
32. Cummings SR, Kelsey JL, et al. Epidemiology of osteoporosis and osteoporotic fractures. Epidemiology Reviews 1985;7:178–207.
33. Alderman BW, Weiss NS, et al. Reproductive history and postmenopausal risk of hip and forearm fractures. American Journal of Epidemiology 1986;124:262–7.
34. Chan GM, Ronald N, et al. Decreased bone mineral status in lactating adolescent mothers. Journal of Pediatrics 1982;101:767–70.
35. Hartz SC, Blumberg J. Use of vitamin and mineral supplements by the elderly. Clinical Nutrition 1986;5:130–6.

36. Spencer H. Minerals and mineral interactions in human beings. Journal of the American Dietetic Association 1986;86:864–7.
37. Morgan KJ, Stampley GL, et al. Magnesium and calcium dietary intakes of the U.S. population. Journal of the American College of Nutrition 1985;4:195–206.
38. Reinhart RA, Desbiens NA. Hypomagnesemia in patients entering the ICU. Critical Care Medicine 1985;13:506–7.
39. Pilch SM, Senti FR. Assessment of the iron nutritional status of the U.S. population based on the data collected in the second National Health and Nutrition Examination Survey, 1976–1980. Bethesda, MD: Federation of American Societies for Experimental Biology, 1984.
40. Stinson W. Women and primary health care. Salubritas 1985;8:1–3.
41. U.S. Interdepartmental Committee for National Defense. Nutrition Survey of the Armed Forces. Washington, DC: Defense Dept., reports issued 1956–61.
42. Cook JD, Layrisse M. Food iron absorption measured by an extrinsic tag. Journal of Clinical Investigation 1972;51:805–15.
43. Monsen ER, Hallberg M, et al. Estimation of available dietary iron. American Journal of Clinical Nutrition 1978;31:134–41.
44. Hallberg L. The role of vitamin C in improving the critical iron balance situation in women. Internationale Zeitschrift fur Vitamin und Ernahrungsforschung 1985;27:177–87.
45. Herbert V. Recommended dietary intake (RDI) of iron in humans. American Journal of Clinical Nutrition 1987;45:679–86.
46. Moore CV. Iron. In: Goodhart RS, Shils ME, eds. Modern nutrition in health and disease. Philadelphia: Lea and Febiger, 1973:297–323.
47. National Research Council Subcommittee on Iron, Committee on Medical and Biological Effect of Environmental Pollutants. Iron. Washington, DC: National Academy of Sciences, 1979.
48. Trinkoff AM, Baker SP. Poisoning hospitalizations and deaths from solids and liquids among children and teenagers. American Journal of Public Health 1986;76:657–60.
49. Prasad AS. Discovery and importance of zinc in human nutrition. Federation Proceedings 1984;43:2829–34.
50. Solomons NW, Helitzer-Allen DL, et al. Zinc needs during pregnancy. Clinical Nutrition 1986;5:63–71.
51. Patterson KY, Holbrook, et al. Copper and manganese balance in adults consuming self-selected diets. American Journal of Clinical Nutrition 1984;40:1397–1403.
52. Holden JM, Wolf WR, et al. Zinc and copper in self-selected diets. Journal of the American Dietetic Association 1979;75:23–8.
53. Sandstead HH. The role of zinc in human health. In: Hemphill HH, ed. Trace substances in environmental health. V. XII. Columbia, MO: University of Missouri Press, 1978.
54. Chandra RK. Excessive intake of zinc impairs immune responses. Journal of the American Medical Association 1984;252:1443–6.

55. Mehta PS, Mehta SJ, et al. Congenital iodide goiter and hypothyroidism: a review. Obstetrical and Gynecological Survey 1983;38:237–47.
56. Gillie RB. Endemic goiter. Scientific American 1971;93–101.
57. Kochupilla N, Godbole MM. Iodisal oil injections in goiter prophylaxis. NFI Bulletin 1986;7:1–4.
58. Mertz W. The essential trace elements. Science 1981;213:1332–8.
59. Pennington JAT, Young BE, et al. Mineral content of foods and total diets: the selected minerals in foods survey, 1982 to 1984. Journal of the American Dietetic Association 1986;86:876–91.
60. Nagataki S. Effect of excessive quantities of iodide. In: Handbook of physiology. III. Endocrinology. Bethesda, MD: American Physiological Society, 1974:329–44.
61. Leverett OH. Fluorides and the changing prevalence of dental caries. Science 1982;217:26–30.
62. Leske GS, Ripa LW, et al. Dental public health. In: Last JM, ed. Public health and preventive medicine. New York: Appleton-Century-Crofts, 1985:1473–1510.
63. Lu KH, Yen OJ, et al. The effect of a fluoride dentifrice containing an anticalculus agent on dental caries in children. Journal of Dentistry of Children 1985;52:449–51.
64. Schubert A, Holden JM, et al. Selenium content of a core group of foods based on critical evaluation of published analytical data. Journal of the American Dietetic Association 1987;87:285–95.
65. Yang G, Wang S, et al. Endemic selenium intoxication of humans in China. American Journal of Clinical Nutrition 1983;37:872–81.
66. Denton DA. The hunger for salt. An anthropological, psychological and medical analysis. Berlin: Springer-Verlag, 1982:427–35.
67. Shank FR, Park YK, et al. Perspective of the Food and Drug Administration on dietary sodium. Journal of the American Dietetic Association 1982;80:29–35.
68. Fischer DR, Morgan KJ, et al. Cholesterol, saturated fatty acids, polyunsaturated fatty acids, sodium and potassium intakes of the United States population. Journal of the American College of Nutrition 1985;4:207–24.
69. McDonald JT. Vitamin and mineral supplement use in the United States. Clinical Nutrition 1986;5:27–33.
70. GNC expanding at a robust pace by moving to malls. NY Times 1981;November 2:D4 (Column 1).
71. Spence H. Minerals and mineral interactions in human beings. Journal of the American Dietetic Association 1986;86:864–7.
72. O'Neil-Curling NH, Crosby WH. The effect of antacids on the absorption of simultaneously ingested iron. Journal of the American Medical Association 1986;255:1468–70.
73. Farris RP, Cresanta JL, et al. Dietary studies of children from a biracial population: Intakes of carbohydrate and fiber in 10- and 13-year-olds. Journal of the American College of Nutrition 1985;4:539–52.

74. Kaplan NM. Dietary aspects of the treatment of hypertension. Annual Review of Public Health 1986;7:503–19.
75. Calloway CW, McNutt KW, et al. Statement on vitamin and mineral supplements. Journal of Nutrition 1987;117:1649.
76. Hunt JC. Sodium intake and hypertension: a cause for concern. Annals of Internal Medicine 1983;98:724–8.
77. Wigle DT. Contaminants in drinking water and cancer risks in Canadian cities. Canadian Journal of Public Health 1986;77:335–42.

## *Chapter 7: Nutrition and the Prevention and Management of Disease throughout Life*

1. Consensus Development Conference. Osteoporosis. Journal of the American Medical Association 1984;252:799–802.
2. Cauley JA. Endogenous estrogen levels and calcium intakes in postmenopausal women. Relationships with cortical bone measures. Journal of the American Medical Association 1988;260:3150–5.
3. Holbrooke TL, Barrett-Connor E, et al. Dietary calcium and risk of hip fracture: 14-year prospective population study. Lancet 1988;2:1046–9.
4. Sowers MR, Wallace RB, et al. Correlates of mid-radius bone density among postmenopausal women: a community study. American Journal of Clinical Nutrition 1985;41:1045–53.
5. Schwartz M, Anwah I, et al. Variations in treatment of postmenopausal osteoporosis. Clinical Orthopedics, January–February 1985:180–4.
6. Recker RR, Bammi A, et al. Calcium absorbability from milk products, an imitation milk, and calcium carbonate. American Journal of Clinical Nutrition 1988;47:93–5.
7. Castelli WP. Cardiovascular disease in women. American Journal of Obstetrics and Gynecology 1988;158:1553–60.
8. Gordon T, Castelli WP, et al. Diabetes, blood lipids and the role of obesity in coronary heart disease risk for women. Annals of Internal Medicine 1977;87:393–7.
9. Kannel WB, Castelli WP, et al. Serum cholesterol, lipoproteins, and the risk of coronary heart disease. The Framingham Study. Archives of Internal Medicine 1971;74:1–12.
10. Schaefer EJ, Rees DG, et al. Nutrition, lipoproteins, and atherosclerosis. Clinical Nutrition 1986;5:99–111.
11. Blackburn H, Luepker R. Heart disease. In: Last JM, ed. Public health and preventive medicine. Norwalk, CT: Appleton-Century-Crofts, 1985:1159–93.
12. Moore RD. Effect of low-dose alcohol use versus abstention on apolipoproteins A-1 and B. American Journal of Medicine 1988;84:884–90.
13. Grundy SM, Floretin L, et al. Comparison of monounsaturated fatty acids and carbohydrates for reducing raised levels of plasma cholesterol in man. American Journal of Clinical Nutrition 1988;47:965–9.

14. Grundy SM, Bilheimer D, et al. Rationale for the diet-heart statement of the American Heart Association: report of the Nutrition Committee. Circulation 1982;65:839A–54A.
15. Krauss RM, Perlman JA, et al. Effects of estrogen dose and smoking on lipid and lipoprotein levels in post menopausal women. American Journal of Obstetrics and Gynecology 1988;158:1606–11.
16. Questions and answers: endogenous and exogenous risk factors for coronary disease in women. American Journal of Obstetrics and Gynecology 1988;158:1602–5.
17. Seidell JC, Mensink RP, et al. Measure of fat distribution as determinants of serum lipids in healthy volunteers consuming a uniform standardized diet. European Journal of Clinical Investigation 1988;18:243–9.
18. Wood PD, et al. Changes in plasma lipids and lipoproteins in overweight men during weight loss through dieting as compared with exercise. New England Journal of Medicine 1988;319:1173–9.
19. Black MR, Medeiros DM, et al. Zinc supplements and serum lipids in young adult males. American Journal of Clinical Nutrition 1988;47:970–5.
20. Cowan LD, Wilcosky T, et al. Demographic, behavioral, biochemical, and dietary correlates of plasma triglycerides. Lipid Research Clinic Program Prevalence Study. Arteriosclerosis 1985;5:466–80.
21. Mead JF, Alfin-Slater RB, et al. Lipids: Chemistry, Biochemistry and Nutrition. New York: Plenum, 1986.
22. Thorngren M, Nilsson E, et al. Plasma lipoproteins and fatty acid composition during a moderate eicosapentaenoic acid diet. Acta Medica Scandinavica 1986;219:23–8.
23. Kinsella JE. Effects of polyunsaturated fatty acids on factors related to cardiovascular disease. American Journal of Cardiology 1987;60:23G–32G.
24. Kromhout D, Bosschiefer EB, et al. The inverse relation between fish consumption and 20-year mortality from coronary heart disease. New England Journal of Medicine 1985;312:1205–9.
25. Carswell H. Fish oil in Anti-CHD Swim. Medical Tribune, June 18, 1986.
26. Dahl LK. Salt and hypertension. American Journal of Clinical Nutrition 1972;25:231.
27. Health status of minorities and low income groups. Washington, DC: Public Health Service, 1985. (DHHS Publication (HRSA) HRS–P–DV85–1)
28. Kaplan NM. Dietary aspects of the treatment of hypertension. Annual Review of Public Health 1986;7:503–19.
29. Page LB. Nutritional determinants of hypertension. In: Winick M, ed. Nutrition and the killer diseases. New York: John Wiley and Sons, 1981:113–26.

30. Langford HG, Blaufox MD, et al. Dietary therapy slows the return of hypertension after stopping prolonged medication. Journal of the American Medical Association 1985;253:657–64.
31. Meneely G, Battarbee HD. Sodium and potassium. In: Present knowledge in nutrition, 4th ed. Washington, DC: The Nutrition Foundation, 1976.
32. Khaw KT. Dietary potassium and stroke-associated mortality. A 12-year prospective population study. New England Journal of Medicine 1987;316:235–40.
33. Schramm MM, Canley JA, et al. Lack of an association between calcium intake and blood pressure in postmenopausal women. American Journal of Clinical Nutrition 1986;44:505.
34. Thomsen K, Nilas L, et al. Dietary calcium intake and blood pressure in nomotensive subjects. Acta Medica Scandinavica 1987;222:51–6.
35. MacMahon SW, MacDonald GJ, et al. A randomized controlled trial of weight reduction and metoprolol in the treatment of hypertension in young overweight patients. Clinical and Experimental Pharmacology and Physiology 1985;12:267–71.
36. Bazzarre TL, Evans BW, et al. The effects of attendance during a 12-week lifestyle management program on body weight, body fat, cardiovascular performance and blood lipids. Journal of Obesity Weight Regulation 1985;4:274–81.
37. Weinberger MH. Antihypertensive therapy and lipids. Evidence, mechanisms, and implications. Archives of Internal Medicine 1985;145:1102–5.
38. Krakoff LR. Hypertension in women: progress and unsolved problems. Women Health 1985;10:75–83.
39. Beauchamp GK, Bertine M, et al. Modification of salt taste. Annals of Internal Medicine 1983;48:763–9.
40. Public Health Service. Women's Health, Vol. II. Washington, DC: Public Health Service, 1985. (DHHS Publication (PHS) 85–50206)
41. Howe GR. The use of polytomous dual response data to increase power in case-control studies: an application to the association between dietary fat and breast cancer. Journal of Chronic Diseases 1985;38:663–70.
42. Gregorio DI, Emrich LJ, et al. Dietary fat consumption and survival among women with breast cancer. Journal of the National Cancer Institute 1985;75:37–41.
43. Committee on Diet, Nutrition, and Cancer, National Research Council. Diet, nutrition, and cancer. National Academy Press, 1982.
44. Rohan TE, Bain CJ. Diet in the etiology of breast cancer. Epidemiological Reviews 1987;9:120–45.
45. Albanes D. Caloric intake, body weight, and cancer: a review. Nutrition and Cancer 1987;9:1199–217.
46. Godin BR, Adlercreutz H, et al. Estrogen excretion patterns and plasma levels in vegetarian and omnivorous women. New England Journal of Medicine 1982;307:1542–7.

47. Katsouyanni K, Trichopoulos D, et al. Diet and breast cancer: a case-control study in Greece. International Journal of Cancer 1986;15:815–20.
48. Phillips RL, Garfinkel L, et al. Mortality among California Seventh-Day Adventists for selected cancer sites. Journal of the National Cancer Institute 1980;75:1097–107.
49. Schoeff L. Vitamin A. American Journal of Medical Technology 1983;49:447–52.
50. Pastorino U, et al. Vitamin A and female lung cancer. A case-control study on plasma and diet. Nutrition and Cancer 1987;10:171–9.
51. Vitamin E. Nutrition Reviews 1977;35:57–62.
52. Newberne PM, Suphakarin V. Nutrition and cancer: a review, with emphasis on the role of Vitamins C and E and selenium. Nutrition and Cancer 1983;5:107–19.
53. Fukushima S. Promoting effects of sodium L-ascorbate on two-stage urinary bladder carcinogenesis in rats. Cancer Research 1983;43:4454–7.
54. Moertel CG. High dose vitamin C versus placebo in the treatment of patients with advanced cancer who have had no prior chemotherapy. New England Journal of Medicine 1985;312:137–41.
55. Willett WC, Polk BF, et al. Prediagnostic serum selenium and the risk of cancer. Lancet 1983;2:130–4.
56. United Kingdom Prospective Diabetes Study. III. Prevalence of hypertension and hypotensive therapy in patients with newly diagnosed diabetes. A multicenter study. Hypertension 1985;7:8–13.
57. Can strict blood sugar control in diabetes avert or lessen blood vessel damage? NIH Record 1983;35:12.
58. Arky RA. Prevention and therapy of diabetes mellitus. Nutrition Reviews 1983;41:165–73.
59. Nelson RL. Hypoglycemia: fact or fiction? Mayo Clinical Proceedings 1985;60:844–50.
60. Handbook of clinical dietetics, American Dietetics Association. New Haven: Yale University Press, 1981.
61. Human Nutrition Information Service. Nutrition monitoring in the United States. Hyattsville, MD: National Center for Health Statistics, 1986. (DHHS Publication (PHS) 86–1255)
62. Mayer J. Genetic factors in human obesity. Annals of the New York Academy of Science 1965;131:412–21.
63. Stunkard AJ, Sorensen TIA, et al. An adoption study of human obesity. New England Journal of Medicine 1986;314:193–8.
64. Simopoulos AP. Obesity and body weight standards. Annual Review of Public Health 1986;7:481–92.
65. Van Itallie TB. Paper presented at the IV International Congress on Obesity. New York, October 3–5, 1983.
66. Gottlieb NH, Bernstein VR. Sex and age differences in lifestyle risks: implications for health promotion programming. American Journal of Preventive Medicine 1987;3:192–9.

67. Van Itallie TB. Obesity: the American disease. Food Technology, December 1979:43–47.
68. Campbell RG, Hashim SA, et al. Studies of food intake regulation in man: responses to variations in nutritive density in lean and obese subjects. New England Journal of Medicine 1971;285:1402.
69. Porikos KP, Booth G, et al. Effect of covert nutritive dilution on the spontaneous food intake of obese individuals: a pilot study. American Journal of Clinical Nutrition 1977;30:1638.
70. Brownell KD. Public health approaches to obesity and its management. Annual Review of Public Health 1986;7:521–33.
71. Ravich WJ, Bayless TM. Carbohydrate absorption and malabsorption. Clinical Gastroenterology 1983;12:335–57.
72. Smith TM, Kolars JC, et al. Absorption of calcium from milk and yogurt. American Journal of Clinical Nutrition 1985;42:1197–200.

## *Chapter 8: What Works for Weight Control*

1. Jeffery RW, Folsom AR, et al. Prevalence of overweight and weight loss behavior in a metropolitan adult population. American Journal of Public Health 1984;74:349–52.
2. Elliot DL, Goldberg L, et al. Sustained depression of the resting metabolic rate after massive weight loss. American Journal of Clinical Nutrition 1989;49:93–6.
3. National Center for Health Statistics. Survey on Americans' knowledge of health practices. Community Nutrition Institute Newsletter, November 28, 1985.
4. Johnson D, Drenick EJ. Therapeutic fasting in morbid obesity. Archives of Internal Medicine 1977;137:1381–2.
5. Fratelli VP. Deaths associated with the liquid protein diet. FDA Bylines 1979;9:179.
6. Monsen ER. Editorial comment. Journal of the American Dietetic Association 1988;88:904.
7. Wadden TA, Stunkard AJ. Letter to the editor. Journal of the American Dietetic Association 1988;88:905, 982
8. Rock CL, Coulston AM. Weight-control approaches. A review by the California Dietetic Association. Journal of the American Dietetic Association 1988;88:44–8.
9. Raymond JL, Schipke CA, et al. Changes in body composition and dietary intake after gastric partitioning for morbid obesity. Surgery 1986;99:15–9.
10. Pories W. The effectiveness of gastric bypass over gastric partition in morbid obesity. Annals of Surgery, October 1982:389–97.
11. Andersen T, Backer OG, et al. Randomized trial of diet and gastroplasty compared with diet alone in morbid obesity. New England Journal of Medicine 1984;310:352–6.

## Chapter 9: Women Sweat: Nutrition, Physical Fitness, and Performance

1. Nutrition and physical fitness. A statement by the American Dietetic Association. Journal of the American Dietetic Association 1980;76:437–43.
2. Bergstrom J, Hermanson L, et al. Diet-muscle glycogen and physical performance. Acta Physiologica Scandinavica 1967;71:140–50.
3. Hultman E, Bergstrom J, et al. Glycogen storage in human skeletal muscle. Acta Medica Scandinavica 1967;182:109.
4. Elliot D, Goldberg L. Nutrition and exercise. Medical Clinics of North America 1985;69:71–81.
5. Evans WJ, Hupnes VA. Dietary carbohydrates and endurance exercise. American Journal of Clinical Nutrition 1985;41:1146–54.

## Chapter 10: When Slimness Is Everything: Eating Disorders

1. Bruch H. Anorexia nervosa: a review. Feelings and their medical significance. Ross Timesaver 1976;18:29–34.
2. Office of Research Reporting, NICHHD. Facts about anorexia nervosa. Bethesda, MD: National Institute of Health, 1983.
3. Johnson C, Lewis C, et al. The syndrome of bulimia: review and synthesis. Psychiatric Clinics of North America 1984;7:267–73.
4. Feldman W, Feldman E, et al. Culture versus biology: children's attitudes toward thinness and fatness. Pediatrics 1988;81:190–4.
5. Hall A, Delahunt JW, et al. Anorexia nervosa in the male: clinical features and follow-up on nine patients. Journal of Psychiatric Research 1985;19:315–21.
6. Zuckerman DM, Colby A, et al. The prevalence of bulimia among college students. American Journal of Public Health 1986;76:1135–7.
7. Garner DM, Garfinkel PE. Sociocultural factors in anorexia nervosa. Lancet 1978;2:674.
8. Crockett S, Littrell JM. Comparison of eating patterns between diabetic and other college students. Journal of Nutrition Education 1985;17:47–9.
9. Drewnowski A, Halmi KA, et al. Taste and eating disorders. American Journal of Clinical Nutrition 1987;46:442–50.
10. Schwartz DM, Thompson MG. Anorexia nervosa. American Journal of Psychiatry 1981;138:319.
11. Lacey JH, Gibson E. Controlling weight by purgation and vomiting: a comparative study of bulimics. Journal of Psychiatric Research 1985;19:337–41.
12. Rock CL, Coulston AM. Weight-control approaches. A review by the California Dietetic Association. Journal of the American Dietetic Association 1988;88:44–8.
13. Pyle RL, Mitchell JE, et al. Bulimia: a report of 34 cases. Journal of Clinical Psychiatry 1981;42:60–4.

14. Dalvit-McPhillips S. A dietary approach to bulimia treatment. Physiology and Behavior 1984;33:769–75.
15. Drewnowski A, Halmi KA, et al. Taste and eating disorders. American Journal of Clinical Nutrition 1987;46:442–50.
16. Story M. Personal communication, December 1987.
17. Healy K, Contry RM, et al. The prevalence of binge-eating and bulimia in 1,063 college students. Journal of Psychiatric Research 1985;19:161–6.

## *Chapter 11: Nutrition and Reproduction*

1. Antonov AN. Children born during the siege of Leningard in 1942. Journal of Pediatrics 1947;30:250–9.
2. Gruenwald P, Funakawa H, et al. Influence of environmental factors on foetal growth in man. Lancet 1967;1:1026–8.
3. Stein Z, Susser M, et al. Famine and human development: the Dutch hunger winter of 1944–45. New York: Oxford University Press, 1975.
4. Frisch RE. Fatness, menarche, and female fertility. Perspectives in Biology and Medicine 1985;28:611–33.
5. Reindollar RH, Novak M, et al. Adult-onset amenorrhea: a study of 262 patients. American Journal of Obstetrics and Gynecology 1986;155:531–43.
6. Baker ER. Menstrual dysfunction and hormonal status in athletic women: a review. Fertility Sterility 1981;36:691–6.
7. Fries H, Nillius SJ. Dieting, anorexia nervosa and amenorrhea after oral contraceptive treatment. Acta Psychiatrica Scandinavica 1973;49:669.
8. Nelson EM, Fisher EC, et al. Diet and bone status in amenorrheic runners. American Journal of Clinical Nutrition 1986;43:910–16.
9. Kemmann E, Pasquale SA, et al. Amenorrhea associated with carotenemia. Journal of the American Medical Association 1983;249:926–9.
10. Hill PB, Garbaczewski L, et al. Gonadotropin release and meat consumption in vegetarian women. American Journal of Clinical Nutrition 1986;43:37–41.
11. Brooks SM, Sanborn CF, et al. Diet in athletic amenorrhea (letter). Lancet 1984;1:559.
12. Russell-Briefel R, Ezzati T, et al. Prevalence and trends in oral contraceptive use in premenopausal females ages 12–54 years, United States, 1976–80. American Journal of Public Health 1985;75:1173–6.
13. Crook D, Godsland IF, et al. Oral contraceptives and coronary heart disease: modulation of glucose tolerance and plasma lipid risk factors by progestins. American Journal of Obstetrics and Gynecology 1988;158:1612–20.
14. LaRosa JC. The varying effects of progestins on lipid levels and cardiovascular disease. American Journal of Obstetrics and Gynecology 1988;158:1621–9.
15. Forrest JD. The public and the pill: is the pill making a comeback? American Journal of Public Health 1985;75:1131–2.

16. Bamji MS, Prema K, et al. Vitamin supplements to Indian women using low dosage oral contraceptives. Contraception 1985;32:405–16.
17. Shojania A, Hornady R, et al. The effects of oral contraceptives on blood plate metabolism. American Journal of Obstetrics and Gynecology 1982;111:782–91. (See also reference number 15.)
18. Hanson M, Hatcher R, et al. Update on oral contraceptives. Journal of Reproductive Medicine 1985;30:691–713.
19. Brown JE. Weight gain during pregnancy: What is "optimal"? Clinical Nutrition 1988;7:181–90.
20. Shepard MJ, Hellenbrand KG, et al. Proportional weight gain and complications of pregnancy, labor, and delivery in healthy women of normal prepregnant stature. American Journal of Obstetrics and Gynecology 1986;155:947–54.
21. Rosso P, Cramoy C. Nutrition and pregnancy. In: Winick M, ed. Nutrition, pre and postnatal development. New York: Plenum, 1979:133–228.
22. Rosso P, Cramoy C. Nutrition and pregnancy. In: Winick M, ed. Nutrition, pre and postnatal development. New York: Plenum, 1979:133–228.
23. Phillipps C, Johnson NE. The impact of quality of diet and other factors on birth weight of infants. American Journal of Clinical Nutrition 1977;30:215–25.
24. Burke BS, Harding VV, et al. Nutrition studies during pregnancy. IV. Relation of protein content of mother's diet during pregnancy to birth length, birth weight, and conditions of infant at birth. Journal of Pediatrics 1943;23:506–15.
25. Laurence KM. Prevention of neural tube defects by improvement in maternal diet and preconceptional folic acid supplementation. Progress in Clinical Biological Research 1985;163B:383–8.
26. Tierson FD, Olsen CL, et al. Nausea and vomiting of pregnancy and association with pregnancy outcome. American Journal of Obstetrics and Gynecology 1986;155:1017–22.
27. Maternal nutrition and the course and outcome of pregnancy. Washington, DC: National Academy of Sciences, 1970:57.
28. Hytten FE, Leitch I. The physiology of human pregnancy, 2nd ed. Oxford, England: Blackwell Scientific Publications, 1971:167.
29. Food and Nutrition Board, National Research Council. Recommended Dietary Allowances, 9th ed. Washington, DC: National Academy of Sciences, 1980.
30. Puolakka J. Serum ferritin as a measure of iron stores during pregnancy. Acta Obstetrica Gynecologica Scandinavica (Suppl) 1980;95:7–31.
31. Winick M. Nutrition and pregnancy. White Plains, NY: March of Dimes Birth Defects Foundation, 1986.
32. Simmer K, Iles CA, et al. Are iron-folate supplements harmful? American Journal of Clinical Nutrition 1987;45:122–5.
33. Herbert V. Recommended dietary intake (RDI) of iron in humans. American Journal of Clinical Nutrition 1987;45:679–86.

34. Taper LJ, Oliva JT, et al. Zinc and copper retention during pregnancy: the adequacy of prenatal diets with and without supplementation. American Journal of Clinical Nutrition 1985;41:1184–92.
35. Apgar J. Zinc and reproduction. Annual Review of Nutrition 1985;5:43–68.
36. Pike RL, Smiciklas HA. A reappraisal of sodium restriction during pregnancy. International Journal of Gynaecology and Obstetrics 1972;10:1–8.
37. Anderson AS, Wichelow MJ. Constipation during pregnancy: dietary fibre intake and the effect of fibre supplementation. Human Nutrition Applied Nutrition 1985;39:202–7.
38. Worthington-Roberts B. The role of nutrition in pregnancy course and outcome. Journal of Environmental Pathological Toxicology and Oncology 1985;5:1–80.
39. Cochrane WA. Overnutrition in prenatal and neonatal life: a problem? Canadian Medical Association Journal 1965;93:893–9.
40. Davis MK, Savitz DA, et al. Infant feeding and childhood cancer. Lancet 1988;1:365–8.
41. Borch-Johnsen K, Joner G, et al. Relation between breastfeeding and incidence rates of insulin-dependent diabetes mellitus: a hypothesis. Lancet 1984;2:1083–6.
42. McTiernan A, Thomas DB. Evidence of a protective effect of lactation on risk of breast cancer in young women. American Journal of Epidemiology 1986;124:358–3.
43. Barron SP, Lane HW, et al. Factors influencing duration of breast feeding among low-income women. Journal of the American Dietetic Association 1988;88:1557–61.
44. Simopoulos AP, Grave GD. Factors associated with the choice and duration of infant-feeding practices. Pediatrics (Suppl) 1984;74:603–14.
45. Chan GM, Ronald N, et al. Decreased bone mineral status in lactating adolescent mothers. Journal of Pediatrics 1982;101:767–70.
46. Wardlaw GM, Pike AM. The effect of lactation on peak adult shaft and ultra-distal forearm bone mass in women. American Journal of Clinical Nutrition 1986;44:2836.
47. Jelliffe DB, Jelliffe EFP. The volume and composition of human milk in poorly nourished communities. A review. American Journal of Clinical Nutrition 1978;31:492–515.
48. Chappell JE, Clandinin MT, et al. Trans fatty acids in human milk lipids: influence of maternal diet and weight loss. American Journal of Clinical Nutrition 1985;42:49–56.
49. Lonnerdal B. Effects of maternal dietary intake on human milk composition. Journal of Nutrition 1986;116:499–513.
50. Scrimshaw NS. Nutrition and preventive medicine. In: Last JM, ed. Public health and preventive medicine, 12th ed. Norwalk, CT: Appleton-Century-Crofts, 1986:1515–42.

51. Watkinson B, Fried PA. Maternal caffeine use before, during and after pregnancy and effects upon offspring. Neurobehavioral Toxicology and Teratology 1985;7:9–17.
52. Worthington-Roberts B. Personal communication, 1988.
53. Whalen RP. Statement before the Subcommittee on Health and Scientific Research, Committee on Human Resources, United States Senate, June 8, 1977.
54. Schwartz PM, Jacobson SW, et al. Lake Michigan fish consumption as a source of polychlorinated biphenyls in human cord serum, maternal serum, and milk. American Journal of Public Health 1983;73:293–6.
55. Miller SA, Chopra JG. Problems with human milk and infant formulas. Pediatrics (Suppl) 1984;74:639–47.
56. Strode MA, Dewey KG, et al. Effects of short-term caloric restriction on lactational performance of well-nourished women. Acta Paediatrica Scandinavica 1986;75:222–9.
57. Update on diet and premenstrual syndrome. Tufts University Diet and Nutrition Letter 1985;3:1.
58. Price WA, Dimarzio LR, et al. Biopsychosocial approach to premenstrual syndrome. American Family Physician 1986;33:117–22.
59. Woods NE, Faan AM, et al. Prevalence of perimenstrual symptoms. American Journal of Public Health 1982;72:1257–64.
60. American Council of Science and Health. Premenstrual syndrome. July 1985.
61. Smith SL, Sauder C. Food cravings, depression, and premenstrual problems. Psychosomatic Medicine 1969;31:281.
62. Abraham GE. Nutritional factors in the etiology of the premenstrual tension syndrome. Journal of Reproductive Medicine 1983;28:446–59.
63. Dalton K, Dalton MJT. Characteristics of pyridoxine overdose neuropathy syndrome. Acta Neurologica Scandinavica 1987;76:8–11.
64. Miller DR, Hayes KC. Vitamin excess and toxicity. In: Hathcock JN, ed. Nutritional toxicology. New York: Academic Press, 1982:81–133.
65. Rossignol AM, et al. Tea and premenstrual syndrome in the People's Republic of China. American Journal of Public Health 1989;79:67–9.


## *Chapter 12: Diagnosing Nutrition Misinformation*


1. Fratelli VP. Deaths associated with the liquid protein diet. FDA Bylines 1979;9:179.
2. The confusing world of health foods. FDA Consumer. Washington, DC: Food and Drug Administration, 1980. (DHEW Publication (FDA) 79–2108)
3. U.S. News and World Report, February 15, 1988:86.
4. Prasad AS, Miale A, et al. Zinc metabolism in patients with the syndrome of iron deficiency anemia, hepatosplenomegaly, dwarfism, and hypogonadism. Journal of Laboratory and Clinical Medicine 1963;61:537–41.
5. Stare FJ. Marketing a nutritional "revolutionary breakthrough." New England Journal of Medicine 1986;315:971–3.

# Index

# *Index*

*Compiled by Eileen Quam and Theresa Wolner*

## *A Unique Offer on High-Quality Discounted Dietary Analysis Software!*

Now, to add to what you've learned from this book, you can use computer analysis of what you eat to help you make well-informed decisions about improving your diet. A special edition of DAS™ (Diet Analysis and Assessment Software) is available to purchasers of *Everywoman's Guide to Nutrition* through an exclusive arrangement with Nutrition Support Headquarters, Inc. DAS allows you to take an in-depth look at the quality of your diet and to monitor the results of changes you make to modify the fat, cholesterol, sodium, or caloric content of your diet—to name just a few of the possibilities.

DAS is easy to use, complete, and up-to-date. Using a database of more than a thousand foods (including brand-name foods, ethnic foods, and fast foods) the program analyzes your diet for twenty-six nutrients, for the percentage of calories from carbohydrates, protein, and fat, and by the seven basic food groups. The program also can be used to calculate the nutrient content of recipes.

The DAS software program runs on IBM personal computers and true compatibles that have at least one floppy disk drive and 256K bytes of memory.

To order DAS and the User's Manual, complete the form on the reverse side and include it with your check or money order made payable to Nutrition Support Headquarters, Inc. Do not send cash. Allow 4 weeks for delivery. U.S. deliveries only.

*Order Form*

☐ Yes! I wish to own this special edition of DAS software and the accompanying manual. (This offer is for single orders only.)

Send me 1 copy @ $14.95 (includes shipping and handling) $________

Minnesota residents add 6% tax ($0.90) ________

Minneapolis residents add 6.5% tax ($0.97) ________

Amount enclosed $________

☐ I prefer a 3.5-inch diskette

☐ I prefer a 5.25-inch diskette

(If you do not indicate a preference, you will receive a 5.25-inch diskette.)

PLEASE PRINT

NAME

ADDRESS AREA CODE / PHONE NUMBER

CITY STATE ZIP CODE

Mail check or money order (payable to Nutrition Support Headquarters, Inc.) and this order form (**not a facsimile**) to:

**Nutrition Support Headquarters, Inc.**
**P.O. Box 141067**
**Minneapolis, MN 55414**

*About the Author*

**Judith Brown** is professor of nutrition in the School of Public Health of the University of Minnesota. She is a registered dietitian and holds a master's degree in public health from the University of Michigan and a doctorate in nutrition from Florida State University. Dr. Brown has worked as a clinical dietitian and is a nutrition researcher and teacher at Minnesota. She has published extensively in the scientific literature and popular press and has received major research grants for studies on the nutrition and health of women and children.

The development of *Everywoman's Guide to Nutrition* has given Dr. Brown the opportunity to pursue intensively one of her favorite activities—the communication of timely and useful nutrition information to those who can benefit from it most. Minnesota also publishes Dr. Brown's *Nutrition for Your Pregnancy*.